OXFORD MEDICAL PUBLICATIONS

Emergencies in Anaesthesia

Second edition

Published and forthcoming titles in the Emergencies series:

Emergencies in Anaesthesia
Edited by Keith Allman, Andrew McIndoe, and Iain H. Wilson

Emergencies in Cardiology
Edited by Saul G. Myerson, Robin P. Choudhury, and Andrew Mitchell

Emergencies in Clinical Surgery
Edited by Chris Callaghan, J. Andrew Bradley, and Christopher Watson

Emergencies in Critical Care
Edited by Martin Beed, Richard Sherman, and Ravi Mahajan

Emergencies in Nursing
Edited by Philip Downing

Emergencies in Obstetrics and Gynaecology
Edited by S. Arulkumaran

Emergencies in Oncology
Edited by Martin Scott-Brown, Roy A.J. Spence, and Patrick G. Johnston

Emergencies in Paediatrics and Neonatology
Edited by Stuart Crisp and Jo Rainbow

Emergencies in Palliative and Supportive Care
Edited by David Currow and Katherine Clark

Emergencies in Primary Care
Chantal Simon, Karen O'Reilly, John Buckmaster, and Robin Proctor

Emergencies in Psychiatry
Basant K. Puri and Ian H. Treasaden

Emergencies in Radiology
Edited by Richard Graham and Ferdia Gallagher

Emergencies in Respiratory Medicine
Edited by Robert Parker, Catherine Thomas, and Lesley Bennett

Head, Neck and Dental Emergencies
Edited by Mike Perry

Medical Emergencies in Dentistry
Nigel Robb and Jason Leitch

Emergencies in Anaesthesia

Edited by

Keith G. Allman MD FRCA

Consultant Anaesthetist,
Royal Devon and Exeter NHS Foundation Trust, UK

Andrew K. McIndoe FRCA

Consultant Anaesthetist and Senior Clinical Lecturer,
University Hospitals Bristol NHS Foundation Trust, UK

Iain H. Wilson FRCA

Consultant Anaesthetist,
Royal Devon and Exeter NHS Foundation Trust, UK

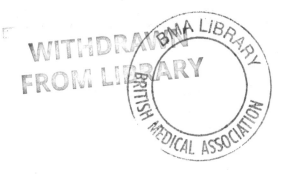
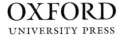

OXFORD
UNIVERSITY PRESS

OXFORD
UNIVERSITY PRESS

Great Clarendon Street, Oxford OX2 6DP

Oxford University Press is a department of the University of Oxford.
It furthers the University's objective of excellence in research, scholarship,
and education by publishing worldwide in

Oxford New York

Auckland Cape Town Dar es Salaam Hong Kong Karachi
Kuala Lumpur Madrid Melbourne Mexico City Nairobi
New Delhi Shanghai Taipei Toronto

With offices in

Argentina Austria Brazil Chile Czech Republic France Greece
Guatemala Hungary Italy Japan Poland Portugal Singapore
South Korea Switzerland Thailand Turkey Ukraine Vietnam

Oxford is a registered trade mark of Oxford University Press
in the UK and in certain other countries

Published in the United States
by Oxford University Press Inc., New York

British Library Cataloguing in Publication Data
Data available

Library of Congress Cataloging in Publication Data
Oxford handbook of emergencies in clinical surgery

Typeset by Cepha Imaging Private Ltd., Bangalore, India
Printed in China
on acid-free paper through
Asia Pacific Offset

ISBN 978–0–19–956082–0

10 9 8 7 6 5

Preface

Welcome to the second edition of *Emergencies in Anaesthesia*. We were delighted with the feedback from the first edition and have incorporated many of the suggestions and comments into this updated text.

The successful management of an emergency arising during anaesthesia depends on the anaesthetist and their team reacting in a calm and logical way. Our ability to do this is much improved by experience, training and preparation of both the individual and the team.

Preparation for emergencies includes gaining the correct knowledge, skills, equipment and help. Protocols provide a structure, which help us to focus and treat the likeliest causes, whilst remembering to exclude the rare.

When all personnel work as a team in a practised approach, and are led effectively, patient risk is minimised. Teamworking helps reduce the chance of human factors interfering with performance. There are a number of ways to prepare for managing emergencies including reading, seminars and simulation.

Emergencies in Anaesthesia has been written to help anaesthetists anticipate different emergency situations that may arise in various areas of anaesthesia. We have described topics that may need to be managed immediately or as soon as practicable. These include problems that may arise in theatre, preoperatively or in recovery. Each emergency has a description of the most common presentations, immediate action required, other potential diagnoses to exclude, and further care required.

We hope that *Emergencies in Anaesthesia* will stimulate readers to reflect on their knowledge and readiness to deal with any of the situations discussed. Additionally, since dealing with emergencies requires all members of the team to help, and for the theatres to be properly equipped, this book may serve to remind us what developments we need in our workplace. Dealing with the unexpected is always made easier by effective planning.

We look forward to feedback on the book, good and bad — please post any comments via the OUP website: www.oup.com/uk/medicine/handbooks

We would especially like to thank all our authors for their excellent work and our families for their continued support.

Keith G Allman
Andrew K McIndoe
Iain H Wilson

March 2009

Note on drug dosages

Some of the drugs and dosages are suggested outside of those stated in the BNF because the book describes the use of drugs in specialist situations. Always refer of the BNF and product literature before using any drug with which you are unfamiliar.

Contents

Abbreviations

1°	primary
2°	secondary
A–a	Alveolar–arterial
AAA	abdominal aortic aneurysm
AAGBI	Association of Anaesthetists of Great Britain and Ireland
ABC	Airway, Breathing, Circulation
ABGS	arterial blood gases
A&E	accident and emergency
ACE	angiotensin-converting enzyme
ACh	acetylcholine
AChE	acetylcholinesterase
ACS	acute coronary syndrome
ACTH	adrenocorticotrophic hormone
ADH	antidiuretic hormone
ADP	accidental dural puncture
AEDS	automated external defibrillators
AF	atrial fibrillation
AFE	amniotic fluid embolus
AHF	acute heart failure
AIDS	acquired immune deficiency syndrome
ALI	acute lung injury
ALS	advanced life support
ALT	alanine aminotransferase
APL	automatic pressure limiting
APTR	activated partial thromboplastin ratio
APTT	activated partial thromboplastin time
ARDS	acute respiratory distress syndrome
ARF	acute renal failure
ASA	American Society of Anesthesiologists
ASAP	as soon as possible
AST	aspartate transaminase
ATN	acute tubular necrosis
AV	atrioventricular/arteriovenous
AVM	arteriovenous malformation
AXR	abdominal X-ray
BAL	bronchoalveolar lavage

BB	bronchial blockers
BCIS	bone cement implantation syndrome
bd	twice daily
BE	base excess
BiPAP	biphasic positive airway pressure
BLS	basic life support
BM	'blood sugar'
BMI	body mass index
BNP	b[rain]-natriuretic peptide
BP	blood pressure
BPF	bronchopleural fistula
bpm	beats per minute
BSA	body surface area
BURP	Backwards, Upwards, Rightwards Pressure
CBF	cerebral blood flow
CCF	congestive cardiac failure
CCU	coronary care unit/critical care unit
CEA	carotid endarterectomy
CI	cardiac index
CICV	can't intubate … can't ventilate
CK	creatine kinase
CK-MB	creatine kinase MB isoenzyme
CMV	cytomegalovirus
CNS	central nervous system
CO	cardiac output
COHb	carboxyhaemoglobin
COPD	chronic obstructive pulmonary disease
CPAP	continuous positive airways pressure
CPB	cardiopulmonary bypass
CPP	cerebral perfusion pressure
CPR	cardiopulmonary resuscitation
CRP	C-reactive protein
CS	Caesarean section
CSE	combined spinal/epidural
CSF	cerebrospinal fluid
CSM	Committee on Safety of Medicines
CT	computed tomography
CTPA	computed tomography pulmonary angiogram
CV	central venous
CVC	central venous catheter
CVE	cerbrovascular episode

CVP	central venous pressure
CVS	cardiovascular system
CXR	chest X-ray
DBS	double-burst stimulation
DC	direct current
DDAVP	1-deamino-8-D-arginine vasopressin
DHI	dynamic hyperinflation
DI	diabetes insipidus
DIC	disseminated intravascular coagulation
DKA	diabetic ketoacidosis
DLT	double-lumen tube
DNAR	do not attempt resuscitation
DVT	deep vein thrombosis
ECG	electrocardiogram
ECM	external cardiac massage
ECMO	extracorporeal membrane oxygenation
ECT	electroconvulsive therapy
ED	external diameter; emergency department
EDTA	ethylenediamine tetra-acetic acid
EEG	electroencephalogram
EMLA	eutectic mixture of local anaesthetics
ENT	ear, nose, throat
ET	endotracheal
$ETCO_2$	end-tidal CO_2
ETT	endotracheal tube
EU	European Union
EUA	examination under anaesthetic
FB	foreign body
FBC	full blood count
FEV_1	forced expiratory volume in 1 second
FFP	fresh frozen plasma
FGF	fresh gas flow
FiAA	inspired fraction of anaesthetic agent
FiO_2	inspired fraction of O_2
FOB	fibreoptic bronchoscope
FOI	fibreoptic intubation
FRC	functional residual capacity
FT_C	corrected flow time
GA	general anaesthesia
G&S	group and save
GCS	Glasgow coma scale

GI	gastrointestinal
G-6-PD	glucose-6-phosphate dehydrogenase
GTN	glyceryl trinitrate
GU	genitourinary
Hb	haemoglobin
HDU	high dependency unit
HIB	*Haemophilus influenzae b* (vaccine)
HIV	human immunodeficiency virus
HME	heat and moisture exchanger
HR	heart rate
IA	intra-arterial
IAP	intra-abdominal pressure
ICD	implantable cardioverter defibrillator
ICP	intracranial pressure
ICS	Intensive Care Society
ICU	intensive care unit
ID	internal diameter
I:E ratio	inspiratory:expiratory ratio
IHD	ischaemic heart disease
ILMA	intubating laryngeal mask airway
IM	intramuscular(ly)
INR	international normalized ratio
IO	intraosseous
IPPV	intermittent positive pressure ventilation
ITU	intensive therapy unit
IU	international units
IV	intravenous
IVC	inferior vena cava
IVCT	*in vitro* contracture testing
IVI	intravenous infusion
IVRA	intravenous regional anaesthesia
JVP	jugular venous pressure
LA	local anaesthetic/left atrium
LBBB	left bundle branch block
LFT	liver function test
LMA	laryngeal mask airway
LMWH	low molecular weight heparin
LOC	loss of consciousness
LSCS	lower segment Caesarean section
LVAD	left ventricular assist device
LVF	left ventricular failure

LVH	left ventricular hypertrophy
LVSWI	left ventricular stroke work index
MA	mean acceleration
MAC	minimum alveolar concentration
MAOIs	monoamine oxidase inhibitors
MAP	mean arterial pressure
MC&S	microscopy, culture and sensitivity
MDI	metered dose inhaler
MEN	multiple endocrine neoplasia
metHb	methaemoglobin
MH	malignant hyperthermia
MHRA	Medicines and Healthcare products Regulatory Agency
MI	myocardial infarction
MRI	magnetic resonance imaging
MSU	midstream urine
NAI	non-accidental injury
NG	nasogastric
NHS	National Health Service
NIBP	non-invasive blood pressure
NIDDM	non-insulin-dependent diabetes mellitus
NSAIDs	non-steroidal anti-inflammatory drugs
NSTEACS	non-ST segment elevation acute coronary syndromes
NSTEMI	non-ST elevation myocardial infarction
od	once daily
OLV	one-lung ventilation
OMV	Oxford Miniature Vaporizer
PA	pulmonary artery
PABA	para-aminobenzoic acid
PAC	pulmonary artery catheter
$PaCO_2$	partial pressure arterial CO_2
PACU	post-anaesthetic care unit
PAFC	pulmonary artery flotation catheter
PALS	paediatric advanced life support
PaO_2	partial pressure arterial O_2
PAP	positive airways pressure/pulmonary artery pressure
P_{aw}	airway pressure
PAWP/ PAOP	pulmonary artery wedge pressure/ pulmonary artery occlusion pressure
PBLS	paediatric basic life support
PCA	patient-controlled analgesia
PCI	percutaneous coronary intervention

PCV	pressure-controlled ventilation
PCWP	pulmonary capillary wedge pressure
PDPH	postdural puncture headache
PE	pulmonary embolism/phenytoin equivalents
PEA	pulseless electrical activity
PEEP	positive end-expiratory pressure
PEFR	peak expiratory flow rate
PEP	postexposure prophylaxis
PICC	peripherally inserted central catheter
PiCCO	pulse contour cardiac output
PICU	paediatric intensive care unit
PIH	pregnancy-induced hypertension
PLMA	ProSeal LMA
PO	by mouth
PO_2	partial pressure O_2
PONV	postoperative nausea and vomiting
PR	*per rectum*
prn	when required
PT	prothrombin
PTH	parathyroid hormone
PUD	peptic ulcer disease
PTT	partial thromboplastin time
PV	peak velocity
PVR	pulmonary vascular resistance
qds	four times daily
RA	right atrium
RAE	Ring–Adair–Elwyn
RBBB	right bundle branch block
RBC	red blood cell(s)
rF	recombinant factor
RS	respiratory system
RSI	rapid sequence induction
RTA	road traffic accident/motor vehicle accident
RUL	right upper lobe
RV	right ventricle
SAG-M	saline adenine glucose–mannitol
SAH	subarachnoid haemorrhage
SaO_2	arterial oxygen saturation
SBCU	special baby care unit
SC	subcutaneous(ly)
SCI	spinal cord injury

ScvO$_2$	central venous O$_2$ saturation
SD	stroke distance
SHOT	Serious Hazards of Transfusion
SIADH	syndrome of inappropriate antidiuretic hormone secretion
SIRS	systemic inflammatory response syndrome
SL	sublingual
SLE	systemic lupus erythematosus
SNP	sodium nitroprusside
SpO$_2$	peripheral oxygen saturation
SSRI	selective serotonin-reuptake inhibitor
STEMI	ST elevation myocardial infarction
SV	stroke volume
SVC	superior vena cava
SVI	stroke volume index
SVR	systemic vascular resistance
SVRI	systemic vascular resistance index
SVT	supraventricular tachycardia
T$_3$	tri-iodothyronine
T$_4$	thyroxine
TB	tuberculosis
TBW	total body water
TCA	tricyclic antidepressants
TCI	target controlled infusion
Tc/Xe	technetium/xenon
tds	three times daily
TFTs	thyroid function tests
TIVA	total intravenous anaesthesia
TMJ	temporomandibular joint
TOE	transoesophageal echocardiography
TOF	train-of-four
t-PA	tissue plasminogen activator
TPN	total parenteral nutrition
TRALI	transfusion-related acute lung injury
TSH	thyroid stimulating hormone
TURP	transurethral resection of the prostate
U	unit
U&Es	urea and electrolytes
USS	ultrasound scan
UTI	urinary tract infection
VATS	video-assisted thoracoscopy

VEs	ventricular ectopics
VF	ventricular fibrillation
VP	ventriculoperitoneal (shunt)
VSD	ventricular septal defect
Vt	tidal volume
VT	ventricular tachycardia
VTE	venous thromboembolism
WPW	Wolff–Parkinson–White (syndrome)
YAG	yttrium–aluminium–garnet (laser)

Contributors

Dr Davinia Bennett
Consultant Anaesthetist
(Hepatobiliary and Liver
Transplant Surgery), University
Hospital Birmingham NHS
Foundation Trust, Birmingham

Colin Berry
Consultant Anaesthetist, Royal
Devon and Exeter NHS Foundation
Trust, Devon

Dr Hannah Blanshard
Consultant Anaesthetist,
University Hospitals Bristol,
Bristol

Dr Tim Cook
Consultant in Anaesthesia and
Intensive Care, Royal United
Hospital, Bath

Dr Jules Cranshaw
Consultant in Anaesthesia and
Intensive Care Medicine,
Royal Bournemouth Hospital,
Bournemouth

Dr Gerard Gould
Consultant Anaesthetist,
Conquest Hospital, Hastings,
East Sussex

Dr Matt Grayling
Consultant in Anaesthesia,
Royal Devon and Exeter
NHS Foundation Trust, Exeter

Dr Kim J Gupta
Consultant in Anaesthesia and
Intensive Care Medicine, Royal
United Hospital, Bath

Dr Katharine Hunt
Consultant in Anaesthesia,
National Hospital for Neurology
and Neurosurgery, London

Dr John Isaac
Consultant Anaesthetist,
University Hospital, Birmingham

Dr Stephen Michael Kinsella
Consultant Obstetric Anaesthetist,
St Michael's Hospital,
University Hospitals Bristol,
Bristol

Dr Daniel Lutman
Consultant for the Children's
Acute Transport Service,
Great Ormond Street Children's
Hospital and Consultant
Anaesthetist, Barts and the
London NHS Trust, London

Dr Bruce McCormick
Consultant Anaesthetist,
Royal Devon and Exeter NHS
Foundation Trust, Exeter

Dr Jerry Nolan
Consultant in Anaesthesia and
Intensive Care Medicine, Royal
United Hospital, Bath

Dr Adrian Pearce
Consultant Anaesthetist,
Guy's and St. Thomas' Hospital,
London

Dr Neil Rasburn
Specialist Registrar, Bristol School
of Anaesthesia, Bristol

Dr Richard Riley
Clinical Associate Professor of
Anaesthesia, University of
Western Australia, Australia

Dr Nicky Ross
Specialist Registrar, Department
of Anaesthesia, Royal Devon and
Exeter NHS Foundation Trust,
Exeter

Dr Mark Scrutton
Consultant Obstetric Anaesthetist,
St Michael's Hospital University
Hospitals Bristol NHS Foundation
Trust, Bristol

Dr Martin Smith
Consultant in Neuroanaesthesia
and Neurocritical Care, Honorary
Reader in Anaesthesia and
Critical Care, The National
Hospital for Neurology and
Neurosurgery, University College
London Hospitals, London

Dr Mark Stoneham
Consultant Anaesthetist and
Honorary Clinical Senior Lecturer,
Nuffield Department of
Anaesthetics, Oxford

Dr Benjamin Walton
Consultant in Anaesthesia,
Frenchay Hospital, Bristol

David Wilkinson
Physician's Assistant (Anaesthesia),
Royal Devon and Exeter NHS
Foundation Trust, Devon

Chapter 1

Cardiovascular

Jerry Nolan

☠ Asystole

Definition
Cardiac arrest associated with the absence of cardiac electrical activity.

Presentation
- No electrical activity on the ECG—the baseline usually undulates slowly on the monitor.
- No palpable central pulses (carotid or femoral).
- Occasionally, atrial electrical activity continues in the absence of ventricular electrical activity. This 'P-wave asystole' may respond to electrical pacing.

Immediate management

(See Figs 1.1, 1.2 (BLS and ALS algorithms, respectively), pp3, 5)
- Stop any surgical activity likely to be causing excessive vagal stimulation (e.g. traction on peritoneum).
- Establish clear airway and ventilate with 100% oxygen. Intubate, but do not let this delay chest compressions.
- Give chest compressions at 100 per min—do not interrupt compressions for ventilation.
- Give atropine IV—according to universal ALS algorithm, 3 mg is given as a single dose. If asystole has been caused by surgical stimulation of the vagus, it is more appropriate to give atropine in increments of 0.5 mg.
- Give adrenaline 1 mg if asystole is not immediately resolved by stopping surgical activity or injecting atropine. Repeat this dose of adrenaline every 3 min until spontaneous circulation is restored.

Subsequent management
- Exclude or treat reversible causes of asystole.
- Rapid infusion of fluid (including blood if severe haemorrhage).
- Complete heart block or Möbitz type II second-degree heart block will require pacing. This can be achieved using a transcutaneous pacer while awaiting someone skilled in transvenous pacing.
- If resuscitation is successful, life-saving surgery (e.g. to control haemorrhage) should be completed. Unless the period of CPR has been very brief (perhaps less than 3 min), the patient should remain intubated and be transferred to the critical care unit. Following prolonged cardiac arrest, if there is a possibility of neurological injury, consider inducing mild hypothermia (32 °C–34 °C)—see below.
- Obtain a CXR, 12-lead ECG, arterial blood gases, and plasma electrolyte analysis.

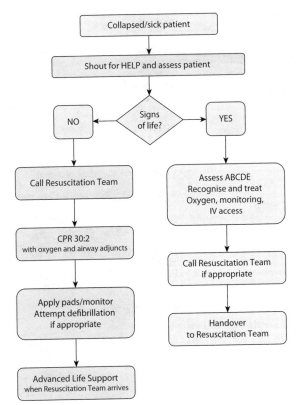

Fig. 1.1 Adult basic life support.[1]

1 With permission of the Resuscitation Council, UK.

Investigations
U&Es, ABGs, ECG, CXR

Risk factors
- Procedures associated with excessive vagal activity, e.g. gynaecological/eye surgery
- Pre-existing complete heart block, second-degree heart block, or trifascicular heart block

Exclusions
- Disconnected ECG lead—this appears on the monitor as a completely straight line
- Excessively low gain on ECG—there is usually some evidence of very small electrical complexes on the monitor
- Hypoxia—obstructed airway, oesophageal intubation, bronchial intubation, oxygen failure
- Hypovolaemia—haemorrhagic shock (particularly with induction of anaesthesia), anaphylaxis
- Hypo/hyperkalaemia and metabolic disorders—renal failure, suxamethonium-induced hyperkalaemia after burns
- Hypothermia—unlikely
- Tension pneumothorax—especially in the trauma patient or after central venous catheter insertion
- Tamponade—after penetrating trauma
- Toxic/therapeutic disorders—after drug overdose (self-inflicted or iatrogenic)
- Thromboembolism—massive pulmonary embolus

Paediatric implications
- The same principles apply to the treatment of asystole in children.
- Hypoxia is more likely as prime cause.
- Refer to Paediatric ALS for drug doses (pp118–20).

Special considerations
- Asystole associated with excessive vagal stimulation or injection of suxamethonium will usually resolve spontaneously on stopping the cause. However, atropine (0.5–1 mg) or glycopyrronium (200–500 μg) should be given and occasionally a brief period of chest compressions is required.
- Under these conditions, follow-up investigations are usually unnecessary.
- In other circumstances asystole is associated with a poor prognosis unless there is a potentially reversible cause that can be treated immediately.

Further reading
Nolan, J., Soar, J., Lockey, A. et al. (2005). *Advanced Life Support Course Provider Manual*, (5th edn). Resuscitation Council (UK), London.

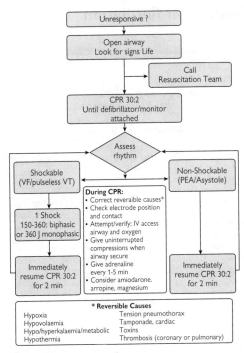

Fig. 1.2 Advanced life support (adults).[1]

☠ **Ventricular fibrillation**

Definition
Cardiac arrest associated with an irregular, chaotic, broad-complex, fast rhythm on the ECG.

Presentation
- Characteristic appearance of VF on ECG
- No palpable central pulses (carotid or femoral)

Immediate management

(See ALS algorithm, p5)
- Call for help and defibrillator—the chance of successful defibrillation reduces considerably with time.
- Precordial thump—if this is done immediately it may successfully restore a perfusing rhythm.
- Attempt electrical defibrillation as soon as possible—the success rate is high if the first shock can be delivered in less than 3 min. If a modern biphasic defibrillator is used, give a single shock of 150–200 J followed by immediate resumption of chest compressions, regardless of outcome. Subsequent biphasic shocks are given at 150–360 J according to the manufacturer's recommendations. If an older, monophasic defibrillator is used give all shocks at 360 J.
- If a defibrillator is not immediately available, start chest compressions and ventilation with 100% oxygen. Intubate but do not allow this to delay start of chest compressions. Do not interrupt chest compressions during ventilation.
- Resume chest compressions immediately following defibrillation without reassessing the rhythm or feeling for a pulse.
- Continue CPR for 2 min, then pause briefly to check the monitor.
- Give adrenaline 1 mg IV if VF/VT is still present during the rhythm check before the 3rd shock.
- Repeat the adrenaline every 3–5 min thereafter (every other cycle).

Subsequent management
- Give amiodarone 300 mg IV if VF persists after delivery of 3 shocks. In an emergency, amiodarone can be given through a peripheral vein and should be followed by a fluid flush.
- Exclude potentially reversible causes if VF persists.
- If resuscitation is successful, life-saving surgery (e.g. to control haemorrhage) should be completed. Unless the period of CPR has been very brief (perhaps less than 3 min), the patient should remain intubated and be transferred to the critical care unit. Consider inducing mild hypothermia (32 °C–34 °C)—see below.

Investigations
U&Es, ABGs, ECG, CXR

Risk factors
- Recent myocardial infarction
- Ischaemic heart disease
- Excessive endogenous or exogenous catecholamines
- Hypokalaemia
- Irritation of myocardium by guidewire during insertion of central venous catheter

Exclusions
- Artefact on the ECG—interference from diathermy or patient movement.
- Polymorphic ventricular tachycardia—in the absence of a pulse, treatment is still defibrillation.
- Atrial fibrillation in the presence of atrioventricular accessory pathway—often capable of conducting very rapidly.

Paediatric implications
- VF cardiac arrest is unusual in children.
- The same principles apply to the treatment of VF in children.
- Refer to Paediatric ALS for appropriate shock energies and drug doses—(pp118–20).

Special considerations
- Electrical defibrillation can be accomplished using self-adhesive patches or, less commonly, manual paddles and gel pads. One electrode is applied just below the right clavicle and the other in the left mid-axillary line in approximately the 5th intercostal space. Self-adhesive patches can be applied prophylactically to those patients deemed to be at very high risk of VF intraoperatively.
- The treatment of pulseless ventricular tachycardia is the same as for VF.
- Automated external defibrillators (AEDs) or shock-advisory defibrillators (with a manual override function) are deployed commonly outside of critical care areas. The need to stop chest compressions while these devices analyse the rhythm is a significant disadvantage and anyone capable of rhythm interpretation should operate these devices in manual mode.

Further reading
Nolan, J., Soar, J., Lockey, A. *et al.* (2005). *Advanced Life Support Course Provider Manual*, (5th edn). Resuscitation Council (UK), London.

☼ Intraoperative arrhythmias: bradycardia

Definition
Ventricular rate <60 bpm. Absolute bradycardia (<40 bpm); relative brady-cardia (heart rate inappropriate for haemodynamic state of patient). May be sinus or associated with AV block/sick sinus syndrome.

Presentation
- Ventricular rate <60 bpm
- 12-lead ECG to define rhythm

Immediate management
(See Fig. 1.3, 'Bradycardia algorithm', p10)
- Urgent correction of any hypoxaemia.
- May not need any action in absence of cardiovascular compromise (blood pressure is acceptable and peripheral perfusion is adequate).
- Correct other underlying causes—stop surgical stimulation likely to be increasing vagal activity.
- Atropine (500 µg increments up to 3 mg), glycopyrronium (200–600 µg) or ephedrine (6–9 mg).
- Consider isoprenaline (0.5–1.0 µg/min) or adrenaline (2–10 µg/min) if persistent.
- External transcutaneous pacing if fails to respond to drug treatment—this is used until a temporary transvenous pacing wire can be inserted. When initiating external transcutaneous pacing the typical current required to achieve electrical capture is 50–100 mA.

Subsequent management
- Treat precipitating reversible causes (electrolyte abnormalities in the presence of a prolonged QT interval). Stop drugs that prolong QT interval, e.g. amiodarone, sotalol, erythromycin, disopyramide, procainamide, quinidine, haloperidol, chlorpromazine.
- In patients with persisting bradycardia, a 12-lead ECG will enable assessment of heart block.

Investigations
ECG, U&Es, ABGs

Risk factors
Sinus bradycardia may be caused by:
- Vagal stimulation during surgery
- Drugs (beta-blockers, digoxin, amiodarone, anticholinesterases, suxamethonium)
- Sick sinus syndrome
- Myocardial infarction
- Raised intracranial pressure
- Hypothermia

Third-degree atrioventricular block and second-degree Möbitz type II AV block will result in significant bradycardia, haemodynamic instability, and the possibility of asystole. Other significant risk factors associated with the risk of asystole include a recent episode of asystole or ventricular pauses of >3 s.

Severe hypoxaemia will cause bradycardia.

Exclusions

Appropriate sinus bradycardia associated with adequate cardiac output—check history and current medication (patient taking beta-blockers, athletic patients).

Paediatric implications

In children, bradycardia is usually secondary to hypoxia and adequate oxygenation must be restored immediately.

Special considerations

Indications for referral for preoperative pacing:
- Second-degree AV block—Möbitz type II or 2:1 (intermittent failure of conduction)
- Complete heart block
- Symptomatic sinus node disease
- Asymptomatic bundle branch block, bifascicular, trifascicular and first-degree heart block are not indications for preoperative pacing. Pacing is not usually required for Möbitz type I second-degree AV block (Wenckebach) unless the patient is symptomatic.

Further reading

ACC/AHA/NASPE (2002). Guideline update for implantation of cardiac pacemakers and antiarrhythmia devices. A report of the American College of Cardiology/American Heart Association Task Force on Practice Guidelines (ACC/AHA/NASPE Committee on Pacemaker Implantation). www.americanheart.org

Nolan, J., Soar, J., Lockey, A. et al. (2005). *Advanced Life Support Course Provider Manual*, (5th edn). Resuscitation Council (UK), London.

If appropriate, give oxygen, cannulate a vein, and record a 12-lead ECG

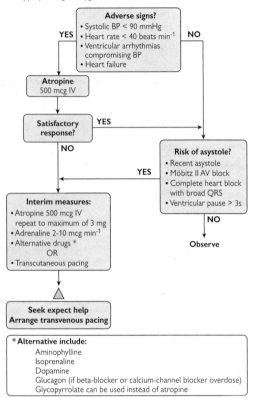

Fig. 1.3 Bradycardia[1] (includes rates inappropriately slow for haemodynamic state).

① Intraoperative arrhythmias: atrial fibrillation

Definition
Chaotic and uncoordinated atrial depolarization and an *irregularly irregular* ventricular rate.

Presentation
- An irregularly irregular QRS complex on the ECG associated with rapid chaotic atrial activity with deflections in size and rate but without visible P waves. A 12-lead ECG provides the best opportunity to confirm AF.
- The refractory period of the AV node determines the ventricular rate. In the absence of drug treatment or disease the ventricular rate will be 120–200 bpm.

Immediate management
(See Fig. 1.4, 'Tachycardia algorithm', p13)
- Treatment of AF depends on whether it is paroxysmal or persistent. If the onset of AF is recent (within 48 h) and is associated with significant cardiovascular compromise (hypotension, rate >150 bpm, cardiac failure, associated valve disease), treatment should include:
  - attempted restoration of sinus rhythm by electrical synchronized cardioversion starting with 120–150 J biphasic or 200 J monophasic. If the first shock does not terminate the arrhythmia, give up to two more shocks of increasing energy up to the maximum setting of the defibrillator
  - immediate correction of precipitating causes, such as electrolyte abnormalities
- If electrical cardioversion fails, attempt chemical cardioversion with amiodarone 300 mg IV over 1 h followed by 900 mg IV over 23 h. Amiodarone will slow the ventricular rate even if it fails to restore sinus rhythm
- In patients with a life-threatening deterioration in haemodynamic stability following the onset of AF, emergency electrical cardioversion should be performed, irrespective of the duration of the AF.
- In patients with non-life-threatening haemodynamic instability, if the AF has been present for more than 48 h, anticoagulation is required before attempting cardioversion (risk of embolizing any blood clot in the atrium):
  - rate control can be achieved with an intravenous beta-blocker, such as esmolol, atenolol, or metoprolol
  - a rate-controlling calcium antagonist is a good option but the best of these drugs, diltiazem, is not available for IV use in the UK
  - in the presence of heart failure, rate control can be achieved with digoxin 500 μg IV, repeated after 2–4 h

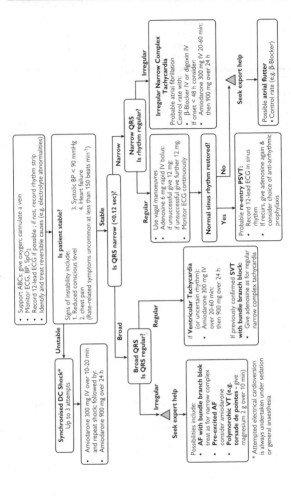

Fig. 1.4 TACHYCARDIA[1]

The flow chart contains the following text:

Top box:
- Support ABCs; give oxygen; cannulate a vein
- Monitor ECG, BP, SpO₂
- Record 12-lead ECG if possible : if not, record rhythm strip
- Identify and treat reversible causes (e.g. electrolyte abnormalities)

Is patient stable?
Signs of instability include:
1. Reduced conscious level
2. chest pain
3. Systolic BP < 90 mmHg
4. Heart failure
(Rate-related symptoms uncommon at less than 150 beats min⁻¹)

Unstable

Synchronised DC Shock*
Up to 3 attempts

- Amiodarone 300 mg IV over 10-20 min and repeat shock; followed by:
- Amiodarone 900 mg over 24 h

* Attempted electrical cardioversion is always undertaken under sedation or general anaesthesia

Stable

Is QRS narrow (<0.12 sec)?

Broad

Broad QRS Is QRS regular?

Irregular

Seek expert help

Possibilities include:
- AF with bundle branch blok treat as for narrow complex
- Pre-excited AF consider amiodarone
- Polymorohic VT (e.g. torsade de pointes - give magnesium 2 g over 10 min)

Regular

If **Ventricular Tachycardia** (or uncertain rhythm):
- Amiodarone 300 mg IV over 20-60 min; then 900 mg over 24 h

If previously confirmed SVT **with bundle branch block**:
- Give adenosine as for regular narrow complex tachycardia

Narrow

Narrow QRS Is rhythm regular?

Regular

- Use vagal manoeuvres
- Adenosine 6 mg rapid IV bolus; if unsuccessful give 12 mg; if unsuccessful give further 12 mg.
- Monitor ECG continuously

Normal sinus rhythm restored?

Yes
Probable **re-entry PSVT:**
- Record 12-lead ECG in sinus rhythm
- If recurs, give adenosine again & consider choice of anti-arrhythmic prophylaxis

No

Seek export help

Possible **atrial flutter**
- Control rate (e.g. β-Blocker)

Irregular

Irregular Narrow Complex Tachycardia
Probable atrial fibrillation
Control rate with:
- β-Blocker IV or digoxin IV
If onset < 48 h consider:
- Amiodarone 300 mg IV 20-60 min; then 900 mg over 24 h

Subsequent management

- Treat precipitating reversible causes (electrolyte abnormalities, hypovolaemia, sepsis). If digoxin is used, ensure therapeutic levels (1–2 ng/mL). Anticoagulate unless contraindicated.
- Patients remaining in AF require 3 weeks of full anticoagulation before attempting cardioversion. In patients with persistent AF, a rate-control strategy is the preferred initial option for those:
  - over 65
  - with coronary artery disease
  - with contraindications to anti-arrhythmic drugs
  - without congestive heart failure
- Patients in AF started on amiodarone to control rate must be converted to an alternative drug (e.g. beta-blocker or diltiazem) for rate control (long-term complications associated with amiodarone).
- The goals for rate control are to produce a resting heart rate of 60–90 bpm and not >110 bpm after slight exercise.

Investigations

ECG, U&Es, ABGs, TFTs

Risk factors

Common causes of atrial fibrillation (AF) include:
- Myocardial ischaemia
- Sepsis
- Rheumatic heart disease
- Electrolyte abnormalities (especially hypokalaemia or hypomagnesaemia)
- Hypertension
- Thoracic surgery

Exclusions

- Frequent atrial ectopic beats can give the appearance of AF.
- Other supraventricular tachycardias are regular—but at very fast rates it can be difficult to distinguish these from AF.
- Atrial flutter is characterized by rapid and regular atrial activity with a rate of 250–350 bpm. This creates characteristic saw-tooth flutter waves on the ECG best seen in leads II and V_1. There is usually AV block of between 2:1 and 8:1. Thus, atrial flutter at 300 bpm and a 2:1 block will result in a ventricular rate of 150 bpm.

Special considerations

Long-term anticoagulation is normally recommended for patients over 65 years with AF, or those with large atria. In these patients the risk of an embolic event is 6% per year. Anticoagulation to an INR of 2.0–4.0 reduces this risk by 70%.

Further reading

Nathanson, M.H., Gajraj, N.M. (1998). The peri-operative management of atrial fibrillation. *Anaesthesia*, **53**, 665–76.

National Institute for Health and Clinical Excellence. NICE clinical guideline 36. Atrial Fibrillation. The management of atrial fibrillation. June 2006.

☩ Intraoperative arrhythmias: narrow-complex tachycardia

Definition
Regular, narrow-complex (QRS <0.12 s duration) tachycardia arising from above the ventricles. Includes sinus tachycardia, atrial tachycardia, junctional tachycardia, and atrial flutter.

Presentation
- ECG demonstrating narrow-complex tachycardia (QRS <0.12 s) with rate 100–300 bpm.
- Presence of normal P wave implies sinus tachycardia.
- Flutter waves (typically 300 bpm) present in atrial flutter. A 2:1 block is common and results in a ventricular rate of 150 bpm.
- During a junctional tachycardia the P waves may be hidden behind the QRS complexes or, if they are visible, they are often inverted or of abnormal morphology.
- A 12-lead ECG taken during sinus rhythm may reveal evidence of an accessory pathway:
  - short PR interval
  - slurred upstroke on the R wave (the delta wave).

Immediate management
(See Fig. 1.4, 'Tachycardia algorithm', p13)
- If sinus tachycardia, treat underlying causes (see below).
- Having excluded sinus tachycardia, attempt vagal manoeuvres such as carotid sinus massage.
- Give adenosine 6 mg by rapid bolus, followed if necessary by up to 2 doses of 12 mg. Adenosine may terminate the arrhythmia or will temporarily slow the ventricular rate, enabling the diagnosis of the underlying rhythm (e.g. flutter waves may become more visible). Avoid adenosine in asthmatic patients—side-effects include flushing, dyspnoea, and headache.
- If cardiovascular compromise (systolic blood pressure <90 mmHg, heart failure, reduced conscious level, evidence of myocardial ischaemia), attempt electrical synchronized cardioversion using 70–120 J biphasic or 100 J monophasic. If the first shock does not terminate the arrhythmia, give up to two more shocks of increasing energy up to the maximum setting of the defibrillator.
- If cardioversion is not achieved, give amiodarone 300 mg IV over 10–20 min, then repeat shock. Follow this with amiodarone 900 mg IV over 23 h.
- In the absence of cardiovascular compromise, there are several options for drug treatment that will control ventricular rate and may produce cardioversion to sinus rhythm (e.g. amiodarone 300 mg IV over 20–60 min followed by 900 mg IV over 23 h, esmolol 50–200 µg/kg/min, or verapamil 5–10 mg IV).

Subsequent management
- Treat precipitating reversible causes (electrolyte abnormalities, hypovolaemia, sepsis). Look for evidence of an accessory pathway.
- Patients with evidence of an accessory pathway will need referral to a cardiologist.

Investigations
ECG, U&Es, ABGs, TFTs

Risk factors
Common causes of sinus tachycardia include:
- Inadequate anaesthesia and/or analgesia
- Hypovolaemia
- Hypoxaemia
- Hypercapnia
- Sepsis

Supraventricular tachycardias may be caused by an atrioventricular accessory pathway causing a pre-excitation antidromic (re-entry) arrhythmia, e.g. Wolff–Parkinson–White (WPW) syndrome.

Exclusions
- Awareness/light anaesthesia—check delivery of inhalational/intravenous agent to the patient.
- Ventricular tachycardia will cause broad QRS complexes (>0.12 s).
- Fast atrial fibrillation can appear regular, but close inspection of a 12-lead ECG should enable the correct diagnosis.

Special considerations
Supraventricular tachycardias associated with aberrant conduction pathways will produce wide-complex tachycardias resembling *ventricular* tachycardia. If the patient is severely compromised, the appropriate treatment is as for ventricular tachycardia (see 'Broad-complex tachycardias', pp18–9).

Further reading
Nolan, J., Soar, J., Lockey, A. et al. (2005). *Advanced Life Support Course Provider Manual*, (5th edn). Resuscitation Council (UK), London.

Thompson, A., Balser, J.R. (2004). Perioperative cardiac arrhythmias. *British Journal of Anaesthesia*, **93**, 86–94.

Intraoperative arrhythmias: road-complex tachycardia

Definition

Tachycardia arising from the ventricles (ventricular tachycardia, (VT) or a supraventricular tachycardia associated with aberrant conduction. QRS >0.12 s. duration. Torsade de pointes is a specific polymorphic form of VT.

Presentation

- Broad-complex tachycardia with rate >100 bpm.
- History of ischaemic heart disease, visible independent P waves, fusion or capture beats imply VT rather than SVT.
- In the patient without haemodynamic compromise, adenosine (6 mg by rapid bolus followed if necessary by up to 2 doses of 12 mg) can be used to differentiate VT from SVT with aberrant conduction.
- Causes of an irregular broad-complex tachycardia include torsades de pointes, pre-excited AF, and AF with bundle branch block. Torsade de pointes is a polymorphic form of VT characterized by beat-to-beat variation, a constantly changing axis, and a prolonged QT interval.

Immediate management

(See Fig. 1.4, 'Tachycardia algorithm', p13)
- Feel for pulse—if pulseless VT, treat as for VF with immediate attempted defibrillation. Give unsynchronized shocks—see p6.
- In the presence of cardiovascular compromise (systolic blood pressure <90 mmHg, heart failure, reduced conscious level, evidence of myocardial ischaemia), attempt electrical *synchronized* cardioversion using 120–150 J biphasic or 200 J monophasic. If the first shock does not terminate the arrhythmia, give up to two more shocks of increasing energy up to the maximum setting of the defibrillator.
- Correct any electrolyte abnormalities such as hypokalaemia or hypomagnesaemia. If the patient is taking a regular diuretic, assume the presence of hypomagnesaemia and give magnesium 2 g IV.
- If attempted electrical cardioversion fails, give amiodarone 300 mg over 10–20 min IV and repeat attempted electrical cardioversion.
- In the absence of haemodynamic compromise, correct any electrolyte abnormalities and attempt chemical cardioversion with amiodarone 300 mg IV over 20–60 min—follow with electrical cardioversion if necessary.
- If torsade de pointes is present, give magnesium 2 g IV and correct any electrolyte abnormalities such as hypokalaemia.

Subsequent management

- Treat precipitating reversible causes (e.g. electrolyte abnormalities in the presence of a prolonged QT interval). Stop drugs that prolong the QT interval.

- Persistent or recurrence of a broad-complex tachycardia will necessitate urgent referral to a cardiologist—may use alternative anti-arrhythmic drugs or overdrive pacing.

Investigations
ECG, U&Es, ABGs

Risk factors
Causes of VT include:
- Ischaemic heart disease
- Ventricular scarring after myocardial infarction or previous cardiac surgery
- Right ventricular failure
- Electrolyte abnormalities in patients with prolonged QT interval (tricyclic antidepressants, antihistamines, phenothiazines; or Brugada syndrome). These conditions may also precipitate torsade de pointes
- Supraventricular tachycardias caused by an atrioventricular accessory pathway causing a pre-excitation antidromic (re-entry) arrhythmia, e.g. Wolff–Parkinson–White (WPW) syndrome, may cause a broad-complex tachycardia.

Exclusions
- Supraventricular tachycardia with aberrant conduction—in an emergency the treatment is as for ventricular tachycardia.
- Sinus tachycardia with bundle branch block—P waves will precede each QRS complex.

Special considerations
Lidocaine (50 mg IV over 2 min repeated every 5 min to a maximum of 200 mg) was previously the drug of choice for treating broad-complex tachycardias. Although amiodarone is now more popular, lidocaine remains a suitable alternative.

Further reading
Nolan, J., Soar, J., Lockey, A. et al. (2005). *Advanced Life Support Course Provider Manual*, (5th edn). Resuscitation Council (UK), London.

Thompson, A., Balser, J.R. (2004). Perioperative cardiac arrhythmias. *British Journal of Anaesthesia*, **93**, 86–94.

✪ Intraoperative hypotension

Definition
Systolic arterial blood pressure <20% preoperative value.

Presentation
- Hypotension detected by non-invasive or invasive blood pressure monitoring.
- Assess peripheral circulation:
  - warm peripheries imply vasodilatation—consider overdose of anaesthetic (check end-tidal volatile) or high regional block, sepsis (fever, tachycardia, precipitating cause), histamine releasing drugs
  - cold peripheries imply hypovolaemia or pump failure
- A tachycardia will accompany most causes of hypotension (hypovolaemia, sepsis, cardiogenic shock). A bradycardia may be the primary cause—it will also accompany a high neuraxial block. Spinal cord injury is a rare cause of hypotension accompanied by bradycardia.

Immediate management
- ABC ... Ensure adequate oxygenation and ventilation—increase FiO_2 if required.
- Check for blood loss and ensure that venous return is not being impaired inadvertently by surgeons, e.g. direct compression of the inferior vena cava, excessive intra-abdominal pressure during laparoscopic surgery.
- Consider excessive 'third space' losses and quickly assess peripheral perfusion.
- Give fluid bolus of 10 mL/kg crystalloid/colloid to optimize filling pressure and assess response (heart rate, blood pressure, CVP if available). A head-down or legs-up position will rapidly increase venous return while fluid is being given.
- Reduce volatile if appropriate.
- Consider vasoconstrictor or inotrope:
  - if peripherally vasodilated and response to fluid challenge is poor, give a bolus of vasoconstrictor, e.g. metaraminol 0.5–1.0 mg IV or phenylephrine 0.25–0.5 mg IV
  - after an appropriate fluid challenge, if peripheral perfusion is poor and the cardiac output is likely to be low, give ephedrine 6 mg IV and consider starting an infusion of an inotrope such as dobutamine (5–10 µg/kg/min) or adrenaline (0.1–0.2 µg/kg/min)

Subsequent management
If hypotension persists, further management may include:
- Insertion of a central venous catheter to assess CVP
- Further fluid resuscitation as indicated by CVP
- Check urine output to assess renal perfusion
- Infusion of noradrenaline (0.1–0.2 µg/kg/min or more as required) if hypotension persists and the patient remains vasodilated, e.g. septic shock
- Infusion of dobutamine (5–10 µg/kg/min) if poor cardiac output and hypotensive despite adequate fluid volume. A persistent metabolic

acidosis and rising serum lactate may also imply inadequate cardiac output and oxygen delivery
- If available, measurement of cardiac output non-invasively (e.g. oesophageal Doppler or pulse contour analysis) will help to guide fluid resuscitation, inotropes, and vasopressors. Patients with persistent hypotension, oliguria, and significant acidaemia will need admission to a critical care unit postoperatively

Investigations

ECG, CXR, ABGs, haemoglobin (HemoCue® if available), cardiac enzymes

Risk factors

Causes of intraoperative hypotension include:
- Hypovolaemia
  - haemorrhage
  - capillary leak (septic shock, anaphylaxis)
  - dehydration (diarrhoea and/or vomiting)
- Obstructed venous return (tension pneumothorax, compression of IVC)
- Vasodilatation
  - high spinal or epidural block
  - excessive anaesthetic or other vasodilating drugs
  - anaphylactic or anaphylactoid reaction, or septic shock
  - Addisonian crisis
- Obstructive shock
  - pulmonary embolism
  - air embolism
- Pump failure
  - left and/or right ventricular failure
- Arrhythmia

Exclusions

- Measurement errors:
  - damped arterial line measurement errors
  - interference with non-invasive blood pressure cuff
- Hypovolaemia—will usually be accompanied by tachycardia, cool peripheries, collapsed veins (low CVP), and an arterial trace with a marked respiratory swing.
- Suspect dehydration—if the patient has been thirsty, has a dry tongue and sunken eyes, and has elevated urea and creatinine.
- Pulmonary/gas embolism—suspect if the patient had a pre-existing low CVP and open venous bed. Signs include a decrease in end-tidal CO_2, decrease in SaO_2, and increase in CVP.
- Suspect microembolism—from intramedullary cavity in the presence of long-bone fractures or intramedullary surgery.
- Cardiac failure—suspect if the patient has distended neck veins (high CVP), tachycardia, cool peripheries, pulmonary oedema (hypoxaemia, fine crackles on auscultation of the lungs), and ischaemic changes on the ECG.
- Anaphylaxis—will be accompanied, variably, by tachycardia, erythema, rash, urticaria, wheeze, and angioedema.

Paediatric implications
- The same principles apply to the treatment of hypotension in children.
- Fluid boluses of 10 mL/kg should be used and repeated as necessary.
- Inotropes are rarely required.

Special considerations
- Patients on beta-blockers will not mount an appropriate tachycardia.
- In young, healthy patients a short period of hypotension is unlikely to be harmful as long as cardiac output is well maintained. Patients with ischaemic heart disease and/or chronic hypertension will require a higher blood pressure to maintain vital organ perfusion.

☼ Intraoperative hypertension

Definition
Blood pressure >15% above baseline; systolic >160 mmHg; or diastolic >100 mmHg.
Severe hypertension: systolic >180 mmHg or diastolic >110 mmHg.

Presentation
- Hypertension detected by non-invasive or invasive blood pressure monitoring.
- Hypoxia/hypercapnia—ABC ... check SpO_2 and end-tidal CO_2.
- Inadequate depth of anaesthesia—check end-tidal volatile anaesthetic concentration, check TIVA pump and IV cannula.
- Inadequate analgesia—if in doubt, give alfentanil 10–20 µg/kg or remifentanil 0.5 µg/kg and observe effect.
- Measurement error—repeat non-invasive BP while palpating distal pulse (return of pulse approximates systolic pressure); check transducer height if using invasive blood pressure monitoring.
- Iatrogenic drug response—re-check ampoules (e.g. cocaine or ephedrine given instead of morphine) and confirm dilution of vasopressors or inotropes.
- Pre-eclampsia—if the patient is over 20 weeks' pregnant, check for proteinuria, platelet count, clotting studies, and liver function tests.
- Intracranial hypertension—check for Cushing response (hypertension and bradycardia) and dilated pupil.
- Thyroid storm causing elevated T_4 and T_3 levels.
- Phaeochromocytoma causing elevated plasma noradrenaline levels.

Immediate management
- ABC ...
- Consider potential causes. Stop surgery until controlled. Increase FiO_2 if required. Increase ventilation if hypercarbic. Confirm readings. Increase depth of anaesthesia. Give analgesia. Give vasodilator and/or beta-blocker and/or alpha-blocker.
- Assuming this is not a physiological response to a correctable cause, the aim of symptomatic management is to prevent myocardial ischaemia/infarction or hypertensive stroke. In addition to increasing the depth of anaesthesia and giving more analgesia, treatment options include:
  - vasodilators:
    - hydralazine 5 mg slow IV every 15 min
    - GTN (50 mg/50 mL starting at 3 mL/h and titrate to effect)
    - sodium nitroprusside for resistant hypertension (0.5–1.5 µg/kg/min)
  - beta blockade, particularly if hypertension is accompanied by tachycardia:
    - metoprolol 1–2 mg increments
    - labetalol 5–10 mg increments (beta:alpha block ratio 7:1)
    - esmolol 0.5 mg/kg loading dose followed by an infusion of 50–200 µg/kg/min

Subsequent management

- Remifentanil 0.25–0.5 µg/kg/min will provide intense analgesia and will help if surgical stimulation is difficult to overcome by other means.
- Check 12-lead ECG postoperatively and cardiac troponin after 12 h if there is thought to have been severe myocardial ischaemia or infarction.
- Close monitoring of blood pressure. Treat any underlying chronic cause (essential hypertension, hyperthyroidism, phaeochromocytoma).

Investigations

ECG, troponin, thyroid function tests, 24 h urinary catecholamine excretion

Risk factors

- Untreated essential hypertension or 'white coat' hypertension preoperatively (increased lability).
- Aortic surgery—cross-clamping, particularly above the renal arteries, greatly increases systemic vascular resistance.
- Pregnancy-induced hypertension.
- Drugs—MAOIs (+ pethidine), ketamine, ergometrine, systemic absorption of adrenaline-containing solutions, phenylephrine eyedrops, cocaine.
- Family history of multiple endocrine neoplasia (type 2) syndrome, medullary thyroid carcinoma, Conn's syndrome.
- Acute head injury.

Exclusions

- Inadequate depth of anaesthesia/analgesia
- Essential hypertension
- Hypercapnia
- Hypoxia
- Tracheal intubation/extubation
- Drugs
- Aortic clamping
- Pregnancy-induced hypertension
- Raised intracranial pressure
- Malignant hyperthermia
- Thyroid storm
- Phaeochromocytoma
- Measurement errors:
  - interference with non-invasive blood pressure cuff
  - transducer for non-invasive blood pressure too low in relation to the patient's heart

Special considerations

If hypertension is thought to reflect intracranial hypertension, undertake a CT scan of the brain to exclude pathology amenable to neurosurgical intervention. Ensure that MAP is maintained >80 mmHg, head-up tilt, unobstructed SVC drainage, and normocapnia. Consider mannitol and temporary period of hyperventilation (see pp180–1).

☼ **Intraoperative myocardial ischaemia**

(See also pp318–20)

Definition
Inadequate myocardial oxygen supply in relation to demand.

Presentation
- ECG displays ST segment depression (ischaemia) or ST segment elevation (evolving acute myocardial infarction). These changes can be analysed properly only by looking at more than one lead. Ideally, obtain a 12-lead ECG immediately, especially if there is suspicion of ST elevation.
- Impaired myocardial function may cause hypotension and/or pulmonary oedema—assess peripheral perfusion, auscultate for fine crackles that signify left ventricular failure and pulmonary oedema.
- Ischaemia of the cardiac conduction system may cause severe ventricular arrhythmias—these will exacerbate myocardial ischaemia.
- Echocardiography will show a non-contracting ischaemic region of the myocardium bulging outward during systole (dyskinesis).
- Myocardial infarction will be accompanied by an increase in cardiac troponin— a significant increase in this cardiac marker in the absence of ST segment elevation implies non-ST elevation myocardial infarction (NSTEMI). A reliable value for troponin can be achieved only after 12 h.

Immediate management
- ABC … restore oxygen delivery to the myocardium:
  - increase FiO_2 if required
  - give fluid if hypovolaemic, and blood if severely anaemic—myocardial oxygen extraction is normally very high, a combination of coronary artery disease and severe acute anaemia will quickly cause myocardial ischaemia which can be reversed by restoring an adequate haemoglobin concentration (7–9 g/dL)
  - central venous catheter may guide fluid replacement
  - if ischaemic changes persist despite restoration of adequate volume, consider vasopressor if hypotensive or an inodilator (e.g. dobutamine) if blood pressure adequate but cardiac output is poor
- Reduce myocardial oxygen demand:
  - if tachycardia is present, reduce heart rate with beta-blocker and/or analgesia (metoprolol 1–2 mg increments, esmolol 0.5 mg/kg loading dose followed by an infusion of 50–200 µg/kg/min)
  - treat tachyarrhythmias as appropriate (see treatment of supraventricular and ventricular arrhythmias, pp16–17, 18–19)
  - if hypertensive, treat underlying cause and consider GTN infusion to reduce afterload (50 mg/50 mL starting at 3 mL/h and titrate to effect). In the first instance, to hasten delivery, GTN can be sprayed under the patient's tongue
- If ST segment elevation, get immediate 12-lead ECG—if acute myocardial infarction confirmed, consider urgent transfer for percutaneous coronary intervention (thrombolysis will be contraindicated by the surgery)—give aspirin (300 mg chewed/NG).

Subsequent management

- Postoperatively—repeat 12-lead ECG, give supplementary oxygen and maintain adequate mean arterial blood pressure. If myocardial ischaemia persists, continue intravenous nitrate and, depending on the risk from postoperative bleeding, fully heparinize. Request urgent cardiac echo to assess myocardial function.
- Persistent myocardial ischaemia despite optimizing preload, afterload and myocardial contractility will necessitate full anticoagulation with heparin (unless absolutely contraindicated) and referral to a cardiologist for further investigation.
- Measurement of cardiac troponin will enable risk assessment (which will direct further treatment) and exclusion or confirmation of myocardial infarction.
- In the presence of an evolving ST elevation myocardial infarction (STEMI), every effort should be made to achieve coronary revascularization as rapidly as possible. Thrombolysis is contraindicated in the patient who has just undergone surgery, but it may be possible to undertake percutaneous coronary intervention (PCI) in the form of angioplasty with or without coronary stenting.

Investigations

ECG, troponin (12 h after the event)

Risk factors

- Pre-existing coronary artery disease:
  - in the presence of coronary artery disease, hypotension, hypovolaemia or anaemia is more likely to cause myocardial ischaemia
  - spontaneous plaque rupture with partial or total occlusion of a coronary artery may also be the primary cause of myocardial ischaemia or infarction
- Incorrectly placed ECG electrodes during surgery—always place in standard position before induction and assess the normal trace. Changes are more likely to be seen and be significant.

Exclusions

Conduction abnormalities, such as bundle branch block, may be confused with ST segment changes that accompany myocardial ischaemia or infarction.

Special considerations

If the patient is conscious, myocardial ischaemia and/or infarction is likely to be accompanied by angina.

✛ Cardiac tamponade

Definition
Low cardiac output state from mechanical compression of heart.

Presentation
- Typically after penetrating chest trauma or cardiac surgery
- Systemic hypotension with elevated and equalized ventricular filling pressures (RA (CVP) and LA (PCWP)); decreased pulse pressure; raised JVP; pulsus paradoxus; no prominent 'y' descent on central venous pulse wave
- Oliguria. Poor peripheral perfusion, cyanosis, metabolic acidosis, hypoxaemia
- Dyspnoea
- Sudden decrease/cessation of chest drainage in patient previously bleeding heavily after cardiac surgery
- Cardiac arrest

Immediate management
- ABC … 100% O_2.
- Assess vital signs.
- Establish adequate IV access if necessary; give IV fluids, inotropic support.
- Post cardiac surgery—strip/'milk' chest drains; attempt to clear clots from drains by sucking inside them with soft-tip suction catheter. Call for surgical help; alert theatres; prepare to open chest (on cardiac recovery area if necessary).
- Do NOT remove penetrating foreign body if present.
- Unless in cardiac arrest, anaesthetize before chest opening: choose technique which minimizes vasodilatation; intubation and ventilation will be required as chest will be opened; be prepared to open chest (wire cutters) immediately after induction.
- Open chest immediately if haemodynamics cannot be controlled.
- If in cardiac arrest caused by cardiac tamponade following penetrating thoracic trauma, immediate resuscitative thoracotomy is required.
- Pericardiocentesis may gain time and lessen the haemodynamic insult of anaesthesia (rarely used in acute situation).
- Request blood, and clotting factors as necessary.

Subsequent management
- Maintain filling pressures and sympathetic tone; avoid bradycardia.
- Anticipate blood pressure overshoot immediately on chest opening and relief of tamponade; usually rapid recovery of haemodynamic stability following mediastinal evacuation.
- Ensure surgeon identifies bleeding point and clears drains of clots.
- Correct metabolic acidosis.
- Positive pressure ventilation will worsen tamponade and hypotension.
- Repeat antibiotics if chest re-opened.

Investigations
- Chest X-ray (widened mediastinum)
- ECG (low voltage, electrical alternans, T-wave abnormalities)
- Echocardiogram/TOE (pericardial fluid collection, small non-filling ventricles)

Risk factors
- Chest trauma (particularly penetrating)
- Recent cardiac surgery, especially if:
  - heavy bleeding through chest drains postoperatively
  - pleurae NOT opened perioperatively
  - re-operations
- Coagulopathy (both hyper- and hypocoagulable)
- Hypothermia

Exclusions
- Tension pneumothorax
- Cardiogenic shock/myocardial failure/MI
- Pulmonary embolus
- Overtransfusion, fluid overload
- Anaphylaxis

Paediatric implications
- Cardiac tamponade can occur with very low volumes of shed blood in the mediastinum.
- Can be very sudden and present as cardiac arrest.
- Increased risk with cyanotic conditions, complex re-operations and impaired coagulation associated with hepatic congestion.

Special considerations
- **Electrical alternans**—beat-to-beat shift in QRS axis associated with mechanical swinging of the heart in a large accumulation of fluid. Virtually pathognomonic of cardiac tamponade, though not always seen.
- High index of suspicion for cardiac tamponade after cardiac surgery.
- Only *definitive* diagnosis is made by opening chest—even small pericardial collections on echocardiography can have large haemodynamic consequences if pressing on the right atrium.
- Diagnosis can be very difficult, especially if possible failure/overload.
- If severe, impaired coronary flow may cause myocardial ischaemia, further complicating diagnosis.
- Presentation can be slow or very rapid.
- Hypocoagulable patients are more likely to bleed into the pericardium.
- Hypercoagulable patients are more likely to clot off chest drains.
- Patients with cardiac tamponade caused by penetrating trauma, including stabbed hearts and gunshot wounds, should be taken to theatre immediately and a pericardial exploration performed. Patients in cardiac arrest following penetrating thoracic trauma require immediate resuscitative thoracotomy (usually in the emergency department). Percutaneous pericardial drainage (pericardiocentesis) is usually ineffective and should not be performed unless surgery is unavailable.

:☼: Pulmonary embolus

Definition
Obstruction of pulmonary circulation by thromboembolus.

Presentation
- Chest pain (typically pleuritic). Dyspnoea, tachypnoea, haemoptysis.
- Hypoxaemia or increased A–a PO_2 gradient.
- Hypotension, tachycardia, dysrhythmia, cyanosis, poor peripheral perfusion, raised JVP/CVP, decreased end-tidal CO_2.
- Oliguria.
- Cardiovascular collapse, cardiac arrest.

Immediate management
- ABC ... 100% O_2, intubation/ventilation if arrested/*in extremis*.
- Define severity:
  - non-massive PE—no RV dysfunction
  - submassive PE—right ventricular dilation and hypokinesis without systemic hypotension. Symptoms of chest pain and dyspnoea
  - massive PE—severe haemodynamic and ventilatory impairment with increased RV afterload

Medical treatment
- *Non-massive and submassive PE*
- Anticoagulation—therapeutic dose of low molecular weight heparin, e.g. enoxaparin 1.5 mg/kg every 24 h is first choice. Unfractionated heparin (10 000 units load, then 1500–2000 units/h aiming for APTT 1.5 – 2.5 × normal) is preferred if severe renal impairment, for those at high risk of bleeding, the elderly, or those extremely under- or overweight.

Massive PE
- Wide-bore IV access, fluid resuscitation, central access.
- Monitor vital signs (including invasive arterial and central venous pressure if massive PE).
- Inotropic support as required.
- Thrombolysis (alteplase rt-PA 10 mg over 1–2 min then 90 mg over 2 h; tenecteplase, t-PA 30–50 mg bolus). Surgery within the previous 1–2 weeks is a relative contraindication to thrombolysis. Thrombolysis is also considered in some cases of submassive PE.
- Consider surgical embolectomy if thrombolytic therapy is contraindicated.

Subsequent management
- Consider insertion of inferior vena cava filter if anticoagulation is contraindicated.
- Surgical embolectomy—if severe, deteriorating state, failed medical treatment, collapse, arrest, and in a centre that has this facility.
- Transvenous embolectomy (in a centre with this facility).

Investigations
- Arterial blood gases (hypoxaemia, hypercapnia or respiratory alkalosis, metabolic acidosis)

- Immediate transthoracic echocardiography
- Chest X-ray (oligaemic lung fields, prominent PA)
- ECG:
  - 'S$_I$ Q$_{III}$ T$_{III}$' 20–50%
  - T-wave inversion anteriorly 85%
  - right heart strain 75%
- CT pulmonary angiogram (CTPA)
- Troponin—an elevated value may identify those with submassive PE who may benefit from thrombolysis.

Risk factors

- Prolonged stasis/immobility; paralysis; recent air travel
- Postoperative patients (classically 10 days), especially following prolonged and extensive pelvic/abdominal dissections; vascular damage
- Previous history of DVT/thromboembolism
- Hypercoagulability, obesity, oral contraceptives, malignancy, elderly
- Heart failure

Exclusions

- Myocardial infarction
- Respiratory tract infection, pneumonia
- Pneumothorax
- Cardiac tamponade
- Bronchial neoplasm; acute airway obstruction
- Sepsis

Special considerations

Anaesthetic management for emergency surgical embolectomy
- Avoid hypotension on induction ('fixed cardiac output'— decreased ventricular loading can lead to arrest).
- Have wide-bore intravenous, central venous, invasive arterial access established and surgical team scrubbed before induction.
- Consider femoral vessel cannulation under LA.
- General aim is to maintain low PVR to offload right ventricle (but NOT cause excessive systemic vasodilatation), maintain cardiac output, and maintain coronary flow.
- If inotropes required, adrenaline may be the best compromise.
- Aggressive fluid therapy to maintain circulating blood volume (increased central blood volume causes pulmonary dilatation; little risk of pulmonary oedema but further RV failure possible).
- Avoid hypoxaemia and hypercapnia (more important than the increase in intrathoracic pressure during IPPV) as this will reduce PVR.
- Gentle hand ventilation during pulmonary arteriotomy on bypass to massage clots back out of PA.
- Manage pulmonary haemorrhage (may be copious bleeding from tracheal tube):
  - crossmatch blood, order clotting factors—especially if prior use of thrombolysis
  - frequent ETT suction
  - PEEP
  - consider double-lumen endobronchial tube if side known
  - may require pneumonectomy

Further reading

Konstantinides, S.V. (2008). Acute pulmonary embolism revisited. *Heart*, **94**, 795–802.

Tapson, V.F. (2008). Acute pulmonary embolism. *New England Journal of Medicine*, **358**, 1037–52.

✣ Cardiac trauma

Definition
Blunt or penetrating injury to heart or great vessels.

Presentation
- Chest bruising, shock, hypotension, hypovolaemia, hypoxaemia.
- Poor peripheral perfusion, unequal/absent peripheral pulses, dysrhythmia, cardiac tamponade. Haemothorax—dull chest percussion, decreased breath sounds.
- May be coexisting injuries of other thoracic structures:
  - chest wall trauma (rib fracture, sternal fracture, sucking wound, flail segment)
  - pulmonary contusion (haemoptysis, haemothorax, hypoxaemia)
  - tracheobronchial rupture (stridor, dyspnoea, pneumothorax, hypoxaemia)
  - diaphragmatic rupture (dyspnoea, hypoxaemia, chest 'bowel' sounds)
  - oesophageal rupture (pain, dysphagia, mediastinal air on CXR)

Immediate management
- General management strategy as for all trauma cases. Neck immobilization.
- ABC … 100% O_2.
- Wide-bore intravenous access, fluid resuscitation.
- Intubate/ventilate if necessary.
- Rapidly establish nature and extent of injuries—cardiac contusion is notoriously difficult to diagnose, rarely an isolated injury, sternal/rib fractures are a common though not essential association.
- Have high index of suspicion in all cases of blunt chest injury. Critical factor is adequacy of cardiac function.
- If penetrating implement in place, do not remove.
- Haemodynamic instability/inadequacy may be hypovolaemia, cardiac tamponade (see pp28–9), blunt thoracic aortic injury or primary myocardial dysfunction.
- Central venous access, invasive arterial monitoring (right arm).
- Chest drain if haemothorax/pneumothorax; observe rate of bleeding/air leak (theatre if excessive).
- Order blood and clotting factors, organize theatres.
- Analgesia.
- If blunt aortic injury is suspected, in the absence of head injury, aim for a systolic blood pressure of 80–90 mmHg until definitive repair/stenting is achieved.

Subsequent management
- Anaesthetic considerations. Assume full stomach; obtain control of airway and ventilation; if airway cannot be controlled (e.g. lower tracheal rupture) urgent bypass may be the only option.
- Cardiac contusion:
  - monitor haemodynamics and ECG

- inotropes and antidysrhythmics as required
- remember to treat other injuries
- coronary artery injury very rare but may require coronary grafting
- Cardiac or great vessel rupture/perforation:
  - ongoing resuscitation
  - theatre for urgent surgical repair
  - order blood and clotting factors
  - like aortic dissection, blunt thoracic aortic injury can present with proximal hypertension
  - typically median sternotomy
  - cardiorrhaphy may be performed on beating heart without bypass; if intracardiac damage, bypass will be required. Remember to give heparin (300 units/kg) before aortic/femoral cannulation. Bleeding may be brisk when chest is opened, requiring chest sucker-to-femoral artery bypass
  - two-thirds of blunt thoracic aortic injuries are now managed with endovascular stent grafts
- Cardiac tamponade—see pp28–9.
- Aortic dissection—see pp36–9.
- Antibiotics, tetanus.

Investigations

- Chest X-ray (rib/sternal fractures, widened mediastinum, haemothorax)
- ECG (dysrhythmia, non-specific or ST segment changes)
- Echocardiogram; CT scan (contrast, spiral); aortogram
- Troponin

Risk factors

- Travel, notably road traffic crash (RTC)
- Use of seatbelts important factor in car accidents
- Velocity of impact

Exclusions

- Haemorrhage from other sites
- Cardiac tamponade
- Aortic dissection
- Primary myocardial dysfunction
- May be coexisting injuries besides thorax (neck, head, abdomen, limbs)

Classification

- Blunt (non-penetrating):
  - blunt cardiac injury ('cardiac contusion')
  - cardiac rupture
  - aortic dissection
  - great vessel tear/rupture
- Penetrating—implement may or may not be in place
  - cardiac perforation
  - great vessel perforation

:⚙: Thoracic aortic dissection

Definition
Intimal tear creates a false lumen in the wall of the aorta.

Presentation
- Sudden-onset 'tearing' chest pain radiating to back.
- Severe hypertension; differential blood pressure in different limbs (some may be hypotensive/pulseless).
- Signs of acute aortic regurgitation (wide pulse pressure, collapsing pulse). Areas of poor peripheral perfusion. Oliguria.
- May present in cardiovascular collapse/cardiac arrest as:
  - cardiac tamponade (if ruptured into pericardium)
  - haemothorax (if ruptured into pleural space).
- When on cardiopulmonary bypass, presents as sudden decreased venous return and mean arterial pressure, with increased arterial 'line pressure' (i.e. pressure measured by perfusionist in arterial tubing returning blood from pump).

Immediate management
- ABC … 100% O_2.
- Wide-bore peripheral IV access.
- Invasive arterial monitoring, central intravenous access, urinary catheter.
- Control BP—decrease myocardial contractility (essential) ± vasodilatation (helpful). Aim for systolic arterial pressure ≤110 mmHg.
  - α_1/β_1-blockade (e.g. labetalol 5 mg boluses or infusion 2 mg/min until satisfactory response; max dose 200 mg)
  - sodium nitroprusside infusion (initially 0.3 µg/kg/min, increasing to max of 1.5 µg/kg/min until satisfactory response)
  - analgesia (e.g. IV morphine)
- Monitor all pulses; neurological examination (?cerebral and spinal cord perfusion).
- Arrange theatres or transfer.

Subsequent management

Classification
- Type 'A'—involving ascending aorta (i.e. proximal, regardless of possible distal extension):
  - urgent surgical management
  - median sternotomy approach
  - usually associated with aortic valve regurgitation (disrupted aortic annulus)
- Type 'B'—involving descending thoracic aorta only (i.e. distal, not involving ascending aorta):
  - usually initial conservative medical management but may proceed urgently to theatre if complicated (rupture, uncontrollable BP, distal vascular compromise), or for endovascular stenting
  - lateral thoracotomy approach
  - often associated with spinal cord ischaemia

Anaesthetic considerations
Type 'A' dissection

- Surgical procedure is interposition of a tubular graft of the ascending aorta and resuspension of aortic valve; occasionally, valve/aortic root must be replaced and coronaries reimplanted (same anaesthetic management) *or* surgery involves arch (requires deep hypothermic circulatory arrest for cerebral protection). Usually no coronary angiogram available and therefore state of coronary arteries is unknown in these patients.
- Use right radial/brachial artery for monitoring; if dissection involves this limb, it will be pulseless, therefore use left arm.
- Wide-bore IV access/central IV access/PAFC introducer pre-induction. Nasopharyngeal, rectal, and peripheral temperature probes. PA flotation catheter useful but don't delay surgery for placement.
- Maintain BP control (aim for systolic arterial pressure of 80–90 mmHg):
  - particularly avoid BP rise (may cause aortic rupture) on intubation, induction, and sternotomy (fentanyl, esmolol)
  - use volatile anaesthetic/labetalol/vasodilator infusion to maintain pressure reduction
- Manage aortic regurgitation—avoid bradycardias (isoprenaline, atropine), decrease afterload (isoprenaline, vasodilators), avoid severe diastolic hypotension (reduction in coronary perfusion).
- Femoral artery cannulation for bypass, usually *before* sternotomy.
- Remember to give heparin before cannulation (300 units/kg). Anticipate major blood loss and coagulopathy—crossmatch blood (6 units), order clotting factors, consider aprotinin.
- Anticipate myocardial dysfunction (myocardial hypertrophy, prolonged bypass and cross-clamp times, dissection involving coronaries).
- Be aware that false lumen may have been cannulated—attempt to verify correct location by monitoring nasopharyngeal ('brain') and rectal ('core') temperatures during start of hypothermia on bypass—head temperature MUST cool with rectal temperature; check pupils; urine output.
- If surgery involves arch, deep hypothermic circulatory arrest will be required (cerebral and renal protection, e.g. thiopental 10 mg/kg; mannitol 0.5 g/kg; methylprednisolone 30 mg/kg).
- Anticipate hypotension on decannulation of femoral artery (lactate release)—sodium bicarbonate 50–100 mmol.

Type 'B' dissection
- Left lateral thoracotomy; double lumen endobronchial tube.
- Not performed on bypass but:
  - one-lung ventilation
  - aorta cross-clamped with severe proximal hypertension (BP control) and haemodynamic upset on unclamping ($NaHCO_3$, inotropes)
  - use right radial/brachial artery for invasive BP monitoring in case left subclavian artery is clamped
  - consider renal protection before aortic cross-clamp applied
  - risk of spinal cord ischaemia (consider steroid, barbiturate, spinal drain for spinal cord protection)
- Severe bleeding common—crossmatch blood (6 units), clotting factors, aprotinin, use cell saver if available.

Investigations
- Chest X-ray (widened mediastinum; loss of aortic knuckle; displacement of intimal calcification)
- ECG (hypertrophy, strain, myocardial ischaemia if coronary involvement)
- CT scan (intimal flap, true and false lumen)—*commonest*
- MRI scan (intimal flap, true and false lumen)
- Aortogram (intimal tear, distal flow)—*definitive*
- Echocardiogram
- ABGs (metabolic acidosis: mesenteric ischaemia?)

Risk factors
- Hypertension
- Marfan's syndrome, connective tissue disease, cystic medial necrosis
- Chest trauma
- Atherosclerosis
- Cardiac surgery (intraoperative complication)

Exclusions
- Myocardial infarction
- Pulmonary embolus
- Acutely extending thoracic aortic aneurysm

Transferring thoracic aortic rupture to a cardiac centre

- Stabilize patient, wide-bore intravenous access, oxygen.
- Analgesia (morphine, fentanyl).
- Monitor cardiorespiratory status (BP, ECG, SpO_2).
- Intubate and ventilate if necessary (cardiostable induction).
- Maintain haemodynamic stability—control systolic arterial pressure between 80 and 90 mmHg (e.g. labetalol infusion). Avoid overtransfusion with intravenous fluids.
- Ensure receiving hospital is fully notified. Transfer rapidly.
- Take blood with patient; maintain monitoring, BP control, and analgesia/sedation.

Respiratory

Tim Cook and Benjamin Walton

☼ Hypercapnia

Definition
$PaCO_2 > 6.3$ kPa (50 mmHg).

Presentation
Raised end-tidal CO_2 or $PaCO_2$.

Immediate management

- Increase inspired O_2 to maintain $SpO_2 > 95\%$.
- Check/increase minute ventilation. If patient is breathing spontaneously, then exclude excessive depth of anaesthesia and consider starting assisted ventilation.
- Compare measured inspired/expired tidal volumes for evidence of circuit leaks leading to reduced V_t. Check ETT or LMA cuff pressure.
- Examine the capnography trace to exclude rebreathing of CO_2. If detected, increase fresh gas flow or change CO_2 absorbent in circle system.
- Check for disconnections within the breathing system that increase dead space (e.g. internal limb of a Bain circuit).
- Ensure expiratory valves of circle system are not sticking.
- If safe functioning of the circuit is in doubt, change to alternative means of assisted ventilation. Remember to maintain adequate anaesthesia.
- Examine patient for signs of inadequate anaesthesia and deepen if necessary.

Subsequent management
If $PaCO_2$/$ETCO_2$ continues to rise, exclude malignant hyperthermia or thyroid storm.

Investigations
ABGs to confirm elevated $PaCO_2$, and check for base deficit suggestive of metabolic problem. K^+ and CK if MH suspected.

Risk factors

- Increased CO_2 production—including pyrexia, sepsis, malignant hyperthermia, neuroleptic malignant syndrome, serotonin syndrome, reperfusion injury, thyroid storm.
- Decreased CO_2 excretion—respiratory depression, bronchospasm, inadequate minute volume during IPPV, inappropriate or faulty breathing system, partial airway obstruction, ineffective breathing during SV, excessive dead space.
- Increased CO_2 delivery to the lungs—abdominal insufflation with CO_2, capnothorax.
- Rebreathed CO_2—exhausted soda lime, inadequate FGF in partial rebreathing system, circuit valve fault, CO_2 in the fresh gas mixture.

Exclusions

- Malignant hyperthermia.
- A degree of hypoventilation is common under anaesthesia with SV.

Paediatric implications

Small increases in equipment dead space may significantly compromise the elimination of expired carbon dioxide.

Special considerations

- The vast majority of cases of intraoperative hypercapnia is not clinically significant in the absence of dysrhythmias or raised intracranial pressure, and specific treatment is not needed.
- The toxic child/adolescent with sepsis may have a very high metabolic rate and raised CO_2. If MH needs to be ruled out, investigate as above (see also pp262–4).

☼ Hypocapnia

Definition
$PaCO_2$ <4.5 kPa (35 mmHg).

Presentation
Reduced end-tidal CO_2 or $PaCO_2$.

Immediate management

No $ETCO_2$
- Check patient, monitors, connections, and ventilator at the same time as switching to 100% O_2 and confirming presence of a pulse.
- If cardiac arrest confirmed, perform advanced life support (see p5).
- Hand ventilate on 100% O_2 looking for chest movement (remove drapes if necessary). This eliminates circuit disconnection and airway/circuit obstruction.
- If cardiac output is present but unable to ventilate, check position of ETT/LMA. Consider passing suction catheter down ETT/LMA to confirm patency. Exclude complete laryngospasm, foreign body, or displacement. If in doubt remove airway device and replace.
- Change to self-inflating bag with 100% O_2 if circuit obstruction confirmed and not remedied immediately. Keep $ETCO_2$ monitoring if possible (e.g. attach side stream analyser to a new HME filter).

Low $ETCO_2$
- Check patient's vital signs (pulse, SpO_2, BP, temperature) and monitors.
- Look for causes of low cardiac output (e.g. reduction in venous return due to caval compression or concealed blood loss).
- Is the patient being overventilated—is the respiratory rate high?
- Consider possibility of air/gas embolism (pp62–3). If likely, ask the surgeon to compress any bleeding points or irrigate wound.
- Check ABGs. Does the $PaCO_2$ correlate with the $ETCO_2$? If not, does $ETCO_2$ monitor need replacing/recalibrating?

Subsequent management
- If equipment problem detected, ensure this is corrected for subsequent cases.
- Compromised elderly patients may have low metabolic rates. Adjust ventilation to produce normal $ETCO_2$ as excessive cerebral vasoconstriction may result.
- Hypothyroidism is a rare underlying cause.

Investigations
- ABGs

Risk factors
Elderly patients undergoing major surgery (hypovolaemia, hypothermia, metabolic rate).

Exclusions
- **No ETCO$_2$**—implies analyser disconnected/faulty, no ventilation or no cardiac output. Check CO$_2$ analyser and connection, pulse/SpO$_2$, airway, and circuit. Is the ventilator on? Remember oesophageal intubation and accidental extubation.
- **Low ETCO$_2$**—consider rate of fall.
  - patient—reduced cardiac output or CO$_2$ production (hypothermia/hypotension/anaphylaxis/embolism). Impaired gas exchange or compensated metabolic acidosis. Obstructing airway
  - anaesthetic—hyperventilation, anaesthesia too deep
  - equipment—monitor, sampling

Special considerations
Beware the elderly, hypotensive, hypovolaemic patient. A low PaCO$_2$ will further compromise cerebral circulation. Reduce ventilation and resuscitate.

✹ Hypoxaemia during anaesthesia

Definition
Inadequate arterial oxygen content.

Presentation
- SaO_2 <90% with good perfusion. Cyanosis.
- Bradycardia in children.

Immediate management
- Change to 100% oxygen—confirm with oxygen analyser. Change oxygen source if doubt.
- Ventilate manually with large tidal volumes—check chest movement.
- If possible circuit leak or obstruction, switch to a self-inflating bag or remove airway components until problem disappears.
- If circuit is patent but ventilation is obstructed, suction down ETT/LMA to clear—replace and use facemask if necessary.
- If chest movement or auscultation is asymmetrical, consider possibility of pneumothorax (especially tension) or bronchial intubation.
- Listen for added sounds suggesting bronchospasm, oedema, or aspiration.
- Check pulse and blood pressure—exclude hypovolaemia/heart failure.
- If atelectasis is suspected (elderly, smokers, obese, supine), alveolar recruitment may be achieved by CPAP of 30 cmH_2O for 30 s. PEEP during IPPV may reverse atelectasis and prevent recurrence.

Subsequent management
- CXR postoperatively (or on table).
- Impact of a low SaO_2 is worsened by anaemia, hypovolaemia, carbon monoxide poisoning, sickle cell disease.
- Severe right to left shunt may present as hypoxia.

Investigations
ABGs, CXR, bronchoscopy

Risk factors
- Reduced FiO_2—anaesthetic gas failure.
- Reduced alveolar ventilation—depressed respiration, neuromuscular blockade, airway failure, circuit obstruction, oesophageal intubation, accidental extubation, or bronchial intubation.
- Increased ventilation/perfusion mismatch—chronic lung disease, interstitial lung problem (oedema, infection), PE, aspiration, airway collapse, atelectasis.

Exclusions

- Faulty SpO_2 probe or poor position, surgical diathermy, or excessive patient movement, e.g. shivering or seizure activity. Check trace as well as the number, reposition the probe to obtain a better trace—if doubt, check ABGs. Oximeters also may misread during poor perfusion: check blood pressure.
- Anaphylaxis may present as hypoxia—hypotension will usually be a feature.
- Methaemoglobinaemia. Pulse oximetry readings falsely low due to the misinterpretation of methaemoglobin for deoxyhaemoglobin by pulse oximeter (typically reads approximately 85%).
- Methylene blue [methylthioninium chloride] injection (e.g. for parathyroid/renal surgery) and patent blue (for sentinel node identification in breast surgery) have similar effects.
- Carboxyhaemoglobin produces a falsely high pulse oximeter reading in the presence of normal ABGs. Exclude by bench oximetry readings from ABGs.

Paediatric implications

- Due to higher oxygen consumption and reduced FRC, rapid desaturation is more likely.
- The infant lung is more susceptible to both mucus obstruction and atelectasis, so frequent tracheal suctioning and administration of PEEP may be beneficial.
- Congenital heart disease. Treat aggressively with 100% oxygen to reduce PVR. Adrenaline and IV fluid to increase SVR, thus diminishing right to left shunt. Seek expert advice.

Special considerations

Cyanosis is only clinically detectable when the amount of deoxygenated haemoglobin is greater than 5 g/dL. An anaemic patient may therefore be extremely hypoxic yet not appear cyanosed.

✪ **Non-tension pneumothorax**

Definition
Air in the pleural space.

Presentation
- Dyspnoea, cough, pleuritic chest pain, hypoxia.
- Asymmetric chest expansion with reduced air entry and hyper-resonance on percussion. Increased airway pressures during IPPV.
- Erect CXR—absent lung markings lateral to lung edge. Diagnosis more difficult with supine CXR. Anterior pneumothorax may occur in trauma/ICU—needs CT for diagnosis.

Immediate management
- High flow 100% oxygen. IV access.
- Exclude tension pneumothorax (hypotension, significant respiratory distress). Tracheal deviation and jugular venous distension are late signs and often absent—see pp50–1.
- If tension pneumothorax is suspected, perform needle decompression (2nd intercostal space mid-clavicular line) followed by intercostal drain insertion.
- Nitrous oxide will worsen pneumothorax and should not be used.

Subsequent management
- Patients on IPPV should have an intercostal drain inserted unless immediate weaning from IPPV is possible.
- 1° pneumothorax—if symptomatic and/or >2 cm: needle aspiration. If unsuccessful, try one repeat aspiration, then insert intercostal drain. If asymptomatic and <2 cm—observe.
- 2° pneumothorax—if symptomatic, >2 cm, or patient >50 years old: intercostal drain, otherwise try aspiration.
- Persistent air leak—consider applying suction after 48 h (high volume/low pressure, 10–20 cmH$_2$O). Refer to thoracic surgery for further treatment (e.g. pleurodesis or pleurectomy).

Investigations
CXR, CT for complex cases

Risk factors
- Secondary pneumothorax—associated with medical conditions: emphysema, Marfan's and Ehlers–Danlos syndromes.
- High-speed trauma—exclude pneumothorax before anaesthesia or IPPV. Prophylactic chest drain advised.
- Procedures—CV line, percutaneous tracheostomy, regional anaesthesia, post-CPR. May present some hours after procedure.
- IPPV-related—COPD, asthma, ARDS.
- Surgery-related—laparoscopic surgery, thoracic surgery, nephrectomy, percutaneous nephrolithotomy.

Exclusions
- Tension pneumothorax, lung bulla, major PE, lung collapse (opposite side). Diaphragm rupture (stomach in chest).
- During IPPV—bronchial intubation, pulmonary collapse.
- Bronchopleural fistula (post thoracic surgery/severe trauma).

Special considerations
- Rapid re-expansion of the collapsed lung may be associated with pulmonary oedema. Monitor closely.
- Chest drain insertion, pp448–50.
- Clamping chest tubes before removal: contentious. No evidence that clamping the drain improves re-expansion rates after drain removal. May detect small air leaks.
- Clamping for transfer is rarely, if ever, indicated. Clamping creates the risk of re-accumulation of a simple pneumothorax and converting a simple pneumothorax into a tension pneumothorax.
- Morbidity due to pain associated with intercostal drains is underestimated. Injection of interpleural local anaesthetic through the chest drain (e.g. 20 mL 0.25% bupivacaine 8 hourly prn) reduces pain without significant morbidity.

Further reading

Hendy, M., Arnold, T., Harvey, J. (2003). BTS guidelines for the management of spontaneous pneumothorax. *Thorax*, **58**, ii39–ii52.

☣ Tension pneumothorax

Definition
Accumulation of air under pressure in the pleural space.

Presentation
- Dyspnoea, cough, chest pain, hypoxia/cyanosis. Asymmetric chest expansion with reduced air entry and hyperresonance on percussion. Tracheal deviation away from the affected side.
- Hypotension and tachycardia, neck vein distension. Airway pressures increased on IPPV.
- CXR—pneumothorax with deviation of mediastinal structures. Occasionally bilateral tension pneumothoraces occur—difficult to diagnose. Clinically resembles severe asthma.

Immediate management
- High flow 100% oxygen. IV access.
- Needle decompression in the 2nd intercostal space, mid-clavicular line of the affected side. Seeker needle to confirm, then a large-bore cannula of sufficient length to reach the pleural space (e.g. 16G or larger in adults), see p450.
- Listen for audible hiss of air under pressure. The cannula should remain in place and open to atmospheric pressure until an intercostal drain is inserted.

Subsequent management
- Intercostal drain insertion on the side of the needle decompression, see pp448–50.
- If decompression did not confirm tension pneumothorax, an inter-costal drain may still be required, as a pneumothorax may develop after needle decompression.

Investigations
Clinical diagnosis but CXR is diagnostic.

Risk factors
- Trauma (blunt or penetrating)—often associated with rib fractures. CPR.
- Prolonged IPPV particularly in ARDS.
- CVC placement, regional anaesthesia (may occur some hours after insertion).
- Simple pneumothorax may become tension pneumothorax—IPPV, N_2O, or inappropriate clamping of intercostal drains.
- Surgery-related—laparoscopic surgery, thoracic surgery, nephrectomy, percutaneous nephrolithotomy.

Exclusions
- Airway obstruction.
- Bronchial intubation.
- Asthma, bronchospasm, and anaphylaxis may present with both respiratory and cardiovascular collapse, but respiratory signs are likely to be bilateral.

Paediatric implications
Small children are particularly at risk, especially if meconium aspiration or IPPV. Tension pneumothorax may present as hypoxia, hypotension, or bradycardia.

Special considerations
- Bronchopleural fistula, see pp216–7.
- The development of tension in a pneumothorax is not dependent on the size of the pneumothorax.
- Avoid N_2O in patients at risk.

Further reading
Laws, D., Neville, E., Duffy, J. (2003). BTS guidelines for the insertion of a chest drain. *Thorax*, **58**, ii53–ii59.

☼ Pulmonary oedema

Definition
Increased extracellular pulmonary fluid.

Presentation
- Dyspnoea, hypoxia, sweating, tachycardia, pink frothy sputum, elevated JVP, gallop rhythm. Lung auscultation—fine inspiratory crepitations and quiet bases.
- Decreasing compliance on IPPV, high CVP/PCWP.
- CXR—pulmonary oedema (classical bat's wing), cardiomegaly.

Immediate management
- 100% O_2 and sit patient up if practical. IV access.
- Furosemide 50 mg IV and diamorphine 1.5–5 mg IV.
- If BP >100 mmHg systolic—GTN (50 mg in 50 mL at 0–10 mL/h).
- Consider CPAP (5–10 cmH$_2$O) or PEEP.

Subsequent management
- Intubation and IPPV if not responding.
- If hypotension (<100 mmHg systolic) consider inotropic support (commonly dobutamine 1–15 μg/kg/min).
- Repeat furosemide, urinary catheter.
- If acute MI, consider emergency angiography or thrombolysis—see pp26–7.
- Intra-aortic balloon counter pulsation.

Investigations
- ECG (tachycardia, ischaemia, myocardial infarction, LVH), CXR, ABGs.
- Echocardiography will detail valve function and contractility.

Risk factors
- Fluid overload
- Increased capillary permeability (sepsis/ARDS)
- Neurogenic
- Aspiration
- Heart failure
- Following airway obstruction

Exclusions
- Chest infection, severe asthma, anaphylaxis, pulmonary embolus, aspiration.
- Distinguish between high venous pressure (heart failure) and capillary leak (ARDS).

Paediatric implication

In children non-cardiac causes (e.g. obstructive airway problems) are more common than in adults.

Special considerations

- LVF is commonest cause of pulmonary oedema.
- Opioids and furosemide also act as vasodilators.
- Differentiating between ARDS and cardiogenic pulmonary oedema is difficult. ARDS is likely with trigger events causing SIRS, e.g. sepsis/major trauma/pancreatitis, etc. Usually normal ECG and CXR showing diffuse bilateral shadowing without cardiomegaly or upper lobe pulmonary venous distension. If PCWP <18 mmHg, a diagnosis of cardiogenic pulmonary oedema is unlikely.
- LVF in extremis—venesection (250–500 mL) can buy time.

☠ Severe bronchospasm

(See also pp124–5)

Definition
Life-threatening bronchospasm, mucus plugging, and bronchial mucosal oedema.

Presentation
- Tachypnoea, hypoxia, tachycardia, cyanosis, hyperexpanded lung fields, wheeze or silent chest, reduced conscious level, exhaustion, hypotension.
- IPPV—increased airway pressure, up-sloping expiratory capnography trace, slow expiratory phase, wheeze may be audible or absent.

Immediate management
- 100% O_2, IV access.
- Nebulized salbutamol 5 mg. May be given continuously at 5–10 mg/h.
- Nebulized ipratropium bromide 0.5 mg (4–6 hourly).
- IV salbutamol if not responding (250 µg slow bolus then 5–20 µg/min).
- Hydrocortisone 100 mg IV 6 hourly or prednisolone orally 40–50 mg/day.
- In extremis (decreasing conscious level) adrenaline may be used:
  - nebulizer 5 mL of 1 in 1000
  - IV 10 µg (0.1 mL 1:10000) increasing to 100 µg (1 mL 1:10000) depending on response
  - beware arrhythmias in the presence of hypoxia and hypercapnia. If intravenous access is not available, intramuscular administration (0.5–1 mg) may be used
- If bronchospasm follows induction of anaesthesia, stop all potential anaesthetic precipitants (including desflurane), maintain with isoflurane, sevoflurane or TIVA. Try salbutamol inhaler 6–8 puffs through adaptor (see p460).
- Exclude circuit/airway obstruction.

Subsequent management
- CXR—exclude pneumothorax (uncommon but may be fatal).
- If no response to initial management consider:
  - aminophylline (5 mg/kg over 20 min then infusion 0.5 mg/kg/h with ECG monitoring). Omit loading dose if already on maintenance
  - magnesium sulphate (2 g IV over 20 min) (unlicensed use).
- Consider ICU and IPPV.
- Volatile anaesthetics (isoflurane/sevoflurane) and ketamine sometimes help bronchodilatation.

Investigations
- ABGs—rising CO_2 ominous.
- CXR—exclude pneumothorax.
- FBC, U&Es (check K^+ which can fall with β_2 agonist therapy).

Risk factors

- History of asthma (especially poor control/ICU/IPPV).
- Non-compliance with treatment or monitoring.
- May be precipitated by induction of anaesthesia, tracheal intubation, or light anaesthesia. Most bronchospasm in this situation will settle rapidly.
- Administration of inappropriate drug. Use of NSAIDs, atracurium, D-tubocurarine, mivacurium, barbiturates, neostigmine, morphine, and oxytocin in susceptible individuals (only a few asthmatics are sensitive to NSAIDs and they can usually be identified from the preoperative history, but cross-sensitivity does occur within this group).

Exclusions

- Anaphylaxis, laryngospasm, foreign body, aspiration, pneumothorax, pulmonary oedema.
- Circuit or airway obstruction including malpositioned LMA.

Paediatric implications

- Same basic principles as in adults, but more frightening!
- See pp124–5.

Special considerations

- Optimize asthma before anaesthesia.
- Routine prescription of antibiotics is not indicated in acute asthma.
- No single drug is predictably effective in any one patient—treatment is with maximal therapy and then reduce.
- Beware of hypokalaemia caused by repeated beta-agonist therapy.
- Heliox has the theoretical advantage of increasing flow in the airways. However, the reduced FiO_2 (20–30%) is usually too significant for it to have a place in the management of life-threatening asthma.
- During IPPV severe gas trapping may raise intrathoracic pressure, reduce venous return, and impair cardiac output necessitating intermittent disconnection of the circuit from the patient.
- Dehydration is common with severe asthma and, coupled with high airway pressures during IPPV, may lead to marked hypotension.

Initiation of ventilation and ventilation strategy

- Moving critically ill asthmatics is dangerous. Asthma is frequently underestimated, and brittle asthmatics may deteriorate and die in a matter of minutes.
- Indications for ventilation include exhaustion, worsening hypoxia, rising CO_2 (even when still in the normal range), reduced conscious level, and respiratory arrest.
- Whenever possible, induction should take place in ICU with senior staff.
- Use intravenous induction (propofol or ketamine) combined with an opioid and relaxant (vecuronium or rocuronium). RSI if indicated. Sedate with propofol or ketamine infusion. Inhalational agents (sevoflurane or isoflurane) can be used. Muscle relaxants will facilitate IPPV, but are not bronchodilators.
- High airway pressures are inevitable to overcome airways resistance.

- Patients may have high levels of intrinsic PEEP and marked air trapping due to failure of expiration. Alveolar distension can impair venous return and cardiac filling. Long expiratory phases should be used to ensure adequate expiration. If hypotension is a feature, try disconnecting the patient from the ventilator, ventilate manually at 4–5 bpm on 100% oxygen, and observe for lung deflation. Manual chest compression has also been used (to augment lung deflation) but is controversial.
  If necessary, low-pressure PEEP may be tried to open airways and aid expiration. Some ventilators have an intrinsic PEEP function (PEEPi) to assess treatment.
- Permissive hypercapnia is indicated in order to avoid iatrogenic complications of ventilation.

Further reading
BTS/SIGN (2003). British guideline on the management of asthma. *Thorax*, **58**(suppl.1), 91–4. www.bri-thoracic.org.uk

☠ Massive haemoptysis

Definition
Lower airway bleeding causing significant morbidity and/or mortality.

Presentation
- Extensive blood from airway, visible blood in ETT or on tracheal suction.
- Deteriorating gas exchange or pulmonary compliance.
- Cardiovascular instability (unlikely to precede significant disruption of gas exchange).

Immediate management
- ABC … 100% O_2 IV access. Call for help.
- Intubation and IPPV may be required urgently.
- High airway pressures may be required if bleeding is extensive.
- Position patient appropriately—lateral (with bleeding lung dependent).
- Ensure efficient suction is available.
- Volume replacement.
- Crossmatch blood and blood products.
- Early bronchoscopy to identify cause.

Subsequent management
- Dependent on cause—advice from thoracic team and radiology.
- Correct any coagulopathy.
- Intubation technique will depend on the clinical situation and the experience of the anaesthetist. If the source of bleeding is known, then lung isolation (using intentional endobronchial intubation, a double lumen tube or a bronchial blocker) will prevent soiling.
- Rigid bronchoscopy may be needed for surgical treatment.
- Radiological bronchial artery embolization has a high chance of controlling bleeding. Re-bleeding is common and requires expectant post-procedure care.
- Emergency surgery carries a high mortality and should be reserved for patients in whom other measures have failed and those with adequate lung function.

Investigations
FBC, U&Es, coagulation, radiology imaging

Risk factors
- Coagulopathy, acute invasion of blood vessel (e.g. traumatic, neoplastic, abscess), bronchiectasis, pre-existing vascular abnormality (e.g. AVM), pulmonary vasculitis (Wegener's granulomatosis).
- Complication of tracheostomy, or pulmonary artery rupture caused by PAFC.
- Malposition of chest drain.

Exclusions

Gastrointestinal haemorrhage, upper airway bleeding.

Special considerations
- Endobronchial isolation may be lifesaving.
- See also pp452–6, 230–4.

☼ Difficult controlled ventilation

Definition
Unexpectedly high airway pressure needed to generate adequate tidal volume during IPPV.

Presentation
- High airway pressure, low tidal volume. Hypoxia.
- Abnormal capnography.
- Circulatory collapse due either to hypoxia or to impaired venous return secondary to high intrathoracic pressures.

Immediate management
- 100% O_2.
- Consider context in which situation has arisen:
  - has the patient's position changed?
  - is there a pneumoperitoneum?
  - any recent procedure (CV line, regional block)?
  - has difficulty been gradually worsening or is it of sudden onset?
- Examine chest for asymmetry.
- Auscultate lung fields for wheeze and/or decreased air entry. Exclude tension pneumothorax clinically.
- Switch to manual ventilation:
  - if ventilation is easy, look for a ventilator circuit problem
  - if ventilation remains difficult, problem is in the patient circuit, catheter mount, filter, airway device, or patient
  - is the patient interfering with ventilator (coughing/breathing)?
  - slow refilling of the reservoir bag, indicates impaired expiration (e.g. partial airway obstruction or bronchospasm)
- If circuit problem still suspected, change to manual ventilation with self-inflating bag connected directly to the airway device. Remember to maintain anaesthesia.
- Pass a suction catheter down the ETT/LMA to confirm patency. Repeat laryngoscopy and pull ETT back 2 cm and try IPPV again. Replace ETT if necessary.
- The above will isolate the cause to the patient, airway device, or circuitry.

Subsequent management
- Deepen anaesthesia/use muscle relaxant if airway patency confirmed.
- Replace circuit if blocked or broken. Use self-inflating bag until new equipment available.
- If wheeze on auscultation, treat for bronchospasm.
- Exclude anaphylaxis and discontinue potential drug precipitants.
- Bronchoscopy to exclude tracheobronchial obstruction (foreign body/ mucus or blood).

Investigations
CXR to exclude pneumothorax/incorrect ETT position/pulmonary oedema/ ARDS and pulmonary collapse. Treat as appropriate.

Risk factors

Pressure on diaphragm/chest wall—pneumoperitoneum, massive gastric distension, relaxation wearing off, chest wall rigidity (opioids).

Exclusions

- Incorrect ventilator settings (inappropriate alarm settings).
- On some anaesthetic machines, incorrect switch placement between controlled and spontaneous ventilation modes.
- Haemo/pneumothorax, pulmonary oedema, fibrosing alveolitis, ARDS, bronchospasm.
- Airway secretions, blood, foreign body (including aspiration), laryngospasm with LMA.
- Equipment fault—kinked or occluded equipment (especially ETT, or circuit). Endobronchial intubation, cuff herniation, malpositioned LMA, blocked or incorrectly assembled breathing circuit.

Paediatric implications

- Laryngospasm and bronchospasm are far more common. Blockage of small tubes with secretions and endobronchial intubation are also common.
- Oxygen reserves are less, so hypoxia develops rapidly.

Special considerations

- Early identification of the problem is aided by correctly set (and switched on) ventilator alarms.
- Total sudden obstruction is most likely to be blockage of circuit or airway. May be anything from a small cap in filter to kinked tubing. By changing to a self-inflating bag directly attached to the ET, most of the circuit is bypassed. The ETT/LMA can be removed and exchanged for a facemask.
- See also Difficult mask ventilation—pp66–7.

☠: Air/gas embolism

Definition
Presence of gas in the vascular system (arterial, venous, or both).

Presentation
- Sudden decreased or absent $ETCO_2$ trace and decreased SaO_2.
- Tachycardia, hypotension, loss of cardiac output, PEA cardiac arrest.

Immediate management
- 100% oxygen. Discontinue and do not restart N_2O (expands embolus).
- Exclude PEA cardiac arrest and breathing circuit disconnection.
- Stop surgery, compress any bleeding points and flood wound to prevent further air/gas entry.
- Left lateral head-down tilt or lower operation site below the level of the heart.
- Attempt to increase venous pressure with fluids and vasopressors.
- CPAP and PEEP may help by raising venous pressure.
- Decompress pneumoperitoneum if present.
- Aspirate CVP line. Ideally tip of line should be in right atrium (i.e. within the embolus itself). Do not delay resuscitation to site a line, if not already present.

Subsequent management
- Inotropes may help to overcome increased pulmonary vascular resistance.
- Application of bone wax to exposed bone sinuses.
- Hyperbaric oxygen therapy (if practical) with paradoxical arterial emboli.

Investigations
Clinical diagnosis. $ETCO_2$, ABGs (hypoxaemia ± hypercapnia), CXR (pulmonary oedema), ECG (right heart strain and ischaemia).

Risk factors
- Surgery with wound above heart or surrounded by pressurized gas—neurosurgery, spinal surgery, intramedullary nailing, major joint arthroplasty, laparoscopy, endoscopy, vascular surgery, neck surgery, thoracoscopy.
- Anaesthetic—hypovolaemia, air within intravenous sets/pressurized infusions, central venous access and removal of central venous catheters.
- Patient—patent foramen ovale (risk of paradoxical air embolus).

Exclusions
- Hypovolaemia, anaphylaxis, PEA cardiac arrest, breathing circuit disconnection, PE, pneumothorax.

Paediatric implications
Neonates—particular risk of paradoxical embolus via the foramen ovale. Although this closes functionally within 24h of birth, it may not close anatomically until 3 months of age.

Special considerations
- Carbon dioxide is less dangerous than air due to rapid re-absorption.
- CPAP/PEEP increases intrathoracic pressure and CVP and may limit the size and progression of an embolus. However, the rise in right atrial pressure may cause a paradoxical embolus in a patient with a patent foramen ovale (present in 10–15% adults).
- Paradoxical embolus presents with CNS signs.
- No investigation is sensitive and specific. TOE is best. A combination of $ETCO_2$, precordial Doppler, and clinical suspicion most practical.
- Other diagnostic signs include mill-wheel murmur and gas bubbles in retina.

Further reading
Muth, C.M., Shank, E.S. (2000). Primary care: gas embolism. *New England Journal of Medicine*, **342**, 476–82.

Airway

Tim Cook and Jules Cranshaw

☼ Difficult mask ventilation

Definition
Unexpected difficulty in mask ventilation of the anaesthetized patient.

Presentation
- Tight reservoir bag with no chest movement, or mask leak with no chest movement.
- Flat capnograph trace.
- Subsequent oxygen desaturation. This may be delayed by preoxygenation, but will be rapid after falling below 90%.

Immediate management
- Administer 100% oxygen at high flow (assistant to hold flush button).
- Optimize head and neck position. Two-handed jaw thrust with Guedel airway ± (6.0 mm nasal airway), extend neck, improve face-mask seal, assistant to squeeze bag (i.e. two-person technique). Slow inflations are better than rapid high pressures.
- If no improvement (either):
  - deepen anaesthesia (propofol or sevoflurane), particularly if laryngospasm or problem due to light anaesthesia
  - paralyse with suxamethonium (1–1.5 mg/kg) and attempt intubation
  - insert LMA (will rescue >90% of cases)
  - abandon anaesthesia and wake patient up
- If difficulties persist go to:
  - 'Can't intubate … can't ventilate'—see pp76–9.

Subsequent management
- Consider NG tube if gastric distension.
- A nasal airway may help, particularly in lighter planes of anaesthesia, but there is a significant risk of bleeding.
- Fully document difficulties in notes (use airway alert if in use). The patient should be informed of difficulties in writing. Inform databases and GP.

Risk factors
- Anaesthetic inexperience
- Anatomical factors: obesity, snorers, small mandible, beard, edentulous patients, craniofacial abnormalities, reduced neck mobility
- Difficulties in face-mask ventilation may occur as frequently as 1:20 patients. Impossible face-mask ventilation occurs in less than 1:1000

Exclusions
- If reservoir bag fills, but chest does not move on ventilation consider:
  - inadequate positioning of airway—most common
  - blocked anaesthetic circuit, filter, catheter mount, mask, or airway device
  - inadequate depth of anaesthesia—a struggling patient with partially preserved upper airway reflexes is difficult to ventilate

- laryngospasm—see pp94–5.
- unexpected upper airway pathology—tumour, cyst, vascular tissue, or abscess
- lower airway obstruction (e.g. tumour/extrinsic compression)
- bronchospasm
- pneumothorax (including tension ± bilateral)
- If reservoir bag does not fill consider:
  - excessive leak/failure of gas supply
  - have the gases been switched on?
  - usually due to poor facemask seal, but may be from circuit/bag/vaporizer leak
  - airway obstruction leading to poor expiratory tidal flow

Special considerations

- If problem is due to poor facemask seal in a bearded patient, seal can be improved by applying a clear plastic adhesive dressing over the beard. Remember to create a hole for the airway!
- One anaesthetist applying the facemask with an additional anaesthetist providing jaw thrust and neck extension and another ventilating with a correctly located and sized oral airway may provide optimal facemask ventilation (six hands!).
- If tracheal intubation is attempted and is unsuccessful after two attempts, try another airway manoeuvre.
- Difficult facemask ventilation is associated with difficult intubation. This is important as patients who are difficult to ventilate may be harder to rescue by intubation, and conversely if intubation fails the 'Can't intubate … can't ventilate' situation is more common than would be expected.
- The ProSeal and I-gel are alternatives to the LMA in these circumstances.
- See also 'Difficult Controlled Ventilation', pp60–1.

Further reading

Adnet, F. (2000). Difficult facemask ventilation: an underestimated aspect of the problem of the difficult airway? *Anesthesiology*, **92**, 1217–18.

Kheterpal, S. *et al.* (2006). Incidence and predictors of difficult and impossible mask ventilation. *Anesthesiology*. **105**, 885–91.

Langeron, O. *et al.* (2000). Prediction of difficult facemask ventilation. *Anesthesiology*, **92**, 1229–36.

☼ Unanticipated difficult intubation

(Figs 3.1–3.3; See also 'Failed Intubation—Obstetrics', p170–2)

Definition

Unexpected difficult intubation of the trachea during direct laryngoscopy.

Presentation

- Larynx not seen or only the tip of the epiglottis visible. View obstructed by airway pathology. Unable to insert ETT despite adequate view.
- The ASA (1993) defined difficult tracheal intubation as intubation requiring more than 3 attempts at laryngoscopy or taking longer than 10 min.

Immediate management

- Confirm ability to bag and mask ventilate with 100% oxygen.
- If not, call for help and go immediately to 'Can't intubate … can't ventilate' (see p76–9).
- Ask for the emergency intubation equipment/trolley.
- Optimize laryngeal view by:
  - improving neck flexion and head extension
  - asking if the tongue is out of way, if cricoid pressure is impeding the view?
  - trying 'BURP' (backwards upwards rightwards pressure on the thyroid cartilage)
  - trying a longer bladed, straight-bladed, or McCoy laryngoscope
  - bending the ETT, with or without a stylet (tip withdrawn inside the ETT)
  - trying a smaller ETT
  - trying 'taking the epiglottis' deliberately (more common in paediatric practice)
- If you can see the epiglottis make two attempts to pass an 'Eschmann' tracheal tube introducer ('gum elastic bougie') or equivalent into the trachea through the space between the epiglottis and posterior pharyngeal wall:
  - successful insertion is supported by coughing in a partially paralysed patient, feeling the bumps of the tracheal cartilages along the bougie or feeling the end lodge in the bronchi. Bending the tip 60° makes these signs more obvious
  - 'railroading' of an ETT is easier if the laryngoscope is left in the mouth, and the tube is small, reinforced, and rotated 90° anticlockwise
- Successful intubation should be confirmed by two out of:
  - seeing the ETT passing through the glottis
  - six consecutive normal capnograph swings
  - normal inflation of an oesophageal detector
- A fibreoptic laryngoscope may also be used to confirm position.
- If in doubt or intubation remains difficult:
  - oxygenate and ventilate via facemask or LMA
  - confirm ventilation with capnography
  - wake patient up or maintain anaesthesia and wait for help

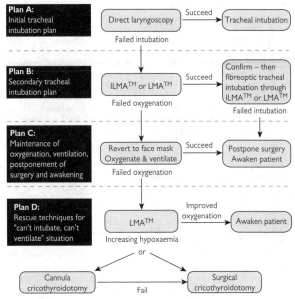

Fig. 3.1 Summary plan for unanticipated difficult intubation.[1]

Subsequent management

- Overall management should be structured as follows:
  - **A** Primary intubation attempt (laryngoscopes ± bougie).
  - **B** Secondary intubation attempt (via LMA or ILMA).
  - **C** Priority is oxygenation and ventilation (abandon intubation).
    Wake patient up unless life-saving surgery or waking is impossible.
  - **D** Invasive tracheal access (life-saving techniques).

  Plan B is not appropriate if intubation is part of RSI. Move directly from Plan A to Plan C (see p72)

- A structured management plan and early recognition of failure will reduce morbidity. After two attempts at one technique use another. Repeated attempts at intubation increase risk of regurgitation and aspiration. A can't intubate, *can* ventilate may progress to CICV.
- Course of action depends on summation risk of several factors:
  - surgery—elective, urgent or emergency/life-threatening
  - aspiration risk—likely full stomach, obstructed bowel, recent meal
  - airway factors—is oxygenation easy or difficult, is it likely to become more difficult?
  - patient factors—obesity, short neck, beard
- As a general rule, patients with a full stomach or those who are difficult to keep oxygenated should be woken at the earliest possible opportunity.
- Consider the risks and benefits of continuing with emergency surgery.
- Postpone elective and non-essential surgery.
- Does patient really need to be intubated? If not, consider a different airway device (LMA, ProSeal, i-gel). If oxygenation and ventilation are adequate with mask ± airway/cricoid pressure this can be continued throughout the operation.
- If the patient is still paralysed with an LMA in place try intubating through this with a 5–6mm ID ETT and fibrescope (ProSeal or ILMA may allow this more easily).
- Techniques using the Aintree Intubating Catheter are an alternative to intubation through the LMA, and enable placement of larger tubes with less difficulty.
- The ILMA allows ventilation in over 95% of cases and tracheal intubation in 75–100% of cases. The LMA restores a clear airway in up to 95% but blind intubation is frequently unsuccessful.
- Record difficult intubation on/in notes; notify GP, databases and patient when fully recovered. Complete 'airway alert' if in use.

Investigations

Capnography, self-inflating bulb (oesophageal detector)

Risk factors

- Inexperienced anaesthetist and unfamiliar equipment.
- Intubation in the emergency medicine and obstetric units.
- Predictors of difficult intubation include obesity, reduced mouth opening and reduced upper cervical spine movement (Mallampati score 3–4), prominent upper incisors, reduced temporomandibular joint mobility, reduced thyromental distance and rheumatoid arthritis.

None are entirely specific or sensitive. 50% of difficult intubations are not predicted.
- Difficult mask ventilation is associated with difficult intubation (and vice versa)

Exclusions
- Poor head and neck positioning.
- Oesophageal intubation.
- Problems with the laryngoscope: blade too short/long; light poor; difficult access; poor insertion—tongue obstructing view.
- Inadequate muscle relaxation.
- Problems with ETT shape or size.

Special considerations
- Patients do not die from failure to intubate—they die from failure to oxygenate. They may die from multiple failed attempts. When intubation fails the priority is establishing a clear airway and oxygenation/ ventilation. If this fails emergency tracheal access may be life-saving and should not be delayed.
- Laryngospasm and inadequate muscle relaxation are possible causes of difficult ventilation (see pp94–5).
- Consider if there will be problems on extubation. Airway trauma may make airway contamination, laryngospasm, and obstruction more likely. Preoxygenate before extubation. Consider the insertion of an airway exchange catheter prior to extubation and have appropriate re-intubation kit and expertise to hand (see pp100–1).
- The ProSeal LMA (PLMA) is an alternative airway through which to ventilate, and offers superior laryngeal seal and protection than an LMA. The oesophageal port can drain regurgitated matter and permits insertion of a gastric tube.
- Even if an LMA does not open the airway sufficiently for ventilation it may provide a route for exhalation, should a cannula cricothyroidotomy be performed.
- It is necessary to briefly release cricoid pressure before siting a laryngeal mask.
- If attempting to pass an ETT through a classic LMA:
  - a size 3/4 should allow a 6 mm ETT
  - a size 5 should allow a 7 mm ETT
  - a standard length ET tube (26–27 cm) passed through an LMA may only reach the vocal cords. Choose a longer tube if possible (flexometallic, nasal RAE, microlaryngeal)
- The Combitube is the most widely quoted alternative to the LMA. However, its use may be associated with airway trauma, and lack of familiarity may lead to potentially fatal incorrect use.

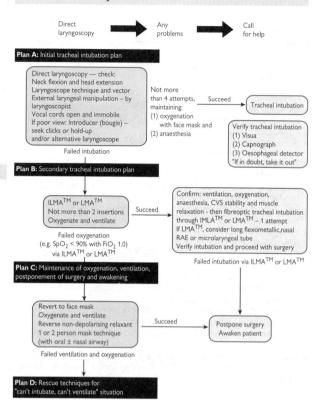

Direct laryngoscopy ➡ Any problems ➡ Call for help

Plan A: Initial tracheal intubation plan

Direct laryngoscopy — check:
Neck flexion and head extension
Laryngoscope technique and vector
External laryngeal manipulation – by laryngoscopist
Vocal cords open and immobile
If poor view: Introducer (bougie) – seek clicks or hold-up and/or alternative laryngoscope

Not more than 4 attempts, maintaining:
(1) oxygenation with face mask and
(2) anaesthesia
→ Succeed → Tracheal intubation

Verify tracheal intubation
(1) Visua
(2) Capnograph
(3) Oesophageal detector
"If in doubt, take it out"

Failed intubation

Plan B: Secondary tracheal intubation plan

ILMA™ or LMA™
Not more than 2 insertions
Oxygenate and ventilate
→ Succeed → Confirm: ventilation, oxygenation, anaesthesia, CVS stability and muscle relaxation - then fibreoptic tracheal intubation through IMLA™ or LMA™ – 1 attempt
If LMA™, consider long flexometallic,nasal RAE or microlaryngeal tube
Verify intubation and proceed with surgery

Failed oxygenation
(e.g. SpO_2 < 90% with FiO_2 1.0) via ILMA™ or LMA™

Failed intubation via ILMA™ or LMA™

Plan C: Maintenance of oxygenation, ventilation, postponement of surgery and awakening

Revert to face mask
Oxygenate and ventilate
Reverse non-depolarising relaxant
1 or 2 person mask technique
(with oral ± nasal airway)
→ Succeed → Postpone surgery
Awaken patient

Failed ventilation and oxygenation

Plan D: Rescue techniques for "can't intubate, can't ventilate" situation

Fig. 3.2 Unanticipated difficult tracheal intubation.[1]

1 With permission of the Difficult Airway Society.

Further reading

Caplan, R.A., Benumof, J.L. *et al.* (1993). Practice guidelines for management of the difficult airway. A report by the American Society of Anesthesiologists' Task force on Management of the Difficult Airway. *Anesthesiology*, **78**, 579–602. (www.asahq.org/publicationsAndServices/Difficult%20Airway. pdf) Last updated Oct 2002.

Combes, X., Le Roux, B. *et al.* (2004). Unanticipated difficult airway in anesthetized patients. Prospective validation of a management algorithm. *Anesthesiology*, **100**, 1146–50.

Cook, T.M., Seller, C., Gupta, K., Thornton, M., O'Sullivan, E. (2007). Non-conventional uses of the Aintree Intubating catheter in management of the difficult airway: fourteen reports. *Anaesthesia*, **62**, 169–74.

Difficult Airway Society, UK Guidelines (www.das.uk.com).

Henderson, J.J., Popat, M.T., Latto. I.P., Pearce, A.C. (2004). Difficult airway society guidelines for management of the difficult airway. *Anaesthesia*, **59**, 675–94.

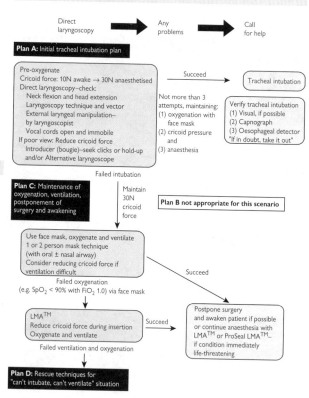

Fig. 3.3 Unanticipated difficult tracheal intubation (rapid sequence induction).[1]

1 With permission of the Difficult Airway Society.

☠: Can't intubate ... can't ventilate (CICV)

(Fig. 3.4)

Definition
Inability to ventilate and oxygenate the patient and inability to intubate.

Presentation
- SaO_2 <90% despite attempts to ventilate with 100% O_2.
- No breath sounds.
- Flat capnograph trace.

Immediate management
- Call for immediate assistance, ideally a more senior anaesthetist.
- Ask for the difficult airway trolley/equipment.
- Administer 100% oxygen at high flow.
- Optimize the airway:
  - reposition head and neck
  - two-handed jaw thrust
  - oral ± nasal airway
  - release or reduce cricoid pressure
- Insert LMA:
  - it will re-establish airway in 95% of cases
  - it may provide some oxygenation during attempts at invasive airway
  - it improves the route for expired gases during jet ventilation
- When necessary, proceed to surgical airway:
  - surgical cricothyroidotomy
  - needle/cannula cricothyroidotomy—see pp432–6.

Subsequent management
- A definitive airway is required. Contact a senior ENT surgeon urgently.
- ICU admission is likely to be required.
- After the definitive airway is placed, a gastric tube should be passed and the stomach drained, as ventilation attempts are likely to have caused gastric distension. If not drained, ventilation may be difficult and aspiration risk is increased.
- Anticipate postobstructive pulmonary oedema.
- Document notes clearly (airway alert if in use). Inform patient of difficulties in writing. Contact databases and GP.

Investigations
CXR to exclude complications (defer until definitive airway established).

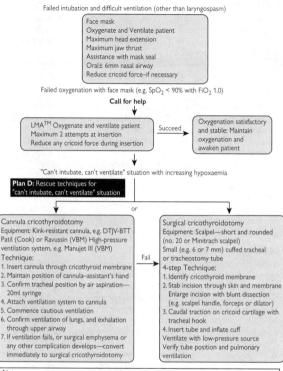

Failed intubation and difficult ventilation (other than laryngospasm)

Face mask
Oxygenate and Ventilate patient
Maximum head extension
Maximum jaw thrust
Assistance with mask seal
Oral± 6mm nasal airway
Reduce cricoid force–if necessary

Failed oxygenation with face mask (e.g. SpO_2 < 90% with FiO_2 1.0)

Call for help

LMA™ Oxygenate and ventilate patient
Maximum 2 attempts at insertion
Reduce any cricoid force during insertion

Succeed → Oxygenation satisfactory and stable: Maintain oxygenation and awaken patient

"Can't intubate, can't ventilate" situation with increasing hypoxaemia

Plan D: Rescue techniques for "can't intubate, can't ventilate" situation

or

Cannula cricothyroidotomy
Equipment: Kink-resistant cannula, e.g. DTJV-BTT Patil (Cook) or Ravussin (VBM) High-pressure ventilation system, e.g. Manujet III (VBM)
Technique:
1. Insert cannula through cricothyroid membrane
2. Maintain position of cannula–assistant's hand
3. Confirm tracheal position by air aspiration—20ml syringe
4. Attach ventilation system to cannula
5. Commence cautious ventilation
6. Confirm ventilation of lungs, and exhalation through upper airway
7. If ventilation fails, or surgical emphysema or any other complication develops—convert immediately to surgical cricothyroidotomy

Fail →

Surgical cricothyroidotomy
Equipment: Scalpel—short and rounded (no. 20 or Minitrach scalpel)
Small (e.g. 6 or 7 mm) cuffed tracheal or tracheostomy tube
4-step Technique:
1. Identify cricothyroid membrane
2. Stab incision through skin and membrane Enlarge incision with blunt dissection (e.g. scalpel handle, forceps or dilator)
3. Caudal traction on cricoid cartilage with tracheal hook
4. Insert tube and inflate cuff
Ventilate with low-pressure source
Verify tube position and pulmonary ventilation

Notes:
1. These techniques can have serious complications—use only in life-threatening situations
2. Convert to definitive airway as soon as possible
3. Postoperative management—see other difficult airway guidelines and flow-charts
4. 4mm cannula with low-pressure ventilation may be successful in patient breathing spontaneously

Fig. 3.4 Can't intubate ... can't ventilate.[1]

Risk factors
- CICV may occur in a normal airway after difficult airway management or prolonged attempts at intubation.
- CICV may also occur after failed facemask ventilation where intubation was not initially planned.
- Patients in whom mask ventilation is difficult (or impossible) are more likely to be difficult (or impossible) to intubate, and vice versa.

Exclusions
- Blocked circuit, mask, or airway device (including foreign body):
  - switch to a self-inflating bag and a fresh mask with a different filter/angle piece. Does this resolve the problem?
- Leaks from airway circuit, mask or airway device (bag collapses).
- Inadequate positioning of airway.
- Inadequate depth of anaesthesia or muscle relaxation.
- Supraglottic airway obstruction.
- Subglottic airway obstruction.
- Severe laryngospasm—see pp94–5.
- Severe bronchospasm—see pp54–6.
- Tension pneumothorax (including bilateral)—see pp50–1.
- Gross aspiration or foreign body.

Special considerations
- Invasive tracheal access should be considered when life-threatening hypoxia continues despite two-person ventilation techniques, Guedel airway/LMA, and conventional intubation attempts having failed.
- Creation of an emergency transtracheal airway is a procedure that should not be undertaken lightly. However, it is likely to take at least 60–120 s from decision to connection time. It is therefore pointless to delay the decision until the patient has a cardiopulmonary arrest. Delays in performing this are common in fatal cases.
- A non-kinking cricothyroid cannula and appropriate equipment to allow ventilation are required—these should be immediately available.
- Specifically designed Seldinger or cannula-over-needle kits are best.
- Problems arise both with insertion of the cannula and more frequently with ventilation. Larger cannulae (≥4mm) lead to more insertion trauma but may allow conventional positive pressure inspiration and passive expiration.
- If the cannula is <4mm ID, a 4 bar (400 kPa) pressure source is required. Jet ventilation or wall oxygen are suitable. The anaesthetic machine is not.
- If an uncuffed cannula of ≥4mm is inserted, conventional ventilation is possible, but may be difficult due to gas escaping via the upper airway—obstruct the mouth and nose to reduce this.
- If dedicated cricothyroidotomy equipment and an oxygen injector are not available and an intravenous (Luer-lock) cannula has been inserted, connection is possible using one of the following methods:
  - remove the plunger from a 10 mL syringe and intubate the barrel with a cuffed ETT
  - insert the connector from a neonatal 3.5 mm ETT into the hub of the needle/cannula

- unscrew capnograph tubing from the monitor, attach the Luer-lock end to the hub of the needle/cannula. Attach the other end (sampling T-piece) to the common gas outlet. Use your thumb to intermittently occlude the other end of the T-piece

Further reading

Cook, T.M., Nolan, J.P., Cranshaw, J., Magee, P. (2007). Needle cricothyroidotomy. *Anaesthesia*, **62**, 289–90.

Crosby, E.T., Cooper, R.M. *et al.* (1998). The unanticipated difficult airway with recommendations for management. *Canadian Journal of Anesthesia*. **45**, 757–76.

Difficult Airway Society, UK Guidelines (www.DAS.uk.com)

☠ Emergency management of the obstructed airway

(See also pp210–1)

Definition
Difficulty predicted in achieving intubation or maintaining ventilation in a patient with an obstructed airway.

Presentation
Soft tissue obstruction or copious blood/debris in the airway.

Immediate management

- Call for senior help (anaesthetic and surgical).
- Assess patient fully, including available CT results.
- Liaise with surgeons to establish urgency and extent of surgery needed, and enrol them in airway management plans. Frequently will need to involve ENT, and occasionally thoracic, surgeons.
- Formulate a primary plan (and a back-up) based on:
  - anatomical level of the lesion
  - degree of obstruction (sitting up and lying flat)
  - ability to oxygenate
  - risk of airway soiling from bleeding or aspiration
  - likely degree of difficulty of surgical access to the trachea

Possible adjuncts
LMA, PLMA, ILMA, cricothyroidotomy kit with appropriate ventilation tools such as oxygen injector, retrograde wire, Heliox, Aintree catheter, airway exchange catheter, cardiopulmonary bypass.

Possible techniques
Inhalational induction with sevoflurane/halothane

- Indications—lesions at or below the vocal cords, inhaled FB.
- Strengths—loss of airway may lead to lightening of anaesthesia, airway tone may be retained longer. SV is more effective than IPPV in partial obstruction of the trachea. Blind nasal intubation possible, upper oesophageal sphincter tone is maintained.
- Weaknesses—achieving adequate depth of anaesthesia in a timely and safe manner.
- Relative contraindications—severe obstruction, especially complete obstruction lying flat.

Awake fibreoptic intubation

- Indications—lesions above the vocal cords.
- Strengths—see round corners. SV is maintained (but not necessarily reflexes).
- Weaknesses—difficult in the presence of copious secretions or dyspnoea.
- Relative contraindications—friable lesions likely to bleed on contact—blood will completely obscure view. May completely block airway with tracheal level obstructions—'cork in a bottle'.

Rigid bronchoscopy and jet ventilation
- Indications—tracheal compression.
- Strengths—allows insertion of a tracheal stent.
- Weaknesses—requires experienced operator (ENT or thoracic surgeon).
- Relative contraindications—severe trismus, cervical spine instability or immobility.

Cricothyroidotomy (needle, cannula, or surgical)
- Indications—severe obstruction above the cricothyroid membrane.
- Strengths—bypasses lesion.
- Weaknesses—complications of insertion (e.g. misplacement, bleeding) and of ventilation (e.g. surgical emphysema, other baro-trauma).
- Relative contraindications—overlying thyroid, presence of tracheal stent, tracheal deviation.

Awake tracheostomy

Subsequent management
Always consider
- Does the patient need general anaesthesia or can regional techniques be used?
- Does the patient need intubation? But beware techniques that leave the airway sub-optimal.
- Is there an aspiration risk? Balance this against the risk of difficult intubation and loss of airway.

Consider your back-up options
- Is oxygenation impaired before starting? (You will have less time).
- Is mask ventilation likely to be difficult?
- Is LMA placement likely to be difficult or ineffective?
- Is cricothyroidotomy/surgical airway likely to be difficult?

In choosing a technique consider the benefits and risks to the patient of
- Awake vs asleep techniques.
- Spontaneous vs controlled ventilation.
- Intubation vs cricothyroidotomy or tracheostomy.

With every patient
- Have a back-up plan.
- Maintain oxygenation and anaesthesia throughout.
- Adopt familiar 'failsafe' techniques wherever possible—waking the patient up will usually be one of the plans, but in life-threatening obstruction even this may not be possible!
- Semi-elective cases—always gain as much information as possible about the lesion (nasendoscopy, CT usually mandatory) and planned surgery before starting.
- Shrink the lesion if time allows by use of steroids, adrenaline, antibiotics (radiotherapy/chemotherapy in less urgent cases), or removal of sutures/clips overlying a compressing haematoma (e.g. bleeding thyroidectomy).

Surgery will not always cure the airway problem and may increase oedema. Retained secretions and bleeding may lead to obstruction during emergence.

Have a management plan for extubation. This may need to be delayed for up to 24h (see 'Difficult extubation', pp100–1).

Investigations
CXR, CT airway, nasendoscopy

Risk factors
- Known pathology (e.g. airway masses).
- Blood or debris in the airway.
- Trauma to the airway.
- External neck masses (bleeding, oedema, etc.).
- All additional factors that increase difficulty of intubation will compound difficulty where obstruction coexists. The obstruction will lead to inefficient preoxygenation and early and more rapid desaturation.

Exclusions
- Identify cases that require awake tracheostomy under local anaesthesia.
- Identify cases that need to be transferred to a specialist cardiothoracic unit.

Paediatric implications
- Awake techniques will be inappropriate for many children.
- The small diameter of paediatric airways and tendency to rapid hypoxia increases the challenge of these cases. Experienced skilled practitioners are required.
- Use of inhalational induction and a dedicated airway for fibreoptic techniques is often appropriate.
- Cricothyroidotomy may be technically demanding and is more hazardous, but the underlying principles are as for adults (see pp432–6).

Special considerations
Lesions impeding intubation rather than gas flow
- Awake techniques are favoured unless impractical. These include fibreoptic intubation, intubation through an LMA, ILMA and PLMA, retrograde intubation, tracheostomy.
- BUT significant bleeding into the upper airway renders fibreoptic techniques useless and awake techniques nearly impossible. Gas induction and maintenance of spontaneous ventilation is usually recommended. Light-guided techniques and retrograde intubation may have a role in the hands of those skilled in the technique. Invasive tracheal access should be considered early.

Obstructing lesions
- These cases are always difficult and if managed poorly will cause life-threatening problems. Their management is controversial. The obstruction is likely to get worse during anaesthesia and airway manipulation due to loss of airway tone, reflex airway responses, trauma, or bleeding.
- Heliox may improve flow through a narrowed airway but reduces the FiO_2. Sevoflurane may be delivered by a drawover vaporizer (e.g. OMV) downstream of a Heliox cylinder, but two in series are needed to achieve adequate anaesthetic concentrations.

- Assess:
  - level of obstruction—oral/supraglottic, laryngeal, mid-tracheal, lower tracheal. Several levels may be affected by one pathology. Inspiratory stridor and voice changes indicate laryngeal obstruction. Intrathoracic obstruction may cause expiratory stridor
  - severity of obstruction—stridor, accessory muscle use, hypoxia, respiratory distress, silent chest, dysphagia, and nocturnal panic all suggest severe obstruction. This may become complete once anaesthetized
  - mobility and friability of lesion
  - effect of patient position (adopt patient's 'best breathing position')
  - neck and trachea for ease of invasive tracheal access

Oral and supraglottic lesions (e.g. trauma, burns, tumour, infective)
- Tracheal access is usually unimpeded and securing tracheal access with the patient awake should be considered (cricothyroidotomy or tracheostomy). Even if this is not plan A, a transtracheal ventilation catheter placed before induction will allow oxygenation and buy time if upper airway obstruction occurs during plan A.
- If awake fibreoptic intubation is used, cricothyroidotomy (or very rapid tracheostomy performed by an experienced surgeon who is scrubbed and prepared) should be plan B in the event of airway obstruction.
- If gas induction is chosen then direct laryngoscopy may be used but cricothyroidotomy (or very rapid tracheostomy) should be plan B in the event of airway obstruction.

Laryngeal (e.g. tumours, infection, burns, haemorrhage into neck)
- Use awake tracheal access for severe airway distortion and fixed friable lesions.
- Consider awake fibreoptic intubation, but avoid if the lesion is very vascular and friable.
- If gas induction is chosen then cricothyroidotomy (or very rapid tracheostomy) should be plan B in the event of airway obstruction. Consider lower trachea access (transtracheal placement below 1st tracheal ring) to avoid the lesion.

Mid-tracheal (e.g. bleeding into goitre/thyroid tumour, trauma)
- Laryngoscopy is likely to be easy (unless coexistent pathology) but tracheal access may be compromised. The site of the lesion may prevent transtracheal access. Attempts may lead to bleeding and complete obstruction.
- Avoid coughing as this may convert partial to complete obstruction with a cycle of decline. In the absence of anticipated upper airway problems this is a reason to avoid local anaesthetic/awake techniques.
- Intravenous induction, neuromuscular blockade, and early passage of a rigid bronchoscope may be favoured. The rigid bronchoscope re-establishes airway patency and is then used as a dedicated airway for further assessment, oxygenation, ventilation, and surgery. Maintain anaesthesia with IV techniques once airway established.
- Gas induction is less advantageous than for supraglottic airway obstruction.

- Bypassing the obstruction from above may require fibreoptic inspection, very small tracheal tube, ventilating catheter, or rigid bronchoscope.
- Surgery may include resection, laser, or insertion of stents.
- Facilities for thoracotomy and cardiopulmonary bypass in the event of complications are the ideal.

Lower tracheal lesions (e.g. tumours, trauma)
- Management may be as for mid-tracheal lesions.
- Invasive tracheal access will not help.
- Transfer to a cardiothoracic centre may be more appropriate for lower airway problems (e.g. bronchial tumour or compression from a retrosternal thyroid). Involve thoracic surgeons.
- Occasionally may require femorofemoral cardiopulmonary bypass. This is a major undertaking and requires full anticoagulation, which may impede surgery.

An alternative to gas induction is a slow induction with increasing levels of target-controlled propofol whilst maintaining spontaneous ventilation. This may provide similar conditions to gas induction without airway irritation. It requires experience and skill. *This is a controversial technique.*

Further reading

Caplan, R.A., Benumof, J.L. et al. (1993). Practice guidelines for management of the difficult airway. A report by the American Society of Anesthesiologists. Task force on Management of the Difficult Airway. *Anesthesiology*, **78**, 579–602.

Conacher, I. (2003). Anaesthesia and tracheobronchial stenting for central airway obstruction in adults. *British Journal of Anaesthesia*, **90**, 367–74.

Mason, R.A., Fielder, C.P. (1999). The obstructed airway in head and neck surgery. *Anaesthesia*, **54**, 625–8.

NCEPOD (1998). The Report of the National Confidential Enquiry into Perioperative Deaths 1996/1997. London.

⑦ **Rapid sequence induction**

Definition
- Intravenous induction of anaesthesia with cricoid pressure followed by rapid intubation of the trachea. Drugs with rapid onset of action are used following thorough preoxygenation.
- Cricoid pressure helps protect the airway during this time.
- Avoidance of manual ventilation of the lungs reduces the possibility of gastric inflation stimulating regurgitation. If intubation difficulty arises, the patient may regain spontaneous ventilation and wake before life-threatening hypoxia occurs: but this must not be assumed.

Presentation
Required for tracheal intubation of patient with significant aspiration risk.

Immediate management
- Skilled assistance is required.
- Check equipment (suction, laryngoscopes, ETTs, cuffs, rescue devices, and capnography).
- A tipping bed or trolley is mandatory.
- Rigid suction catheter is placed under the patient's pillow, at the anaesthetist's right hand.
- The patient's head and neck are placed in the 'sniffing' position.
- A large-bore cannula is sited and fluid infusion started.
- The patient is fully preoxygenated (and therefore denitrogenated).
- Cricoid pressure is partially applied (see below).
- A predefined dose of induction drug is administered (e.g. propofol 1–2.5 mg/kg, thiopental 2–5 mg/kg) followed immediately by suxamethonium 1–1.5 mg/kg.
- No attempts at mask ventilation are made before laryngoscopy.
- Laryngoscopy and intubation are performed 45–60 s after IV suxamethonium.
- Cricoid pressure is maintained until the tracheal tube is inserted, cuff inflated, and position confirmed (bilateral expansion, auscultation, capnography, etc.). If there is difficulty with intubation then cricoid pressure should be reduced or released to improve view: but reapplied if it does not.
- If intubation fails, the anaesthetist should follow a predefined 'failed intubation protocol' (see p72).
- The priority is then oxygenation. Manual ventilation of the lungs should be attempted, while the patient is allowed to wake up. An LMA or PLMA may help if there is airway obstruction, but cricoid pressure will need to be released during insertion then reapplied.
- If intubation *and* ventilation fail, proceed immediately to 'Can't intubate … can't ventilate' (CICV) protocol, see pp76–9.

Subsequent management
- Drain the stomach peroperatively with a large-bore oro/nasogastric tube.
- Following surgery, extubate awake and on side if aspiration risk remains.

Risk factors

RSI is indicated when there is increased risk of regurgitation of gastric contents at induction of anaesthesia (e.g. bowel obstruction, recent meal, symptomatic reflux).

Exclusions

Avoidance of general anaesthesia (e.g. regional techniques) or securing the airway before induction (awake fibreoptic intubation) should be considered, particularly if the patient has features that suggest difficult laryngoscopy.

Paediatric implications

- Young children are unlikely to tolerate preoxygenation and cricoid pressure. They also desaturate rapidly during apnoea.
- Forces required for effective cricoid pressure in children are not established.
- RSI may, therefore, need to be modified with gentle mask ventilation after induction to prevent hypoxaemia before or during laryngoscopy.
- Difficult laryngoscopy and tracheal intubation is much less common in children.
- Use 2 mg/kg suxamethonium in infants; 1.5 mg/kg in older children.

Special considerations

Cricoid pressure

The cricoid cartilage should be identified while the patient is awake. A force of 10 N (1 kg) should be applied as induction begins. This should be increased to 30 N (3 kg) as the patient loses consciousness. Excessive pressure increases intubation difficulty and airway obstruction. If laryngoscopy is difficult cricoid pressure should be reduced or released to improve view: but reapplied if it does not. The BURP manoeuvre (redirecting the pressure backwards, upwards and to the right) may improve the view of the larynx, but increases the risk of airway obstruction. If intubation fails, cricoid pressure should revert to normal. In the rare event of active vomiting (but not regurgitation), cricoid pressure should be released to prevent oesophageal rupture. Cricoid pressure cannot be maintained reliably by one person for more than 5 min. An LMA cannot be correctly placed while cricoid pressure is applied, so it should be released during passage of an LMA.

Preoxygenation (denitrogenation)

This increases the time to hypoxia. Tidal ventilation of 100% oxygen for 3–5 min or until end-tidal oxygen is >90% are ideal. Patients with lung disease require more prolonged preoxygenation. 4 vital capacity breaths (using the oxygen flush) are suitable in extreme emergency. Whichever technique is used, a seal between face and mask is essential.

Head-up tilt of at least 20° also prolongs the time to hypoxia, and can be used routinely.

Use of non-depolarizing muscle relaxant

Some favour rocuronium because of the side-effects of suxamethonium. It must be given in a dose of 0.9–1.0 mg/kg and with an opioid for intubation conditions to approach those of suxamethonium. The patient will remain paralysed for up to 50 min. This approach cannot currently be recommended for routine RSI. If the specific reversal agent suggamadex enters clinical practice this option may become more acceptable.

Use of opioids

The use of opioids at RSI is widespread due to improved haemodynamic stability (e.g. for pre-eclampsia, IHD, raised ICP). The risk is impaired preoxygenation (instruct the patient to breathe) and prolonged apnoea in the event of difficulties. The likelihood of inducing vomiting is small. Alfentanil 10–30 µg/kg is suitable. If intubation fails, reverse with naloxone 400–800 µg.

Nasogastric tube

This should be left *in situ*, but should be aspirated by gentle suction prior to induction and then left open to the atmosphere to normalize intra-gastric pressure. The NG tube tends to be displaced laterally by cricoid pressure and improves occlusion of the oesophagus during induction and intubation.

Airway rescue following failed intubation

The PLMA (which enables ventilation and protects the airway better than a classic LMA) is a more logical rescue device following failed intubation during RSI. It should only be used in the emergency setting by experienced operators.

Evidence-base and safety of RSI

There is little published evidence that RSI improves safety, but it is medi-colegally advisable in cases with a high risk of aspiration. When failed intubation occurs during RSI, life-threatening hypoxia is likely to occur before suxamethonium wears off so the technique cannot be assumed to be safe. RSI must, therefore, only be undertaken when the equipment and skill for airway rescue are immediately available.

Further reading

Benumof, J.L., Dagg, R., Benumof, R. (1997). Critical hemoglobin desaturation will occur before return to an unparalyzed state following 1 mg/kg intravenous succinylcholine. *Anesthesiology*, **87**, 979–82.

Cheng, L.W., Xue, F. S., Xu, Y. C., Liu, Y., Mao, P., Liu, K. P., Yang, Q. Y., Zhang, G. H., Sun, H.T. (2007). Cricoid pressure impedes insertion of, and ventilation through, the ProSeal laryngeal mask airway in anesthetized, paralyzed patients. *Anesthesia and analgesia*, **104**, 1195–8.

Donati, F. (2003). The right dose of succinylcholine. *Anesthesiology*, **99**, 1037–8.

Heier, T., Feiner, J.R., Lin, J., Brown, R., Caldwell, J.E. (2001). Hemoglobin desaturation after succinyl-choline-induced apnea: a study of the recovery of spontaneous ventilation in healthy volunteers. *Anesthesiology*, **94**, 754–9.

Morris, J., Cook, T.M. (2001). National survey of Rapid sequence induction. *Anaesthesia*, **56**, 1090–7.

Vanner, R.G., Asai, T. (1999). Safe use of cricoid pressure. *Anaesthesia*, **54**, 1–3.

☢ Oesophageal intubation

Definition
Placement of ETT in the oesophagus.

Presentation
- Abnormally low, rapidly extinguished or absent $ETCO_2$. Progressive hypoxia following tracheal intubation (delayed by preoxygenation). Absent or equivocal breath sounds on auscultation of the chest. Gurgling breath sounds in epigastrium.
- Abnormal resistance or compliance on hand ventilation (and slow refilling of reservoir bag due to absent expiration). Leak around the ETT despite normal pressure and volume in the cuff.
- Regurgitation of gastric contents up the ETT.

Immediate management
- Stop ventilating down ETT once the diagnosis is suspected.
- Recheck location of ETT by direct laryngoscopy—if in doubt, take it out.
- Ventilate with 100% oxygen by mask and restore oxygen saturation.
- Re-attempt to intubate the trachea and verify tube position by direct observation of passage through the vocal cords, auscultation, and use of a capnograph or Wee detector. Visualize the carina with a fibreoptic scope if available and time allows.
- Secure the ETT.
- If intubation is difficult or fails, maintain oxygenation/ventilation and follow the guidelines for unexpected difficult tracheal intubation, pp68–75.

Subsequent management
Once the airway has been secured, decompress the stomach with an orogastric or nasogastric tube.

Investigations
- An absent capnograph trace following the start of ventilation is typical of oesophageal intubation but a normal then rapidly diminishing capnograph has been observed.
- A Wee's oesophageal detector (a self-inflating bulb or a bladder syringe attached to a catheter mount) may aid in supporting the diagnosis (air cannot be withdrawn if the tube is in the collapsible oesophagus) but is neither 100% sensitive nor specific.
- Position of the ETT can also be confirmed with a fibreoptic scope.

Risk factors
- Difficult intubation:
  - difficulty in visualizing the larynx at intubation
  - difficulty in passing the ETT into the trachea (blind use of gum elastic bougie, adjuncts, or other blind tracheal intubation techniques)
- Intraoperative manipulation of the head or neck
- Surgery involving the shared airway

Exclusions
- Cardiac arrest as cause of 'flat' capnograph.
- Failure of capnography or blocked sampling line.
- Disconnection or leak in the breathing system.
- Ventilator not switched on or working.
- Bronchial intubation.
- Severe bronchospasm (including anaphylaxis).
- Bilateral pneumothoraces.
- Kinked or obstructed ETT.
- Failure to inflate or leak from ETT cuff.
- Unintentional extubation.

Paediatric implications
Neonatal ETTs are prone to displacement within the mouth if unsupported by a Guedel airway. Gastric distension may produce vagal reflexes.

Special considerations
- Auscultation of the chest and epigastrium may be unreliable and may lead to false reassurance.
- Hypoxaemia may be considerably delayed by preoxygenation.
- Late diagnosis of hypoxaemia is more likely in patients with pigmented skin.

Further reading

Caplan, R.A., Posner, K.L., Ward, R.J., Cheney, F.W. (1990). Adverse respiratory events in anesthesia: A closed claims analysis. *Anesthesiology*, **72**, 828–33.

Clyburn, P., Rosen, M. (1994). Accidental oesophageal intubation. *British Journal of Anaesthesia*, **73**, 55–63.

Williamson, J.A., Webb, R.K., Szekely, S., Gillies, E.R., Dreosti, A.V. (1993). The Australian Incident Monitoring Study. Difficult intubation: an analysis of 2000 incident reports. *Anaesthesia and Intensive Care*, **21**, 602–7.

ⓘ **Bronchial intubation**

Definition
Passage of an ETT beyond the carina.

Presentation
- Uneven chest expansion.
- Quieter breath sounds in the unintubated hemithorax.
- Unexpectedly high peak and plateau airway pressures (or reduced tidal volumes in a pressure-limited ventilatory mode).
- Low or falling SpO_2 (but may not be dramatic with a high FiO_2).
- Altered capnography (may be initially low and subsequently high).
- Altered rates of volatile gas exchange and control of anaesthetic depth.

Immediate management
- Increase FiO_2 to 100% if saturations are low or falling.
- Observe the chest and compare auscultation in both axillae.
- Check that the length of the ETT at the teeth is appropriate for the patient.
- Check there are no obstructions or kinks in the ETT.
- Deflate the cuff and withdraw the ETT—best done under direct laryngoscopy or fibreoptic bronchoscopy. Re-inflate the cuff.
- Auscultate the chest for the return of bilateral breath sounds during hand ventilation with relatively large volume but low pressure tidal ventilation.
- Feel and measure the fall in inspiratory pressure.
- Pass a suction catheter through the length of the ETT to verify patency if not responding to ETT withdrawal.
- Re-secure the tube. Note the length of the ETT at the teeth.

Subsequent management
- Ensure adequate re-expansion of previously non-ventilated lung.
- May require hand ventilation, CPAP, PEEP, or recruitment manoeuvres and lateral positioning if bronchial intubation has been prolonged.
- Exclude barotrauma to previously ventilated lung.
- Postoperative chest X-ray if re-inflation clinically incomplete.
- Physiotherapy may be required.

Investigations
- Fibreoptic visualization of carina.
- CXR to establish position of ETT tip and to look for evidence of residual collapse, barotrauma, or acute lung injury.

Risk factors

- Poor intubation technique with inadequate check of ETT depth after intubation. Suspect following emergency intubation by non-anaesthetists.
- Insertion depth—suspect if >21 cm at teeth in small females, >23 cm in larger patients.
- More likely after difficult intubation or intubation with blind techniques (e.g. ILMA, Trachlight).
- Uncut and preformed ETTs (e.g. reinforced and RAE ETTs).
- Manipulation of head or neck during patient positioning. Flexion advances ETT.
- Prone positioning.
- Surgery involving a shared airway.
- Pneumoperitoneum and head-down position. The carina moves cranially relative to the ETT.
- Surgical manipulation of the trachea and bronchi.
- Paediatric patients in inexperienced hands.
- Aberrant tracheal or bronchial anatomy.
- Insertion of an ETT through a tracheostomy or emergency cricothyroidotomy.

Exclusions

- Breathing circuit obstruction—check patency by disconnection.
- ETT obstruction or kinking—pass catheter beyond tip of tracheal tube.
- Bronchospasm—typically bilateral and associated with wheeze and sloping capnography.
- Pneumothorax—check percussion note and position of trachea.
- Complete or partial lung collapse—consider if ETT repositioning does not correct problem.
- Cuff herniation—check cuff pressure. Pass catheter beyond ETT tip.
- Bronchial foreign body (including aspiration)—if appropriate ETT repositioning does not correct problem.

Paediatric implications

- Collapse and hypoxia occur more rapidly than in adult.
- Increased likelihood of bronchial intubation because:
  - absolute length of trachea is reduced
  - uncuffed tracheal tubes may move more
  - formulae for correct length are estimates only
  - RAE tubes often too long

Further reading

Black, A.E., Mackersie, A.M. (1991). Accidental bronchial intubation with RAE tubes. *Anaesthesia*, **46**, 42–3.

Freeman, J.A., Fredricks, B.J., Best, C.J. (1995). Evaluation of a new method for determining tracheal tube length in children. *Anaesthesia*, **50**, 1050–2.

McCoy, E.P., Russell, W.J., Webb, R.K. (1997). Accidental bronchial intubation. An analysis of AIMS incident reports from 1988 to 1994 inclusive. *Anaesthesia*, **52**, 24–31.

:⚙: **Laryngospasm**

Definition
Narrowing or closure of the laryngeal aperture by the action of the laryngeal muscles.

Presentation
- The sound associated with laryngospasm is readily recognizable. Stridor or 'crowing' indicate partial obstruction and are heard during inspiration. During severe laryngospasm the airway is completely obstructed and is silent.
- Respiratory distress, tracheal tug, suprasternal and/or intercostal recession. Abdominal muscles are usually tightly contracted during severe laryngospasm.
- Assisted ventilation may be difficult or impossible with a flat capnograph and rapidly progressive hypoxaemia.

Immediate management
- Stop the stimulus that precipitated laryngospasm.
- Open and clear the airway as much as possible and remove airway devices that may be stimulating the larynx.
- Forcible jaw thrust or anterior pressure on the posterosuperior mandibular rami just anterior to the mastoid process (**Larson's point**) may 'break' laryngospasm due to a combination of stimulation and airway clearance.
- Apply CPAP with 100% oxygen via bag and mask.
- If desaturation continues—call for help. Deepen anaesthesia with an IV agent (propofol 20–40 mg increments) and continue CPAP.
- If arterial saturation continues to decrease, give suxamethonium.
- If ventilation becomes easier, oxygenation improves, and the airway does not require protection, bag and mask ventilation may be sufficient to maintain adequate oxygenation. If not, an airway should be established with an LMA or by intubation.
- In the exceptional case of severe laryngospasm causing life-threatening hypoxaemia despite treatment, or where appropriate intubating drugs are unavailable, cricothyroidotomy or a surgical airway may be life-saving.

Subsequent management
- Monitor for the development of negative pressure pulmonary oedema after a severe episode.
- Consider inserting a nasogastric tube to decompress a stomach inflated by CPAP.
- If intubation was required, determine a plan for extubation in appropriate surroundings with monitoring, personnel, and equipment to manage a recurrence. Insertion of an LMA under deep anaesthesia is one strategy for emergence but will not suit all circumstances.
- Other drugs—doxapram (1–1.5 mg/kg), diazepam (1–2 mg in adults), lidocaine (0.5–1.5 mg/kg) have been recommended to treat laryngospasm, but are probably suitable only for less severe cases.

Investigations

Monitor SaO_2 in case of subsequent pulmonary oedema.

Risk factors

- Light anaesthesia (induction and emergence).
- Soiling of the larynx with secretions/blood/gastric contents.
- Strong stimuli—anal stretch, cervical dilatation.
- Tracheal extubation; particularly in smokers and those with 'irritable airways'.
- Insertion or removal of supraglottic airway devices.
- Movement of head and neck with supraglottic airway devices *in situ*.
- Recurrent laryngeal nerve damage.
- Surgery to the larynx and upper airway.
- Upper respiratory tract infection.
- Paediatric patients.
- Barbiturate induction agents.
- Desflurane > isoflurane > sevoflurane > halothane.
- Anaesthesia in very anxious unpremedicated patients.

Exclusions

- Breathing circuit obstruction (detach it for a moment).
- Supraglottic obstruction due to base of tongue, foreign body (e.g. surgical pack), clot, tumour, angioneurotic oedema.
- Laryngeal obstruction; trauma (dislocated arytenoid cartilage), oedema, haematoma, tumour, vocal cord paralysis (especially bilateral or incomplete recurrent laryngeal nerve damage).
- Infraglottic airway obstruction; foreign body, gastric aspiration, clot, sputum, tumour, bronchospasm, tracheomalacia.
- Residual neuromuscular block.
- Breath-holding.
- Tension pneumothorax.
- Hyperventilation/anxiety.
- Hypocalcaemia.

Special considerations

- Suggested doses of suxamethonium vary from 0.1 to 1.0 mg/kg IV, depending on hypoxaemia severity. If IV access is not immediately available, give 2–4 mg/kg suxamethonium IM/IO or into tongue.
- Have atropine 10–20 µg/kg immediately available to prevent or treat bradycardia, particularly in children.
- Prolonged head-down position, prolonged prone position, massive fluid resuscitation, pre-eclampsia, and anaphylactic reactions are all associated with laryngeal oedema that, on extubation, may resemble refractory laryngospasm.

Further reading

Larson, C.P. (1998). Laryngospasm—the best treatment. *Anesthesiology*, **89**, 1293–4.

① **Aspiration**

Definition

Inhalation or ventilation of foreign material into the respiratory tract.

Presentation

- During intubation—direct visualization of foreign material in oropharynx entering laryngeal inlet.
- Intraoperatively—coughing, laryngospasm, unexpected rise in airway pressure, hypoxaemia, especially with appearance of gastric contents in oropharynx or supraglottic airway.
- Postoperatively—material present on suctioning ETT, unexpected hypoxaemia, tachypnoea/dyspnoea, bronchospasm, intercostal/suprasternal recession. Wheeze, crackles, or reduced air entry, particularly in dependent regions.

Immediate management

- If soiling of the trachea is recognized and material is emerging from the oesophagus or supraglottic airway, immediately apply cricoid pressure to limit further aspiration and remove airway device.
- Clear the pharynx with a rigid sucker.
- Intubate the trachea and pass soft suction catheters via the ETT to clear the trachea.
- Consider replacing the ETT if grossly soiled with particulate matter.
- Do not ventilate during these manoeuvres within the limits of arterial oxygen desaturation.
- If actively vomiting, turn the patient to left lateral position with head-down tilt. Avoid cricoid pressure while vomiting to reduce risk of oesophageal rupture.
- When airway cleared and protected, maintain adequate arterial saturation by ventilating with 100% oxygen.
- PEEP may be required to maintain adequate arterial saturation.
- Empty stomach with large-bore gastric tube.
- Cancel elective surgery.
- Proceed with emergency surgery but complete as quickly as possible.

Subsequent management

- Aspiration of blood rarely causes problems, unaltered gastric acid is high risk.
- Patients with minor aspiration (non-particulate and without marked clinical deterioration) may recover rapidly. These patients may be extubated at the end of surgery and need to be observed for at least 2 h. If they have no symptoms, are well saturated, and the lungs are clear, the likelihood of deterioration is small.
- If aspiration is extensive or particulate, admit to ICU. A few will develop aspiration pneumonitis (ALI/ARDS) and pneumonia. Most have an uncomplicated recovery.
- Supportive care on the ICU:
  - therapeutic bronchoscopy if there is particulate aspiration, focal pulmonary collapse, or CXR evidence of a foreign body.

There is no evidence that lavage of non-particulate aspiration improves outcome. Bronchodilators may help

- the principles of ventilation are centred upon avoiding further harm to the injured lung and avoidance of complications—pneumonia, abscess, empyema, ARDS, barotrauma, and ventilator-induced lung injury
- steroids and blind antibiotic therapy are not helpful in the early phase
- choose antibiotics on the basis of protected catheters/BAL fluid cultures.

Investigations

CXR (often unremarkable within the first few hours). Later films may show streaky/interstitial shadowing and regional or generalized hyperinflation. The right lower lobe is most often affected, but the aspiration pattern may occur in any distribution.

Risk factors

- Full stomach (especially alcohol) or inadequate starvation time.
- Latter half of pregnancy and up to 48 h postpartum.
- Obesity.
- Diabetes mellitus (and other causes of autonomic neuropathy).
- Significant trauma or opioid analgesia after recent ingestion.
- Upper GI bleeding.
- Intestinal obstruction or raised intra-abdominal pressure (e.g. laparoscopic surgery).
- Oesophageal pathology (stricture, malignancy, achalasia, hiatus hernia, incompetent lower oesophageal sphincter). Pharyngeal pouch or web.
- Ineffective cricoid pressure or inexperienced application/premature release.
- Difficult manual ventilation with inflation of the stomach.
- Straining, coughing, and bucking on a supraglottic airway. Hiccups.
- Deep inspiration with surgical stimulation and inadequate depth of anaesthesia.
- Surgery in head-down or lithotomy position.
- Tracheal extubation during light planes of anaesthesia.
- Inadequate reversal of neuromuscular blockade.
- Impaired laryngeal reflexes. Topical anaesthesia of larynx and trachea.
- Neuromuscular disease affecting the larynx and/or the cough reflex.
- Elderly patients with residual anaesthesia or undergoing heavy sedation.
- Antimuscarinic agents.

Exclusions

- Obstruction of breathing system or airway.
- Bronchospasm.
- Foreign body aspiration.
- Acute pulmonary oedema/ARDS.

Special considerations
- Mixed aerobic–anaerobic infections are more common in nosocomial aspiration.
- Ensure adequate starvation time. Use RSI when appropriate. Avoid GA in high-risk situations in favour of regional technique.
- Buffering gastric acid preoperatively with sodium citrate, H_2 receptor antagonists, or proton pump inhibitors do not reduce the risk of aspiration, but may reduce the consequences. This is not true for aspiration of particulate matter.

Further reading

Engelhardt, T., Webster, N.R. (1999). Pulmonary aspiration of gastric contents in anaesthesia. *British Journal of Anaesthesia*, **83**, 453–60.

Ng, A., Smith, G. (2001). Gastroesophageal reflux and aspiration of gastric contents in anesthetic practice. *Anesthesia and Analgesia*, **93**, 494–513.

Vanner, R.G. (1996). Oesophageal sphincter function: regurgitation and its prevention with cricoid pressure. In *International Practice of Anaesthesia* (ed. C. Prys-Roberts and B. Brown), Vol. 2, Ch. 130, 11pp. Butterworth, Heinemann, Oxford.

Warner, M.A., Warner, M.E., Weber, J.G. (1993). Clinical significance of pulmonary aspiration during the peri-operative period. *Anesthesiology*, **78**, 56–62.

⑦ Difficult tracheal extubation

Definition
Extubation where the risk of complications, especially airway obstruction or difficult re-intubation, is high.

Presentation
Based on knowledge of intubation difficulty, trauma, subsequent surgery, or previous extubation difficulty.

Immediate management

- Extubation is not an emergency. Extubate only when safe/optimal conditions, personnel, and equipment available.
- Extubate in an appropriate area for postextubation monitoring.
- Anticipate the potential need for urgent re-intubation.
- Optimize the airway by clearing pharyngeal and tracheal secretions. Empty the stomach if necessary.
- Ensure full reversal of residual neuromuscular paralysis before extubation.
- Perform a 'leak test' before extubation (if there is no leak around the tracheal tube during inflation of the chest with the cuff deflated, extubation is unwise as total obstruction may occur). Consider delaying extubation and transferring to ICU. Dexamethasone (4 mg, 6-hourly) may reduce laryngeal oedema. Topical adrenaline only works briefly and is not recommended as delayed obstruction may occur.
- Consider insertion of an airway exchange catheter prior to extubation (see below).
- Occasionally pre-emptive insertion of a subglottic ventilation catheter or tracheostomy may be required prior to extubation.
- Consider benefits of performing extubation either deep or fully awake. Extubation between these two extremes is often difficult. This may require a change in anaesthetic technique to allow rapid wake-up and return of adequate spontaneous respiration (e.g. use of remifentanil-based anaesthesia).
- Optimize patient position: usually sitting up.
- Preoxygenate fully prior to extubation—do not disconnect the circuit prior to extubation.
- Make efforts to provide oxygenation before, during, and after extubation.
- Monitor after extubation until the risk of airway obstruction has passed.
- If airway irritability is anticipated, consider changing the tracheal tube to an LMA (or PLMA) before waking up.

Subsequent management
- Re-intubate if necessary.
- Consider tracheostomy for weaning.

Investigations
CXR or CT may reveal soft-tissue oedema.

Risk factors

Tracheal extubation may be hazardous when:
- Intubation was difficult or impossible by conventional means.
- Laryngoscopy may have become more difficult as a result of surgery (e.g. surgical fixation of the cervical spine).
- Laryngeal oedema may be present (multiple intubation attempts, anaphylaxis, prolonged prone position or neck surgery, airway burns).
- Extubation has led to complications before (e.g. severe laryngospasm).
- Extubation may cause adverse physiological changes (e.g. raised ICP, severe IHD).

Exclusions

Patients likely to require tracheostomy.

Paediatric implications

- Same underlying principles, but techniques will need to be altered depending on patient's age.
- All but the smallest catheters may obstruct a small child's airway and are unlikely to be tolerated.

Special considerations

Remember that after extubation the patient is likely to have incomplete elimination of the effects of anaesthesia, may be uncooperative, and a high FiO_2 may be difficult to provide. In this respect extubation may be less controlled and potentially more hazardous than difficult intubation.

Airway exchange catheters

An airway exchange catheter (e.g. Cook airway exchange catheter) will allow apnoeic oxygenation, jet ventilation (attachments to allow connection of the catheter to a standard 15 mm connector or jet ventilator are provided), and a route for railroading a tracheal tube. Application of local anaesthetic to the catheter or trachea allows it to be well tolerated. The Frova introducer (resembling a gum elastic bougie with a hole through the middle and also supplied with attachments) is an alternative, but is likely to be less well-tolerated as it is rigid. Alternatives include suction catheters and nasogastric tubes, but these are not designed for this purpose, so cannot be recommended. Extubation over a fibreoptic bronchoscope may be used in a similar manner, but adequate anaesthesia of the airway is required.

Changing to an LMA

Recovery with an LMA in place is associated with reduced coughing, airway irritation, laryngospasm, and cardiovascular stimulation. However, should these problems occur, the airway will be harder to control than with a tracheal tube. The PLMA has potential benefits over the LMA.

Further reading

Cooper, R.M. (1996). Extubation and changing endotracheal tubes. In *Airway Management: Principles and Practice* (ed. J.L. Benumof), pp. 864–5. Mosby Year Book, St Louis.

Crosby, E.T., Cooper, R.M. et al. (1998). The unanticipated difficult airway with recommendations for management. *Canadian Journal of Anesthesia*, **45**, 757–76.

☠ Airway fire

Definition
Ignition of an ETT, tracheal catheter, tissue, or other material during laser surgery or diathermy in the airway.

Presentation
- Visible burning or smoke from the surgical field.
- Usually diagnosed by the surgeon.

Immediate management
- Stop laser or diathermy. Flood area with 0.9% saline.
- Disconnect ETT or catheter from the breathing system.
- Immediately clamp the end to reduce airflow to the burning area.
- Withhold jet and/or mask ventilation to reduce airflow to the burning area.
- Monitor pulse oximetry and re-ventilate when the fire is out.

Fire in the supraglottic airway
- Squirt 0.9% saline onto fire. Syringes containing 0.9% saline (50 mL) should always be available during laser surgery.
- Remove debris with a rigid sucker.
- Remove the ETT. Even if a burned ETT appears intact, it is wise to replace it rather than risk blowing debris into the distal airway or supporting combustion of residual hot spots within the tube. An intact uninvolved ETT may be left in place.
- Once the fire is extinguished, mask-ventilate with enough oxygen to maintain adequate oxygen saturation and maintain anaesthesia intravenously.
- Re-intubate early if there is a risk of losing the airway.

Fire in the infraglottic airway
- Squirt 0.9% saline into the trachea.
- If available, ventilate for a few breaths with nitrogen, CO_2, or helium (not nitrous oxide) to suffocate the fire.
- If the fire involves the ETT remove it.
- Remove debris with a large-bore suction catheter passed into the trachea.
- Once the fire is extinguished, mask-ventilate with enough oxygen to maintain adequate oxygen saturation, and maintain anaesthesia intravenously.
- Re-intubate.
- Early re-intubation will prevent subsequent oedema jeopardizing the airway.
- If re-intubation is impossible, use temporary transtracheal jet ventilation.
- Urgent fibreoptic evaluation of the extent of the burn may be required before proceeding to cricothyroidotomy or tracheostomy.

Subsequent management
- Consider high-dose intravenous steroids (dexamethasone 4–8 mg, 6-hourly) to limit burn oedema.
- Extubation may need to be deferred. Laryngospasm, laryngeal oedema, stridor, and complete airway obstruction are possible complications after extubation. If extubation is planned, ensure this occurs in an appropriate high-care area with suitable monitoring, personnel, and equipment to allow rapid re-intubation if required.
- Intensive care may be required to maintain airway and gas exchange in the early postburn period.
- ALI/ARDS may develop slowly, despite early normal gas exchange.
- Examine the ETT for damage. Missing pieces may still be in the bronchial tree.
- Early referral to a specialist centre for management of scarring and stenosis.

Investigations
Fibreoptic bronchoscopy.

Risk factors
- Fire requires fuel, a gas that supports combustion, and a form of ignition. The fuel is any material that burns, the supporting gas may be oxygen or nitrous oxide, and ignition may be provided by a laser or (rarely) electrodiathermy.
- During laser use the risk is increased by:
  - use of inappropriate equipment (e.g. use of a normal tracheal tube)
  - misuse of appropriate equipment (e.g. use of air rather than 0.9% saline in ETT cuff)
  - high inspired oxygen and nitrous oxide concentrations
  - flammable material in the airway

Exclusions
The normal smoke 'plume' released during laser activity.

Paediatric implications
Relatively little airway oedema can result in a significant reduction in flow.

Special considerations
- Using the lowest FiO_2 and avoiding nitrous oxide during laser use minimizes risks. Use a carrier gas that does not support combustion, such as nitrogen or helium if possible.
- On ignition, an ETT will channel smoke and hot gases into the distal airway. Anticipate significant airway trauma.
- Filling the ETT cuff with 0.9% saline and placing flame-retardant wet packs around uncuffed ETTs before supraglottic surgery may reduce the risk of an airway fire. Protocols should be in place.

- Methylene blue may be added to the 0.9% saline used for ETT cuff inflation. It is then obvious if the cuff is breached by the laser (before the upper airway fills with oxygen-rich gas).
- Practising fire drills may increase the speed of anaesthetic decision-making in a crisis, but efficient communication between the surgeon and the anaesthetist is essential.

Further reading

Kitching, A.J., Edge, C.J. (2003). Lasers and surgery. *British Journal of Anaesthesia. CEPD Reviews*, **8**, 143–6.

Patel, A. (2005). Anaesthesia for endoscopic surgery. *Anaesthesia & Intensive Care Medicine*, **6**, 231–6.

Paediatrics

Daniel Lutman

☠ Neonatal resuscitation

Definition
Resuscitation of the newborn infant at delivery.

Presentation
Floppy, blue or pale newborn, apnoeic or gasping respiration, bradycardia.

Immediate management

(See Fig. 4.1, 'Newborn life support algorithm', p108)
- Dry and wrap baby. Keep warm.
- Assess colour, tone, breathing, heart rate.
- Open airway (neck in neutral position).
- Give five inflation breaths (2–3 s, 30 cmH$_2$O).
- Reassess heart rate, confirm chest movement.
- If ventilation inadequate:
  - reposition airway
  - repeat inflation breaths
  - reassess heart rate
- If still no response:
  - inspect oropharynx and suction if necessary
  - consider intubation
  - repeat inflation breaths
- When ventilation is adequate and heart rate <60 bpm and not increasing:
  - start chest compressions at a rate of 120/min
  - 3 chest compressions to 1 breath
- Reassess heart rate every 30 s.
- If heart rate increasing, stop chest compressions. Continue ventilation if not breathing.
- If heart rate still <60 bpm, continue ventilation and chest compressions.
- If no response, consider giving drugs (see Table 4.1):
  - insert umbilical venous catheter, interosseous, or other venous access
  - give adrenaline IV or IO (0.1–0.3 mL/kg 1:10 000)
  - give sodium bicarbonate intravenously (2–4 mL/kg 4.2%)
  - consider adrenaline via ETT (1 mL/kg 1:10 000) (may not be as effective as IV or IO)
  - if still no response, give glucose IV (2.5 mL/kg 10%)
  - if baby is pale or white, give a rapid infusion of 10–20 mL/kg 0.9% saline or O-neg (CMV-negative) blood as volume expansion

Table 4.1 Doses and routes for resuscitation drugs in the newborn

Drug	Dose	Route
Adrenaline 1:10 000	1 mL/kg	Via ETT
Adrenaline 1:10 000	0.1–0.3 mL/kg	Intravenous
Sodium bicarbonate 4.2% (0.5 mmol/mL)	2–4 mL/kg (1–2 mmol/kg)	
Glucose 10%	2.5 mL/kg	Intravenous
Volume expander (Group O-neg., CMV-neg. blood or 0.9% saline)	10–20 mL/kg	Intravenous

Newborn Life Support

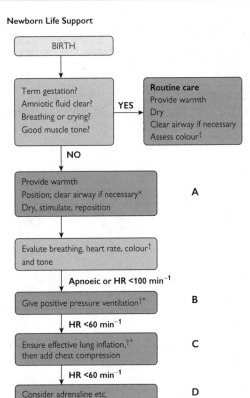

* Tracheal intubation may be considered at several steps
† Consider supplemental oxygen at any stage if cyanosis persists

Fig. 4.1 Newborn life support.[1]

1 With permission of the Resuscitation Council, UK.

Subsequent management

- If the response to resuscitation is prompt and the baby is pink, vigorous, and crying, hand to parents.
- If there are no signs of life after 10 minutes of continuous adequate resuscitation with ventilation, cardiac compressions, drugs, and volume expansion, discontinuation of resuscitation should be discussed with a senior paediatrician.
- Record Apgar scores (Table 4.2).

Risk factors

- Fetal distress, instrumental delivery, meconium-stained liquor.
- Maternal opioid administration, general anaesthetic.
- Multiple births, preterm delivery, shoulder dystocia.

Exclusions

- Hypovolaemia—baby remains very pale despite good ventilation and reasonable heart rate. Give 20 mL/kg O-negative blood via the umbilical vein (0.9% saline if blood not available). May need to be repeated.
- Diaphragmatic hernia—difficult to establish lung inflation, displaced apex, scaphoid abdomen. Pass wide-bore nasogastric tube and empty the stomach. Intubate to avoid further mask ventilation.
- Pneumothorax—tension pneumothoraces can develop during resuscitation. Poor air entry on one or both sides. Heart sounds quiet. If condition too critical to await X-ray, needle anterior chest wall, second intercostal space, mid-clavicular line, aspirating air using 20 mL syringe and three-way tap.
- Hydrops fetalis—many causes of this condition. Infants are born with severe generalized oedema and may have ascites, pleural, or pericardial effusions. Poor response to resuscitation may be improved by draining effusions and ascites with a needle or cannula.
- Congenital complete heart block. Baby has good colour, tone, and respiration but heart rate remains around 60 bpm. Good pulses. No further resuscitation is needed. Transfer to neonatal unit for further investigation.
- Macerated stillbirth. No heart beat detectable at any stage after birth. Skin sloughage, abdominal discoloration. Baby has been dead *in utero* for some time. Further resuscitation is pointless.

Special considerations

Meconium aspiration

- Most infants with meconium-stained liquor are in good condition. If baby is vigorous, no further airway management is required.
- If baby is floppy, with absent or poor respiratory effort, visualize the vocal cords with a laryngoscope and suction trachea below cords under direct vision using a wide-bore catheter (see Table 4.3).
- Repeat suction until airway is clear before applying positive pressure ventilation as required.

Table 4.2 Apgar scores

Clinical feature	Score		
	0	1	2
Colour	Pale/blue	Body pink, extremities blue	Pink
Heart rate	Absent	<100 bpm	>100 bpm
Response to stimulation	Nil	Some movement	Cry
Muscle tone	Limp	Some flexion of extremities	Well flexed
Respiratory effort	Absent	Poor respiratory effort or weak cry	Good

Table 4.3 Endotracheal tube diameters and lengths according to gestation and weight

50th centile weight by gestation		Tube diameter and length at the lip	
Gestation (weeks)	Body weight (kg)	Diameter (mm)	Length (cm)
23/24	0.5	2.5	6
26	0.75	2.5	6.5
27	1.0	2.5	7
30	1.5	2.5	7.5
33	2.0	2.5–3.0	8
35	2.5	3.0	8.5
37	3.0	3.0–3.5	9
40	3.5	3.5	9.5
	4.0	3.5–4.0	10

Prematurity
- Survival of infants <23 weeks' gestation is very poor and resuscitation is not recommended.
- Wrapping a preterm infant in food-grade plastic wrapping immediately after birth greatly reduces the risk of hypothermia.
- For most preterm infants, inflation pressures of 20–25 cmH$_2$O are adequate. Reduce pressure wherever possible to avoid lung injury.
- Most infants of 28 weeks' gestation or less require treatment with surfactant. Early administration is more effective than later treatment.

Maternal opioids
- Naloxone is not a drug of resuscitation.
- Establish effective ventilation first.
- Consider naloxone if infant remains depressed.
- 200 μg (60 μg/kg) dose intramuscularly for term infants.

Oxygen therapy
Ventilation may be initiated with air, if the clinician is concerned regarding the effects of hyperoxia in the preterm infant. Unless the infant responds immediately to air, additional oxygen should be given.

Reasons to transfer to SCBU
- Ongoing requirement for respiratory support
- Major congenital abnormality
- Prematurity

Further reading

Resuscitation Council (UK) (2005). *Newborn Life Support Guideline* Resuscitation Council, London (accessed 29/07/2008 http://www.resus.org.uk/pages/nlsalgo.pdf)

:☠: **Paediatric basic life support**

Definition
- Maintenance of the airway and support of respiration and circulation without the use of equipment:
  - infant—under 1 year
  - child—1 year to puberty

Presentation
- Unresponsive child, signs of breathing and circulation absent.
- Primary cardiac arrest uncommon. Cardiac arrest survival 3–17%.
- Ventricular fibrillation less than 10% of cases.

Immediate management

(See Fig. 4.2, 'PBLS algorithm', p113)
- Check child's responsiveness:
  - gently stimulate, 'Are you alright?' (children with suspected spine injuries should not be shaken)
- If responding:
  - leave in position, check condition, reassess regularly
- If not responding:
  - open airway by tilting the child's head and lifting the chin, do not push on soft tissues under the chin as this may block the airway, avoid head tilt if spinal injury suspected—use jaw thrust.

Airway
Keep airway open. Look, listen and feel for breathing by putting your face to the child's face and looking along the chest.

Breathing (<10 s for assessment)
- If the child is breathing normally, turn on side, watch for continued breathing.
- If not breathing or irregular breathing pattern, remove any obvious airway obstruction, give 2 breaths (up to 5 rescue breaths may be needed to achieve 2 effective breaths).

Circulation pulse (<10 s for assessment)
- Look for signs of movement and check:
  - child—carotid
  - infant—brachial
- If pulse >60 bpm, continue rescue breathing until the child starts to breathe.
- If pulse <60 bpm or absent (or uncertain), start chest compressions and continue rescue breaths.

Subsequent management
- If resuscitation is successful, transfer to hospital/ICU. There may be a continuing risk of further cardiorespiratory arrest *en route*.
- Obtain IV access as soon as is practical.

Risk factors

Primary respiratory and cardiovascular disease, metabolic disease, immersion in water, choking, trauma, haemorrhage, electrocution, sepsis.

Exclusions

Hypoxia—respiratory obstruction, drowning, poisoning, toxic gases, electric shock.

Special considerations

- Immersion in cold water:
  - BLS should be continued until the core temperature is above 32°C
  - VF may be persistent at lower body temperatures

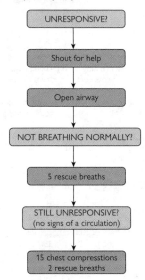

**Paediatric Basic Life Support
(Healthcare professionals
with a duty to respond)**

UNRESPONSIVE?

↓

Shout for help

↓

Open airway

↓

NOT BREATHING NORMALLY?

↓

5 rescue breaths

↓

STILL UNRESPONSIVE?
(no signs of a circulation)

↓

15 chest compresstions
2 rescue breaths

After 1 minute call resuscitation team then continue

Fig. 4.2 Paediatric basic life support.[1]

1 With permission from the Resuscitation Council, UK.

Rescue breaths

Child
- Head tilt and chin lift.
- Pinch nose closed, open mouth, and maintain chin lift.
- Blow steadily into mouth while watching the chest rise.
- Take your mouth away and observe the chest fall—maintain the head tilt and jaw lift.
- Repeat up to 5 times.

Infant
- Head tilt and chin lift.
- Cover the nose and mouth with your mouth. This may be difficult in a larger infant and mouth to nose with the mouth held closed may be more effective.
- Blow steadily into mouth and nose over 1–1.5 s, watching the chest rise.
- Take your mouth away and observe the chest fall—maintain head tilt and jaw lift.
- Repeat up to 5 times to achieve 2 effective breaths.

Chest compressions

Child
- Place the heel of one hand over the lower half of the sternum.
- Lift your fingers to avoid pressing on the child's ribs.
- Keep your arm straight, press vertically down on the sternum.
- Depress the chest by one-third of its depth.
- Release and repeat at a rate of 100 compressions per minute.
- After 15 compressions, tilt the head, lift the chin, and give 2 effective breaths.
- Continue compressions and breaths in a ratio of 15:2.
- Children over the age of 8 may need the adult two-handed compression technique.

Infant
- Place the tips of two fingers one finger breadth below a line between the nipples.
- Press down on the sternum and depress the chest by one-third of its depth.
- Release and repeat at a rate of 100 compressions per minute.
- Continue compressions and breaths at a 15:2 ratio.
- If there is more than one rescuer, then an alternative technique in an infant is:
  - encircle the chest with both hands, placing both thumbs over the lower half of the sternum, one finger's breadth below a line between the nipples
  - press down on the sternum with both thumbs to one-third to one-half the depth of the chest
  - the second rescuer delivers rescue breaths

Foreign body obstruction

(See Fig. 4.3, 'FBAO *algorithm', p116)*

- Encourage coughing because this is the most effective way of relieving obstruction caused by FBs in the airway.
- Active interventions to dislodge an FB are indicated when coughing attempts become ineffective or breathing is inadequate.
- Blind finger sweeps in the mouth are contraindicated as an FB may be impacted/pushed further into the airway.

Conscious with an ineffective cough

- Position the child prone with his head lower than his chest and his airway open
- Deliver up to 5 sharp blows to the middle of the back between the shoulder blades
- If the FB is not dislodged, then proceed to perform 5 anterior thrusts (chest for infants, abdominal for child >1 yr)
- Chest thrust—place the infant supine with the head lower than the chest and the airway open
- Deliver up to 5 sharp chest thrusts to the sternum, using the same technique as for chest compressions
- Abdo thrust—stand or kneel behind child, encircle the torso with your arms, clench your fist and place it between umbilicus and xiphisternum. Grasp your fist and pull inwards and upwards
- The aim is to relieve obstruction with each blow/thrust rather than to deliver all five blows/thrusts
- After chest or abdominal thrusts, check the mouth for evidence of dislodged FB. Remove any debris carefully

Unconscious with ineffective cough

- Open the mouth: attempt removal of an obvious foreign body with single finger sweep.
- Reassess airway and breathing.
- If still obstructed, continue with BLS by opening airway, giving 5 rescue breaths, and commencing CPR (see p114).
- body with single finger sweep
- Reassess airway and breathing:
  - continue with BLS (see p113)

Paediatric FBAO Treatment

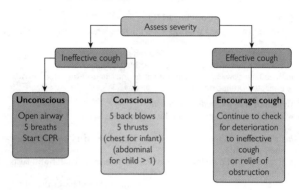

Fig. 4.3 Paediatric foreign body airway obstruction (FBAO) treatment.[1]

Further reading
UK Resuscitation Council Guidelines: www.resus.org.uk

1 With permission from the Resuscitation Council, UK.

☢ Paediatric advanced life support

Definition
Application of advanced skills to support vital organ function.

Presentation
- Asystolic arrest, rarely VF/VT, in response to hypoxia or vagal stimulation.
- Cardiac arrest in children is usually secondary to hypoxia—not an acute primary event.

Immediate management

(See Fig. 4.4, PALS algorithm, p119.)

- Discontinue all vagal stimuli
  - initial management is as BLS (see p108 and Fig. 4.2)
- After establishing CPR and calling for help, assess rhythm using cardiac monitor/defibrillator:
  - infants may need pads or paddles front and back of chest
  - child pads should be placed just below the right clavicle and in left axillary line
- Rhythm is often 'non-shockable' (PEA/asystole) but may be 'shockable' (VF/pulselessVT).
- **Non-shockable (PEA/asystole):**
  - drugs should be given IV/IO rather than by tracheal route
  - adrenaline 10 µg/kg IV/IO (0.1 mL/kg of 1 in 10 000) or 100 µg/kg via ETT (0.1 mL/kg of 1 in 1000)
  - repeat cycles of 10 µg/kg adrenaline/3–5 min CPR
- **Shockable (VF/pulseless VT):**
  - give one defibrillatory shock (4 J/kg)
  - resume CPR immediately for 2 min without reassessing rhythm or feeling for a pulse
  - then pause briefly to check the monitor
  - if still in VF/VT give a second shock (4 J/kg) and resume CPR immediately
  - repeat cycles of defibrillation, CPR, and 10 µg/kg adrenaline every 3–5 min
  - a standard AED may be used for children >8 yr (and if no other defib available >1 yr)
  - no evidence for or against AED use in <1yr.
- **During CPR**—consider reversible causes:
  - hypoxia
  - hypovolaemia
  - hypo/hyperkalaemia
  - hypothermia
  - tension pneumothorax
  - tamponade
  - toxic/drug ingestion
  - thromboemboli

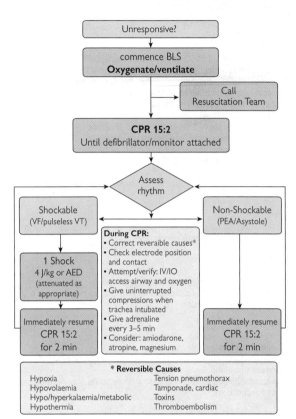

Fig. 4.4 Paediatric advanced life support.[1]

1 With permission of the Resuscitation Council, UK.

Subsequent management
- Effective CPR is a priority.
- Deliver 100% oxygen, aim for normocapnia.
- Hypovolaemia should be treated with 20 mL/kg 0.9% saline.
- Amiodarone (5 mg/kg) consider for VF/pulseless VT after 3 shocks. Given peripherally over 20 min—diluted in 4 mL/kg 5% glucose.
- Lidocaine (1 mg/kg) as alternative to amiodarone.
- Atropine may be considered for persistent bradycardia.
- Magnesium 25–50 mg/kg if 'torsade de pointes'.
- Sodium bicarbonate 1–2 mL/kg 8.4% for a prolonged arrest, hyperkalaemia or tricyclic antidepressant overdose.
- Children with core temp <37.5°C should not be warmed.
- Children with core temp <33°C should be warmed to 34°C
- Survival is unlikely after 20–min of continuous, adequate, APLS; discontinuation of resuscitation should be discussed with a senior paediatrician.

Investigations
ECG, ABGs, FBC, U&Es, glucose, clotting screen, consider COHb and toxicology screen (depending on history).

Risk factors
- Hypoxia
- Vagal stimulation, e.g. surgical traction on the ocular muscles
- Metabolic derangement, e.g. diabetic ketoacidosis, hypothermia
- Pre-existing cardiac disease

Exclusions
- Identify causes of hypoxia and treat immediately.
- Ask surgeons to stop any vagal stimulation.
- Consider access to drugs or toxic substances and seek advice if overdose suspected. Smoke inhalation.
- Suspected inhaled foreign body in an arrested child may need urgent rigid bronchoscopy.

Special considerations
Children with congenital heart defects, e.g. univentricular heart, Fallot's tetralogy, uncorrected VSD, may have large right-to-left shunts as pulmonary pressures rise. Try to maintain systemic pressure.

Intraosseous access
(See also pp470–2.)

All recommended resuscitation drugs can be given by this route. Recommended sites for insertion:
- Anterior surface of the tibia, 2–3 cm below the tibial tuberosity (avoiding the epiphyseal plate).
- Anterolateral surface of the femur, 3 cm above the lateral condyle.

Further reading
UK Resuscitation Council Guidelines: www.resus.org.uk

☠ Drowning and near-drowning

Definition
- **Drowning**—death consequent upon hypoxia due to lack of oxygen or laryngeal spasm after immersion in water or other fluid.
- **Near-drowning**—survival following asphyxia after immersion in a fluid.

Presentation
History of immersion in a fluid with respiratory or cardiorespiratory arrest. May be profoundly hypothermic. There may be associated trauma—involve the paediatric trauma team.

Immediate management

Basic life support
- Assume cervical spine injury. The neck should be immobilized by in-line stabilization.
- If resuscitation equipment available, give oxygen via bag/valve/mask.
- There is a risk of aspiration of gastric contents, early intubation is desirable.
- Consider a rapid sequence induction.
- Pass a gastric tube to decompress the stomach and also allow gastric lavage.

Advanced life support
- If core temperature is <30°C, withhold adrenaline and other resuscitation drugs.
- Core temperature >30°C, use lowest recommended doses and double the dose interval.
- If VF is present, 3 shocks with CPR should be given, but further defibrillation attempts should be withheld until core temperature reaches 30°C.

Active re-warming
Resuscitation is unlikely to be successful unless the core temperature can be increased >32°C. Institute rectal or (preferably) oesophageal temperature monitoring.
- Remove all wet clothing and dry the patient.
- Use forced warm-air blanket and warm all IV fluids.
- If possible, warm the ventilator breathing circuit or use a circle system with soda-lime and low fresh gas flow to warm inspired gas (NB reduced CO_2 production in hypothermia).
- Gastric or bladder lavage with 0.9% saline at 40–42°C.
- Peritoneal lavage with potassium-free dialysate at 40–42°C 20 mL/ kg/15 min cycle.
- Extracorporeal circuit with blood rewarming.

Complete a secondary survey for other injuries.

Subsequent management
- Aim to optimize recovery from the hypoxic CNS injury.
- Manage associated trauma.

- Supportive therapy in an intensive care unit.
- Regular tracheal toilet and culture of aspirate.
- Consider antibiotic therapy.
- Physiotherapy and follow-up chest X-ray.

Investigations
ABGs, blood glucose, electrolytes, core temperature with *low-reading thermometer* (e.g. thermistor probe), CXR, blood cultures, CT cervical spine.

Risk factors
- Children playing near water. Accidental injury resulting in immersion, exposure to poisons (e.g. pesticides or toxic gases) near waterways or farmyard slurry.
- History of non-accidental injury.

Exclusions
- Diving accidents with head injury
- Exposure to toxic waste and chemicals in water
- Poisoning
- Deliberate harm (non-accidental injury)

Special considerations
- Three-quarters of near-drowning victims survive intact if they receive immediate BLS when removed from the water.
- Longer exposures reduce the chance of survival. Survival is unlikely if more than 8 min of immersion has occurred.
- Return of spontaneous ventilatory effort soon (a few minutes) after commencing resuscitation is a good prognostic sign.
- Profound hypothermia (after cold-water immersion) may preserve vital organ function but predisposes to ventricular fibrillation, which may be refractory to treatment until re-warming has occurred to above 32°C.
- The myocardium is unresponsive to drugs at temperatures <30°C, so if core temperature is <30°C withhold adrenaline and other resuscitation drugs. Accumulation of drugs occurs peripherally with standard ALS dose intervals, so >30°C use lowest recommended doses and double the dose interval.
- Submersion causes initial apnoea and bradycardia due to vagal stimulation (diving reflex). Continuing apnoea leads to hypoxia and reflex tachycardia. Continuing hypoxia produces severe acidosis. Eventually breathing resumes (the 'break-point') and fluid is inhaled, causing immediate laryngeal spasm. Eventually this spasm subsides with profound hypoxia; water and debris are inhaled. Continuing hypoxia and acidosis lead to bradycardia and arrhythmia, culminating in cardiac arrest.

Further reading
Mackway Jones, K., Molyneux, E., Phillips, B., Wieteska, S. (ed.) (2001). *Advanced Paediatric Life Support: The Practical Approach*, (3rd edn), BMJ Books, London.

UK Resuscitation Council Guidelines: www.resus.org.uk

☠ Acute severe asthma

(See also pp54–6.)

Definition
Severe bronchospasm with history of asthma.

Presentation
- **Acute severe**—any one of:
  - PEFR 33–50% best or predicted, SpO_2 <92%, pulse >120 bpm (>5 yr) or >130 bpm (2–5 yr), respiration >30 breaths/min (>5 yr) or >50 breaths/min (2–5 yr), use of accessory muscles
- **Life threatening**—any of the following in a patient with acute severe asthma:
  - PEFR <33% best or predicted, SpO_2 <92% or PaO_2 <8 kPa (60 mmHg), normal $PaCO_2$ (4.6–6 kPa (35–45 mmHg)), hypotension, exhaustion, confusion or coma, silent chest, cyanosis, poor respiratory effort
- **Near-fatal**—raised $PaCO_2$ and/or requiring mechanical ventilation
  - confused or drowsy, maximal use of accessory muscles, exhausted, SpO_2 <92% in air, heart rate >140 bpm and unable to talk.

Immediate management
- 100% O_2
- *Acute severe*:
  - salbutamol 10 puffs via inhaler and spacer ± facemask or nebulized salbutamol (2.5–5 mg)
  - prednisolone PO 20 mg (2–5 yr), 30–40 mg (>5 yr) or IV hydrocortisone (<1 yr 25 mg, 1–5 yrs 50 mg, 6–12 yrs 100 mg 4 times daily)
  - repeat salbutamol every 20–30 min, add ipratropium bromide 250 μg nebulized every 20–30 min
- *Life threatening*:
  - salbutamol nebulized 2.5–5 mg
  - ipratropium bromide nebulized 500 μg (2–12 yrs 250 μg)
  - IV hydrocortisone (<1 yr 25 mg, 1–5 yrs 50 mg, 6–12 yrs 100 mg 4 times daily)
  - repeat bronchodilators every 20–30 min
  - consider IV bronchodilators; salbutamol, aminophylline, and magnesium sulphate

Subsequent management
- If improving—monitor SpO_2, nebulizers 3–4 hourly, oral prednisolone for 3 days, transfer to respiratory ward once stable.
- If deteriorating despite medical therapy:
  - salbutamol as a single dose IV (1 month–2 yrs 5 μg/kg; 2–18 yrs 15 μg/kg maximum 250 μg), then infusion 1 month–18 yrs 60–300 μg/kg/hr, dose adjusted according to response and heart rate (doses above 120 μg/kg/hr with close monitoring), monitor for lactic acidosis
  - aminophylline 5 mg/kg loading dose (not if already on theophylline) then 1 mg/kg/h (<9 yrs), 800 μg/kg/h (9–16 yrs) IV infusion
  - continue nebulizers every 20 min
  - IV magnesium sulphate 50 mg/kg (max. 2 g)
- If impending respiratory failure: intubate, ventilate, and transfer to PICU once stable.

Investigations

- SpO_2, peak expiratory flow (PEFR) or FEV_1 (>5 yr)
- If critical: ABGs, CXR, lactate, serum theophylline level

Risk factors

- History of asthma with previous acute admissions
- Respiratory tract infection
- Trigger exposure, e.g. stress, cold, exercise, smoke, allergen
- Prematurity and low birth-weight infants

Exclusions

- Consider other causes of wheeze:
  - bronchiolitis or croup
  - aspiration of foreign body—asymmetry on auscultation
  - epiglottitis—rare since introduction of HIB vaccine
  - pneumonia—primary cause of wheeze or trigger of asthma attack
  - tracheomalacia

Special considerations

- IPPV may be difficult in severe asthma with very high airway pressures ($30–40\,cmH_2O$), sloping expiratory capnograph trace, and small tidal volumes. Hand ventilation may be necessary. Permissive hypercapnia may be indicated.
- Try PEEP $5–7\,cmH_2O$ and slow respiratory rates to avoid dynamic hyperinflation.
- Volatile anaesthetic agents all cause bronchodilatation and may be useful *in extremis*. Attention should be given to scavenging of waste gas.
- These children are usually dehydrated, so induction of anaesthesia for intubation should be preceded with a fluid load of 20 mL/kg of crystalloid. Slow administration of drugs is preferable, but rapid sequence induction may be required in non-fasted patients. Consider ketamine 1–2 mg/kg.
- Avoid histamine releasing drugs like morphine or atracurium.
- If sedation is adequate postintubation physiotherapy can be beneficial.
- *Peak expiratory flow rate in children*—this is a simple method of measuring airway obstruction and will detect moderate or severe disease. It is measured using a standard Wright peak flow meter (see Table 4.4):

$$PEFR\ (L/min) = [height\ (cm) - 80] \times 5.$$

Table 4.4 PEFR by height

Height (cm)	PEFR (L/min)
120	215
130	260
140	300
150	350
160	400
170	450
180	500

Further reading

www.sign.ac.uk

:💀: Stridor

Definition
- Harsh respiratory noise produced by airway obstruction.
- Inspiratory stridor implies laryngeal/nasal/pharyngeal pathology.
- Expiratory stridor implies tracheal/bronchial (intrathoracic).
- Biphasic stridor implies subglottic or glottic pathology.

Presentation
- Stridor, increased work of breathing suprasternal, intercostal, or subcostal recession and increased use of accessory muscles.
- Signs of deterioration and need for urgent intervention—hypoxia, fatigue, or decreasing conscious level, increased work of breathing.
- Impending respiratory failure may also be heralded by a reduction in work of breathing (exhaustion) and less stridor (more complete obstruction).
- Beware the disinterested child.

Immediate management
- Allow the child to sit quietly on the parent's lap in a comfortable position.
- Observe closely without interference.
- Assess severity of respiratory distress and plan for most likely underlying cause.
- Supplemental oxygen can result in falsely reassuring SpO_2 readings in severe obstruction.
- Consider EMLA® or tetracaine gel 4% (Ametop®)for intravenous access.
- Consider nebulizing 0.5 mL/kg 1 in 1000 adrenaline (up to 5 mL)
- If condition deteriorating, consider intubation.

Anaesthesia for the child with the obstructed airway
- Call for senior anaesthetist and senior ENT help.
- Inhalational induction in theatre in a quiet environment.
- Consider antisialagogue (atropine 20 µg/kg IV—min 100 µg, max 600 µg).
- 100% O_2 and sevoflurane (or halothane if experienced in its use; halothane is better for maintaining depth of anaesthesia).
- May induce on parent's lap or sitting if airway best maintained in that position.
- Apply CPAP via facemask once tolerated.
- Adequate depth of anaesthesia will take a long time to achieve!
- Maintain spontaneous breathing but check if you can ventilate with the bag. If yes, *gently* assist inspiration if necessary, but avoid gastric distension.
- Once patient is sufficiently anaesthetized—direct laryngoscopy without muscle relaxant.
- Intubate if possible—may need much smaller tube than anticipated in croup (do not pre-cut the ETT).

- Intubation may be difficult in epiglottitis—look for air bubbles from glottic opening. Use a bougie and railroad tube over it.
- If emergency IV access required remember interosseous route can be quickly established.
- If obstruction persists following successful intubation: try advancing the tube (mediastinal mass/foreign body), consider a blocked tube (tracheitis), try prone ventilation (mediastinal mass).
- The vast majority of children with stridor can be intubated by an experienced anaesthetist; occasionally rigid bronchoscopy in the hands of an experienced ENT surgeon may be life-saving.

Subsequent management

- Once intubated, maintain anaesthesia (IV morphine and midazolam infusion or inhalational agent whilst in theatre).
- Consider dexamethasone 0.6 mg/kg IV if not already given.
- Transfer to PICU.
- Cefotaxime 50 mg/kg IV 6-hourly or ceftriaxone 50 mg/kg IV daily (epiglottitis).
- Extubation: dexamethasone often given (0.25 mg/kg IV 6-hourly 2 or 3 doses) at least 6 h prior to extubation. A small leak around the ET tube at a pressure of 20 cmH$_2$O should be observed before attempting extubation.
- Soft-tissue X-rays usually add no useful information. Even with a leak, oedema may require re-intubation in some cases.

Investigations

Check SpO$_2$ on air and 100% oxygen.

Risk factors

- Croup most likely acute cause in UK.
- High degree of overlap in clinical presentation.
- Supplementary oxygen may be falsely reassuring as a child in severe respiratory distress may be pink in oxygen.

Exclusions

- Croup—harsh barking cough, febrile, miserable but well.
- Epiglottitis—toxic, no cough, low-pitched inspiratory and expiratory stridor, and drooling.
- Foreign body—sudden onset, previously well, coughing, choking, and aphonia.
- Anaphylaxis—swelling of face and tongue, wheeze, urticarial rash.
- Retropharyngeal abscess—high fever, hyperextension of neck, dysphagia, pooling of secretions.
- Bacterial tracheitis—toxic, tender trachea (vigilance is require if intubated—mucopurulent membrane can block ET).
- Pre-existing stridor—congenital abnormality, laryngomalacia, or subglottic stenosis.

☠ Anaphylaxis

(See also pp256–8)

Definition

- A severe, life-threatening, generalized, or systemic hypersensitivity reaction.
- This definition includes IgE- and non-IgE-mediated reactions.

Presentation

- Commonly—stridor, wheeze, cough, desaturation, respiratory distress, ECG changes, cardiovascular collapse, and clinical signs of shock.
- Less commonly—oedema, rash, and urticaria.
- Consider when compatible history of severe allergic-type reaction with respiratory difficulty and/or hypotension, especially if skin changes are present.

Immediate management

- 100% O_2.
- Adrenaline 1 μg/kg slow IV given incrementally with ECG monitoring until hypotension resolves (1:10 000 solution):
  - >12 yrs: 500 μg IM (0.5 mL) i.e. same as adult dose, 300 μg (0.3 mL) if child is small or prepubertal
  - >6–12 yrs: 300 μg IM (0.3 mL)
  - >6 mths–6 yrs: 150 μg IM (0.15 mL)
  - <6 mths: 150 μg IM (0.15 mL)
- IM adrenaline (1:1000 solution) may be safer and less arrhythmogenic:
  - 12 yrs: 500 μg (0.5 mL)
  - 6–12 yrs: 250 μg (0.25 mL)
  - >6 mths–6 yrs: 120 μg (0.12 mL)
  - <6 mths: 50 μg (0.05 mL)
- Antihistamine: chlorphenamine (chlorpheniramine):
  - 12 yrs: 10 mg IM or slow IV
  - 6–12 yrs: 5 mg IM or slow IV
  - 6 mths–6 yrs: 2.5 mg IM or slow IV
  - <6 mths: 250 μg/kg IM or slow IV
- Hydrocortisone:
  - 12 yrs: 200 mg IM or slow IV
  - 6–12 yrs: 100 mg IM or slow IV
  - 6 mths–6 yrs: 50 mg IM or slow IV
  - <6 mths: 25 mg IM or slow IV
- Repeat doses of adrenaline may be given at 5 min intervals as necessary, further fluid boluses may be needed

Subsequent management

- Bronchodilators, e.g. salbutamol inhalers/nebulizers, as per protocol for acute severe asthma (pp124–5) if bronchospasm severe and unresponsive to adrenaline.
- Catecholamine infusion as CVS instability may last several hours—adrenaline or noradrenaline 0.05–0.1 μg/kg/min.
- Check ABGs, consider bicarbonate—up to 1 mmol/kg 8.4% sodium bicarbonate (1 mmol = 1 mL) if pH less than 7.1.

Investigations

Plasma tryptase (early, 1–2 h and 24 h samples)

Risk factors

- Previous allergic reaction; particularly history of increasingly severe reactions.
- History of asthma or atopy.
- Penicillin, radiographic contrast media, some foods (especially nuts). Cross-sensitivity means that previous exposure is not always necessary (e.g. latex and bananas).
- Intravenous administration of antigen increases risk.

Exclusions

- Primary cardiovascular disease (e.g. congenital heart disease in the newborn)
- Sepsis (with rash)
- Latex allergy
- Tension pneumothorax
- Acute severe asthma (history of asthma, previous admissions)
- Airway obstruction (e.g. foreign body aspiration)

Special considerations

- Never give undiluted adrenaline 1:1000 IV. IM adrenaline carries less risk of provoking potentially life-threatening arrhythmias, but may be poorly absorbed if perfusion is compromised, such that the dose may be ineffective. IV adrenaline may cause arrhythmia, but given slowly with full ECG monitoring, may be more effective in profound anaphylactic shock.
- Chlorphenamine and steroids take hours to achieve any benefit— omission in immediate management is acceptable.
- Chlorphenamine is not suitable for neonates.
- Absence of a circuit/airway filter increases the risk of exposure to aerosolized latex particles.
- Report adverse drug reactions to MHRA (www.mhra.gov.uk).
- All patients with anaphylaxis should be referred to an allergy clinic (www.bsaci.org).

Further reading

Association of Anaesthetists of Great Britain and Ireland and British Society for Allergy and Clinical Immunology (2003). *Suspected anaphylactic reactions associated with anaesthesia.* www.aagbi.org

UK Resuscitation Council Guidelines: www.resus.org.uk

✪ Major trauma

Definition
Serious injury to head/chest/abdomen/pelvis/spine.

Presentation
- A history is the key to understanding the severity and pattern of injuries.
- There is considerable time pressure initially and a protocolized multidisciplinary approach, which prioritizes the treatment of immediately life-threatening injuries, has improved outcomes.
- After this initial 'Primary survey' a detailed 'Secondary survey' aims to completely identify all the injuries.
- Children and infants often have a greater compensatory reserve than adults, resulting in a tendency to underestimate the severity of injuries.
- Treatment priorities are a clear airway, adequate ventilation, avoidance of hypoxia and hypotension.

Immediate management
- ABC … 100% O_2.
- Place 2 large-bore cannulae or obtain intraosseous access. Do not waste time if peripheral veins are not available.
- Intubation after rapid sequence induction may be required to protect the airway (GCS <8 or trend in the GCS motor component), and avoid hypoxia (respiratory failure developing). Protect the cervical spine—assume spinal damage and use in-line stabilization or a hard collar.
- Unconscious patients must be ventilated, preferably using muscle relaxants. Aim for normocapnia.
- Hypovolaemia as evidenced by tachycardia and poor capillary refill should be treated with fluid boluses of 20 mL/kg crystalloid (Hartmann's solution or 0.9% saline). Use colloid if the initial response to crystalloid is poor. Blood should be given as the third fluid bolus if there is no improvement.
- Avoid fluid overload in head-injured patients, but ensure perfusion with an adequate mean arterial pressure. There may be large blood loss from scalp wounds or into the subdural space in patients with head injuries, particularly infants.
- Thoracocentesis or pericardiocentesis may be required urgently.
- An orogastric tube and urinary catheter should be placed routinely.

Subsequent management
- Secondary survey looking at all systems for signs of injury. Vital signs and neurological status (disability) should be reassessed continually.
- All patients need ventilation, oxygenation, and cardiac output problems addressed before transfer to CT or PICU. The clinician undertaking a transfer must have a clear understanding of the risk of the journey and the benefit of the transfer in order to make the correct stabilization decisions.
- If non-accidental injury is suspected, contact Child Protection Service (usually via a consultant paediatrician).

Investigations
- FBC, U&Es, glucose, crossmatch ABGs, clotting
- X-ray—C-spine, CXR, pelvis, thoracic/lumbar spine
- Ultrasound—checking for abdominal free fluid
- CT scan
- Peripheral X-rays

Risk factors
- Pedestrians most at risk, then cyclists and vehicle passengers.
- Head injury accounts for 40% of trauma deaths in children.

Exclusions
- Non-accidental injury in cases of apparent accidental trauma, particularly head injury. 'Shaken baby' syndrome.
- Poisoning, deliberate or accidental in cases of coma or fitting.

A = Airway
B = Breathing
C = Circulation
D = Disability (neurological assessment)
E = Exposure (remove clothes to assess—BUT keep warm)

Disability is assessed initially using **AVPU**:

A = Alert
V = responds to Voice
P = responds to Pain
U = Unresponsive

The GCS can be used in children over 4 years of age (p183).

Further reading
Mackway Jones, K., Molyneux, E., Phillips, B., Wieteska, S. (ed.) (2001). *Advanced Paediatric Life Support: The Practical Approach*, (3rd edn). BMJ Books, London.

☼ Burns

Definition

Dry burn or scalding injury ± smoke inhalation.

Presentation

- Obvious thermal injury—remove all clothing where possible.
- Smoke deposits, carbonaceous sputum, airway obstruction, or bronchospasm suggest airway/lung damage, and early intubation should be considered (this may not be possible within hours due to oedema).
- Hypovolaemia soon after burn injury is probably due to other causes, such as bleeding (e.g. from falls, injuries sustained while escaping the fire or blast).
- A multidisciplinary paediatric trauma team should manage all but the most straightforward cases.

Immediate management

- ABC … 100% O_2.
- Airway assessment. If in doubt, intubate. Use uncut ET tube to allow for oedema.
- Analgesia essential—IV morphine 100 µg/kg titrated and repeated as required. Consider ketamine 0.5–1 mg/kg.
- Two large-bore IV cannulae or IO access. Consider femoral central line (avoids risk of pneumothorax). Initially Hartmann's or 0.9% saline 20 mL/kg for hypovolaemia—repeat as required if signs of hypovolaemia (capillary refill >2 s; low blood pressure).Urine output should be >1–2 mL/kg/h. NB Burn fluid formulae are not used at this stage.
- Consider inhalational induction with sevoflurane if airway involvement could make the airway or intubation difficult.

Subsequent management

- Do not rely on pulse oximetry as a guide to oxygenation. Frequent measurement of COHb may be necessary. Prolonged oxygen therapy is required in significant carbon monoxide poisoning. The risk/benefit of hyperbaric oxygen is not clear.
- Cyanide antidote may be required (sodium nitrite 3% solution 4–10 mg/kg, plus sodium thiosulphate 50% solution 400 mg/kg (max 12.5 g)). Monitor methaemoglobin level (should remain <10%).
- Urinary catheter to guide fluid balance (urine output >2 mL/kg/h).
- Wound care—infection is a significant cause of mortality. Keep the burn wound covered with 'clingfilm', sterile towels, or dressings.
- Antibiotic prophylaxis according to local protocol.

Fluid therapy

- Burn depth and area are assessed during the secondary survey.
  This assessment can be used to guide fluid therapy during subsequent
  management. NB Formulae for fluid therapy are only a guide, and frequent
  reassessment of circulatory status and urine output are required.

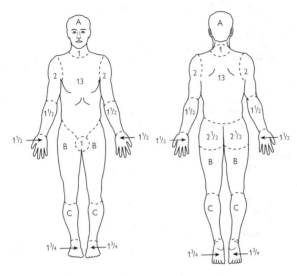

Relative percentage of area affected by growth (age in years)

	0	1	5	10	15	Adult
A: half of head	9½	8½	6½	5½	4½	3½
B: half of thigh	2¾	3¼	4	4½	4½	4¾
C: half of leg	2½	2½	2¾	3	3¼	3½

Fig. 4.5 Assessing extent of burns—Lund and Browder charts (see also p400).

- Special charts that take into account changes in relative surface area with
  age (e.g. Lund and Browder, Fig. 4.5) can be used to assess the burn area.
  The 'rule of nines' (see pp400–3) cannot be applied to children below
  14 years of age. For extensive burns, count unburnt area using the patient's
  palmar surface area (including fingers) = 0.8% body surface area (BSA).
- Dry, waxy/leathery, insensitive burns that DO NOT BLEED on pinprick
  are full thickness. Full-thickness burns can easily be confused with
  normal skin.

- Patients with partial-thickness burns greater than 10% BSA or 5% full thickness require IV fluid in addition to basal fluid requirement. This additional fluid can be calculated using different formulae, or simply as:

    %burn × weight (kg) × 4 mL.

- 50% of this volume is given in the first 8h following the burn injury. Controversy exists as to the relative benefit of crystalloid or colloid, but crystalloid is now more commonly used. Subsequent fluid therapy is guided by urine output.

Investigations
SpO_2, ABGs, Hb, COHb, cyanide level (>100 ppm may be fatal), U&Es, glucose, G&S, myoglobin (particularly in electrical burns), chest radiograph if inhalation.

Risk factors
- 70% are preschool children, greatest risk 1–2 years of age.
- Most fatal burns in house fires are due to smoke inhalation. Other injuries are often sustained while attempting to escape the fire.
- Cyanide poisoning in house fires due to burning plastics and wool.
- Common causes of burns in children include hot drinks, hot baths (infants), cooking oil.
- Electrical burns.

Exclusions
Non-accidental injury (NAI)—burns may have a 'glove or stocking' appearance due to limb, or whole-body, immersion in a hot bath. 'Cold burns' (contact with deep frozen objects), delay in seeking help, vague history, and the combination of healing and fresh injuries should also lead to suspicion of NAI. If NAI is suspected, contact the Child Protection Service (usually via a consultant paediatrician).

Criteria for transfer to a burns unit
- More than 10% partial or any full-thickness burns.
- Burns to special areas, e.g. face, hands, and perineum.
- Lack of facilities to manage burn wounds of <10% BSA.
- Lack of expertise at the receiving hospital (e.g. paediatric team).

Special considerations
- Small area electrical burn—may be internal organ damage and myoglobinuria.
- Psychological damage.
- Forensic evidence in NAI cases.

Further reading
Pediatric burn injuries. www.depts.washington.edu/pccm/3-pediatric%20burns%2011.pps

Peltier, P.J., Purdue, G., Shepherd, J. Burn injuries in child abuse. www.ncjrs.org/txtfiles/91190.txt

:O: Severe sepsis

Definition
- *Severe sepsis*—acute organ dysfunction secondary to infection.
- *Septic shock*—severe sepsis plus hypotension not reversed with fluid resuscitation.

Presentation
- *'Warm' shock*—low blood pressure, especially low diastolic, tachycardia, vasodilated with short capillary refill time, often high cardiac output.
- *'Cold' shock*—normal or low blood pressure, tachycardia, prolonged capillary refill, often low cardiac output state.

Early recognition and fluid administration is the key intervention that improves outcome.

Immediate management
- If the child is febrile and unwell, but conscious with an adequate circulation, give oxygen; obtain vascular access, baseline investigations, give maintenance fluid, and observe for signs of impending septic shock.

Septic shock
- Recognize impaired mental status and perfusion.
- Oxygen and assess airway (BLS).
- 20 mL/kg crystalloid (not containing glucose) or colloid boluses titrated to improvement.
- Correct hypoglycaemia/hypocalcaemia, give antibiotics.
- Contact a PICU for advice as soon as possible. Retrieval of the child may be an option, but he/she will need to be stabilized for transfer.
- If the shock persists—start dopamine (5–15 µg/kg/min—peripherally initially), intubate (ketamine/suxamethonium/fentanyl), establish central and arterial access and give more fluid (up to 100 mL/kg may be required).
- Consider dobutamine (5–15 µg/kg/min) for fluid-loaded cold shock with a normal blood pressure.
- Fluid-refractory, dopamine-resistant shock:
  - warm shock—noradrenaline (0.1–1.0 µg/kg/min)
  - cold shock—adrenaline (0.1–1.0 µg/kg/min)
  - titrate the inotropes to clinical endpoints and ScvO₂ saturations >70%
  - management should be guided by advice from the local PICU

Consider
- Hydrocortisone if there is adrenal insufficiency.
- 4.5% human albumin may be used after initial boluses of crystalloid.
- Profound acidosis should be corrected with 8.4% sodium bicarbonate (4.2% in neonates). Give half the correction based on base deficit (if pH <7.1) and repeat ABGs:

Full correction (mL) = weight × 0.3 × base deficit.
- Avoid hypoglycaemia, but beware of giving 'free water' as dilute glucose solutions. 10 or 20% glucose should be used to correct low blood sugar levels.
- Antibiotics:
  - neonates—ampicillin 30 mg/kg qds (tds,if aged <7 days), plus gentamicin 2.5 mg/kg 8-hourly (12-hourly if aged <7 days); monitor blood levels.
  - older children—cefotaxime 50 mg/kg 6-hourly IV, or ceftriaxone 50 mg/kg daily.

Subsequent management
- Do not perform lumbar puncture if risk of raised ICP.
- If raised ICP is suspected, mannitol (0.5–1.0 g/kg) or furosemide (1 mg/kg) to 'buy time'. The patient should be catheterized.

Investigations
Hb, U&Es, glucose, clotting, ABGs, calcium, magnesium, phosphate, blood cultures

Risk factors
- Exposure to Gram-positive or -negative bacteria, *Listeria spp.*, *Rickettsia spp.*, fungi, and viruses, particularly herpes.
- Immune system deficiency, surgery, and chronic illness.

Exclusions
- Hypovolaemia from any cause.
- Primary cardiac disease (e.g. cardiomyopathy); congenital cardiac defects (e.g. undiagnosed ventricular septal defect with heart failure).
- Anaphylaxis.
- Poisoning.

Special considerations
- The shocked child with no obvious haemorrhage should be treated as sepsis until another cause is found.
- Rash in meningococcal disease does not always develop immediately. A careful survey for purpuric spots is mandatory. A small number of cases have no rash.
- Bleeding into mucosal surfaces may indicate DIC.
- Fever may not be present in babies. A temperature >38°C is significant.
- Deteriorating level of consciousness, irritability, hypertonia/hypotonia warrant immediate investigation.

Meningitis
- A petechial or purpuric rash may occur not only with meningococcal meningitis but also with *Haemophilus spp.* and pneumococcus (*Streptococcus pneumoniae*).

- Meningitis may be bacterial or viral. Bacterial meningitis is more common in neonates and infants. Viral meningitis is usually less severe, with fever, headache, and neck stiffness, but may mimic bacterial meningitis.
  - newborns—Group B beta-haemolytic streptococcus, Gram-negative bacteria (*Escherichia coli*; *Pseudomonas spp.*), *Listeria spp.*
- Infants >3 months and children—*Haemophilus influenzae, Streptococcus pneumoniae, Neisseria meningitidis,* TB, fungi, viruses (usually enteroviruses), coxsackie- and echoviruses.
- Consider meningitis in any infant or child with an altered level of consciousness or coma, particularly with fever and a high white cell count.
- Common signs—fever, lethargy, irritability, decreased appetite, vomiting, headache, photophobia, altered consciousness, convulsions, neck stiffness. Signs of raised ICP—bulging fontanelle, papilloedema, altered pupils. Focal signs (e.g. hemiparesis) suggest tumour or ischaemia.
- Steroids are indicated in *H. influenzae* and *S. pneumoniae* meningitis to reduce hearing loss due to VIIIth nerve damage. There is no indication for routine steroid use in viral meningitis or encephalitis.

Encephalitis
- Rarer than meningitis. Most common presentation is altered level of consciousness/coma, headache, nausea, and vomiting. Herpesvirus infection may present with convulsions, often focal. Fitting may be difficult to control. Varicella infection characteristically involves the cerebellum (ataxia).
- Common pathogens—herpes simplex and zoster, Epstein–Barr virus, cytomegalovirus, measles, mumps, varicella, enteroviruses, adenoviruses.
- If CT scan suggests herpes encephalitis, give aciclovir.

Further reading
Levin, D.L., Morris, F.C. (ed.) (1997). *Essentials of Paediatric Intensive Care*, (2nd edn). Churchill Livingstone, Edinburgh.

Macnab, A.J., Macrae, D.J., Henning, R. (ed.) (2001). *Care of the Critically ill Child*. Churchill Livingstone, Edinburgh.

Surviving Sepsis Campaign: international guidelines for management of severe sepsis and septic shock. (2008). *Critical Care Medicine*, **36**, 296–327.

Useful data

Paediatric ET tube sizes and length

Age	Weight (kg)	ID (mm)	ED (mm)	At lip (cm)	At nose (cm)
Newborn	<0.7	2.0	2.9	5.0	6
Newborn	<1.0	2.5	3.6	5.5	7
Newborn	1.0	3.0	4.3	6	7.5
Newborn	2.0	3.0	4.3	7	9
Newborn	3.0	3.0+	4.3	8.5	10.5
Newborn	3.5	3.5+	4.9	9	11
3 month	6.0	3.5	4.9	10	12
1 year	10	4.0	5.6	11	14
2 year	12	4.5	6.2	12	15
3 year	14	4.5	6.2	13	16
4 year	16	5.0	6.9	14	17
6 year	20	5.5	7.5	15	19
8 year	24	6.0	8.2	16	20
10 year	30	6.5	8.9	17	21
14 year	50	7.5	10.2	19	23

ET tube size: (age/4) + 4
ET tube length (oral): (age/2) + 12
ID, internal diameter; ED, external diameter.

LMA sizes

Weight	Size
<5 kg	1
5–10 kg	1.5
10–20 kg	2
20–30 kg	2.5
30–50 kg	3

Normal values

Age	Weight (kg)	Pulse (bpm)	Mean BP (mmHg)
Term	3.5	95–145	40–60
3 month	6.0	110–175	45–75
6 month	7.5	110–175	50–90
1 year	10	105–170	50–100
3 year	14	80–140	50–100
7 year	22	70–120	60–90
10 year	30	60–110	60–90
12 year	38	60–100	65–95
14 year	50	60–100	65–95

Age <9 years: weight (kg) = (age + 4) × 2
Age >9 years: weight (kg) = approx. 3 × age

Drug formulary

Useful drug doses

Adrenaline	IV: 1 µg/kg (0.01 mL/kg of 1:10000) increments
	IM: 10 µg/kg (0.1 mL/kg of 1:10000 or 0.01 mL/kg of 1:1000)
	ETT: 100 µg/kg (0.1 mL/kg of 1:1000)
	Infusion: 0.05–1 µg/kg/min
Aminophylline (not if on oral theophylline)	Load 5 mg/kg IV over 1 h
Amiodarone	5 mg/kg IV centrally (or peripherally in emergency)
Atracurium	0.5 mg/kg IV then 0.1 mg/kg as required
Atropine	10–20 µg/kg IV (min. 100 µg, max. 600 µg)
Bicarbonate (sodium)	1 mmol/kg IV
Chlorphenamine	1 month–1 year 250 µg/kg (avoid in neonates) IM/Slow IV
	1–5 year 2.5–5 mg IM/Slow IV
	6–12 year 5–10 mg IM/Slow IV
Calcium chloride 10%	0.1–0.2 mL/kg slow IV
Calcium gluconate 10%	0.3–0.5 mL/kg slow IV
Dantrolene	1 mg/kg repeated until improvement (max. 10 mg/kg/24 h)
Dexamethasone	0.1–0.25 mg/kg/dose qds PO/IV
Diazepam	0.3 mg/kg IV/IO; 0.5 mg/kg PR
Fentanyl	1–2 µg/kg
Furosemide	0.5–1 mg/kg
Glucose	Hypoglycaemia: 1 mL/kg 50% glucose or 2.5 mL/kg 20% glucose
	Hyperkalaemia: 0.1 U/kg insulin + 5 mL/kg 20% glucose IV infused over 15 min
Glycopyrronium	5–15 µg/kg IV
Ketamine	Anaesthesia: 1–2 mg/kg IV, 5–10 mg/kg IM
	Sedation/analgesia: 0.5 mg/kg then 4 µg/kg/min IV infusion
Lidocaine	VF: 1 mg/kg IV
	Nerve block: max. 3 mg/kg
Lorazepam	Status epilepticus: 0.1 mg/kg IV
Magnesium	25–50 mg/kg IV slowly
Mannitol	0.25–0.5 g/kg IV

Midazolam	Sedation: 0.1–0.2 mg/kg IV, up to 0.3 mg/kg nasal, 0.5 mg/kg PO (use IV solution in juice or buccal suspension)
Mivacurium	0.1–0.2 mg/kg
Morphine	0.1–0.2 mg/kg IV
Naloxone	Opioid overdose: 100 µg/kg IV/IM/SC/ETT—then 10 µg/kg/h
	Reversal in anaesthesia: 0.5–1 µg/kg IV increments repeated as necessary
Neostigmine	Reversal neuromuscular blockade: 50–100 µg/kg IV
Nitric oxide	1–40 ppm (0.1 L/min of 1000 ppm added to 10 L/min gas = 10 ppm)
Noradrenaline	0.05–0.5 µg/kg/min IV infusion; via a central line
	Can be given peripherally only for very short periods due to profound vasoconstriction
Phenytoin	15 mg/kg IV (therapeutic range = 10–20 mg/L)
Propofol	2–5 mg/kg IV
Remifentanil	Up to 1 µg/kg IV, then 0.05–0.25 µg/kg/min IV infusion
Rocuronium	0.6–1.2 mg/kg IV, then 0.1–0.2 mg/kg IV as required
Salbutamol	2.5 mg nebule 2–6 hourly, 15 µg/kg over 10 min IV then 1–5 µg/kg/min
Suxamethonium	2 mg/kg IV (child), 3 mg/kg (neonate)
Thiopental	2–5 mg/kg IV slowly (up to 7 mg/kg in status epilepticus)
Tramadol	1–2 mg/kg IV
Vecuronium	0.1 mg/kg IV then 20–50 µg/kg IV as required

Infusions

Adrenaline, noradrenaline	300 µg/kg in 50 mL of 5% glucose
	1 mL/h = 0.1 µg/kg/min
	Dose range: 0.05–1 µg/kg/min (0.5–10 mL/h)
	Peripherally in emergency, change to central venous line when available
Dobutamine, dopamine	3 mg/kg in 50 mL of 5% glucose
	1 mL/h = 1 µg/kg/min
	Dose range: 3–20 µg/kg/min (3–20 mL/h)
	Peripherally in emergency, change to central venous line when available
Atracurium	Dose range: 0.5 mg/kg then 300–600 µg/kg/h

Obstetrics

Mark Scrutton and Michael Kinsella

☠️ Maternal collapse

Definition
Acute maternal cardiovascular collapse/respiratory failure after 24 weeks in pregnancy.

Presentation
- Collapse in late pregnancy—usually during labour, postpartum, or intraoperatively.
- Shock, respiratory distress, impaired consciousness, convulsions.

Immediate management
- ABC … 100% O_2
- Position—minimize compression of the inferior vena cava by the uterus. If external cardiac massage (ECM) required, displace uterus to the left by tilting body/pelvis or manually retracting uterus laterally and cephalad; otherwise turn full left lateral unless obstetric management precludes this.
- Intubate as soon as possible to prevent aspiration and ensure effective alveolar ventilation in presence of diaphragmatic splinting. If there is a delay in intubation, consider cricoid pressure.
- Persisting gas exchange impairment in the presence of adequate alveolar ventilation and circulation may indicate pulmonary oedema, pulmonary or amniotic fluid embolus, or pulmonary aspiration.
- Initial rapid intravenous fluid infusion if the diagnosis is unclear. If bleeding is present, do not delay giving blood (O-negative if patient-specific blood not immediately available).
- Vasopressor—consider ephedrine for α- and β-effects, phenylephrine or metaraminol for α-effect—the choice may depend on maternal heart rate. If these do not produce a response use adrenaline 100 µg and then escalating doses. Adrenaline causes placental vasoconstriction but should not be avoided on this account.
- If 5 min of effective CPR has not established adequate circulation, Caesarean section (CS) should be performed.

Subsequent management
- The condition of the fetus, if undelivered, must be assessed as soon as possible. Delivery of a compromised baby must be coordinated with stabilization of the mother.
- Further investigation and treatment, and transfer to operating theatre or ITU, will depend on the cause.

Investigations
ECG, ABGs, U&Es, coagulation tests. If indicated investigate for pulmonary embolus (PE) following local protocol. Echocardiogram.

Risk factors
- Venous return and cardiac output is impaired by haemorrhage, IVC compression, and high regional anaesthesia. These causes augment each other.
- Vasovagal bradycardia and asystole may occur.

Exclusions

- Aortocaval compression—rapid improvement in lateral position.
- Hypovolaemia—obstetric examination to check for internal bleeding (intrauterine or extrauterine); will respond to adequate volume replacement—CVP guidance will help.
- High regional block—check sensory level, arm motor power and breathing; good response to vasopressors but intubation and ventilation may be necessary.
- Eclampsia—cardiovascular system returns to normal or hypertension after convulsion; possible respiratory impairment if pulmonary aspiration has occurred.
- Local anaesthetic toxicity—prodromal symptoms, convulsions; bupivacaine may produce torsade de pointes VT, prolonged cardiac depression. Treat with Intralipid® (see pp236–8).
- Pulmonary embolus—may have history suggestive of DVT or other risk factors; ECG changes ($S_I Q_{III} T_{III}$). Radiological investigations as per local protocol (e.g. V/Q or spiral CT scan).
- Cardiac disease—variable presentation, echocardiogram as soon as possible to identify myocardial dysfunction, valve lesions, establish cardiogenic or non-cardiogenic cause for pulmonary oedema.
- Anaphylaxis—temporal relationship to drug administration; bronchospasm may be prominent; final diagnosis by serum tryptase assay.
- Amniotic fluid embolus; variable presentation but most commonly includes respiratory failure; also cardiovascular collapse, coagulopathy, and convulsions. Diagnosis is by exclusion and lack of response to treatment.

Special considerations

- Cardiac arrest in pregnant women is rare and the anaesthetist is likely to be the team leader during CPR.
- The maximum amount of thoracic tilt consistent with effective ECM is 27°. Whole body tilt to this extent is ideal, otherwise an object under the right hip and/or manual leftwards and cephalad displacement of the uterus should be used.
- Cricoid pressure and early intubation are necessary because of increased risk of aspiration. Normal $PaCO_2$ in term pregnancy is 4.0 kPa. Variable-performance oxygen masks achieve lower FiO_2 in pregnant than non-pregnant women.
- Blood volume is increased by 20% in term pregnancy, therefore blood loss is initially better tolerated than in non-pregnant subjects.
- The use of alpha-adrenergic agonists during resuscitation unresponsive to adrenaline is currently under debate. In the event of cardiovascular collapse after extensive regional anaesthesia, standard resuscitation doses of vasopressors may not be effective.
- CPR provides little blood flow to the fetus, and Caesarean section (CS) within 5 min is recommended to allow fetal survival and enhance maternal resuscitation by relieving IVC compression. The larger the pregnant uterus, the greater the degree of IVC compression. CS should definitely be undertaken at >28 weeks' gestation and possibly between 24 and 28 weeks.

- The postpartum application of abdominal aortic compression should be considered, diverting flow to the brain and heart. It may also help to control uterine haemorrhage.

Treatment of severe local anaesthetic toxicity (see also pp236–8)

- Call for help.
- ABC ... 100% oxygen—early oxygenation essential.
- Control seizures with benzodiazepine, thiopental, or propofol.
- If cardiovascular collapse:
- CPR.
- Give bolus Intralipid® 20% 1.5 mL/kg over 1 min.
- Start IV infusion of Intralipid® 0.25 mL/kg/min.
- If circulation is not restored repeat bolus twice at 5 min intervals then increase infusion rate to 0.5 mL/kg/min.
- Continue infusion until circulation restored and stable.

Further reading

Guidelines for the management of severe local anaesthetic toxicity. www.aagbi.org/publications/guidelines/docs/latoxicity07.pdf

Morris, S., Stacey, M. (2003). Resuscitation in pregnancy. *British Medical Journal*, **327**, 1277–9.

⚙ Intrauterine fetal resuscitation

Definition
Measures to maximize fetal oxygenation in response to acute fetal compromise, usually during labour.

Presentation
- Severity of acute fetal compromise should be communicated to the anaesthetist by the obstetrician.
- Severe compromise needing immediate delivery is associated with sustained fetal bradycardia
- Less severe compromise is associated with:
  - late or complicated variable decelerations
  - sinusoidal heart rate pattern
  - tachycardia with absent variability
  - pH <7.2

Immediate management
- The aim of intrauterine fetal resuscitation is to restore uteroplacental oxygen delivery, produce maternal hyperoxia, and to restore fetoplacental (umbilical) blood flow.
- Turn off oxytocin.
- Full left lateral position; continue for transfer and, on operating table, if fetal heart rate remains low, try right lateral/knee–elbow position for possible cord compression.
- Oxygen maximum flow via tight-fitting Hudson mask with reservoir bag.
- Intravenous Hartmann's 1000 mL stat (unless fluid intake is restricted, e.g. pre-eclampsia).
- Low blood pressure—IV ephedrine (6 mg).
- Tocolysis—terbutaline 0.25 mg subcutaneous. Alternatively, for immediate action: GTN sublingual spray 2 puffs initially, repeat after 1 min until contractions stop (maximum 3 doses).
- NB electronic fetal monitoring should be re-started in theatre and maintained as long as possible.

Subsequent management
- Delivery of the fetus may be necessary if resuscitation is ineffective. The obstetrician will determine whether this is possible vaginally or by CS. Urgency of CS is categorized as either:
  1. immediate threat to life of woman or fetus;
  2. maternal or fetal compromise which is not immediately life-threatening.
- Decision-making on the mode of anaesthesia for category 1 CS will vary case by case and unit by unit (see also 'Category 1 Caesarean section', p164.)

Investigations
- Obstetric examination to assess cervical dilation, cord prolapse.

Risk factors

- Factors associated with irreversible disruption of fetal oxygenation making urgent fetal delivery more likely include:
  - suspected placental abruption/separation
  - fetal haemorrhage, e.g. from vasa praevia
  - uterine scar dehiscence
  - umbilical cord prolapse with abnormal fetal heart rate

Exclusions

- Fetal bradycardia may be an early warning of significant maternal hypotension related to regional analgesia and other rare causes of maternal collapse.

Special considerations

- Care with IV fluid in women with pre-eclampsia.
- Terbutaline may be contraindicated in some women with cardiac disease.
- Maternal cardiovascular compromise that reduces uteroplacental oxygen delivery will affect the fetus. The management is the same as intrauterine fetal resuscitation except for tocolysis.
- Umbilical cord prolapse:
  - maintain manual upward displacement of presenting part
  - reposition into knee–elbow or left semi-prone position
  - gently replace cord into the vagina
  - give oxygen by mask at maximum flow rate
  - give terbutaline 0.25 mg subcutaneously (0.5 mL)
  - if delivery not immediately possible: insert size 14 Foley catheter into the bladder and blow up the balloon; instil 500 mL warmed sterile solution through the catheter and then clamp it (manual displacement may now be discontinued)
  - check fetal heart rate. Prepare for:
    - abnormal—Category 1 CS
    - normal—Category 2 CS

Further reading

Thurlow, J., Kinsella, S.M. (2002). Intra-uterine resuscitation; active management of fetal distress. *International Journal of Obstetric Anaesthesia*, **11**, 105–16.

⊙ Severe haemorrhage

Definition
- *Primary*—acute peripartum blood loss from uterus or genital tract of over 1000 mL.
- *Secondary*—blood loss from uterus or genital tract of over 1000 mL occurring between 24 h and 12 weeks' postpartum.

Presentation
- Hypovolaemic shock—systolic BP <90 mmHg, pulse rate >120 bpm, decreased level of consciousness, decreased peripheral perfusion.
- Blood loss frequently underestimated.
- Total blood volume increases by 20% in pregnancy, so symptoms and signs are often masked, but decompensation may be rapid.

Immediate management
- Call for help.
- ABC ... 100% O_2.
- Establish two 14G IV cannulae.
- 2000 mL IV crystalloid/colloid.
- Group-specific red cells (consider O-negative).
- 'Rub up' a contraction and consider continuous bimanual compression.
- If likely cause is uterine atony or retained products, consider oxytocin 5–10 IU *slow* IV (NB causes vasodilatation that may exacerbate hypovolaemia), ergometrine 500 µg IM, misoprostol 400–1000 µg PR/SL, carboprost 250 µg IM.
- Order coagulation factors—fresh frozen plasma (FFP), cryoprecipitate, and platelets—early, particularly in severe abruption where coagulopathy is out of proportion to blood volume lost.
- Transfer to theatre for EUA while resuscitation is in progress—do not delay, use vasopressors as required (ephedrine 6 mg, phenylephrine 25–50 µg, or adrenaline 5–10 µg).
- General anaesthesia is indicated in haemorrhage—RSI is mandatory. Regional anaesthesia is relatively contraindicated, but occasionally considered in some situations, e.g. epidural *in situ* in a stable patient.

Subsequent management
- Arterial line, central line, and urinary catheter after definitive treatment started.
- Continue to monitor full blood count and clotting.
- Warm fluid (rapid transfusion system mandatory for Delivery Ward operating theatre).
- Warm patient.
- During laparotomy, consider aortic compression if haemorrhage excessive.
- Target Hb may be >7 g/dL in this group due to the fact that re-bleeding within the first 24 h postpartum is not uncommon.
- Once stabilized the patient should be transferred to an obstetric HDU or ITU for further monitoring.

Risk factors
- Antepartum haemorrhage (abruption/placenta praevia)
- Prolonged labour
- Multiparity
- Previous CS, uterine surgery, uterine anomaly (e.g. fibroids)
- Multiple pregnancy, large baby, polyhydramnios
- Previous postpartum haemorrhage
- Coagulation disorder

Exclusions *(see Table 5.1)*
Hypotension associated with vagal stimulation, e.g. uterine inversion or products of conception sitting in the cervical os.

Table 5.1 Oxytocic drugs

Drug	Dose	Side-effects
Oxytocin	5 IU slow IV injection 10 IU/h IV infusion	Vasodilatation → hypotension. Tachycardia. Possibly increased pulmonary vascular resistance
Ergometrine	500 µg IM injection	Vasoconstriction → hypertension. Bradycardia. Nausea and vomiting. Contraindicated in pre-eclampsia
Misoprostol	400–1000 µg PR/SL	Flushing, hyperthermia, diarrhoea
Carboprost	250 µg IM/intrauterine (one dose every 15 min, max. 8 doses)	Hypertension. Bronchospasm (severe if accidental IV injection)

Syntometrine® contains 5 IU oxytocin and 500 µg ergometrine in 1 mL solution. All oxytocic drugs are potentially dangerous in maternal cardiac disease and should only be used with caution.

Special considerations
- Haemorrhage may be concealed or difficult to quantify in obstetrics.
- Following severe abruption or amniotic fluid embolus, fulminant DIC may occur. This will require large quantities of clotting factors. Seek urgent advice from consultant haematologist.
- Consider tranexamic acid 0.5–1 g.
- Recombinant activated factor VII has been used with success in a number of cases of massive obstetric haemorrhage.

Red cell transfusion
- If blood loss exceeds 40%, red cell transfusion is likely to be required.
- Target red cell transfusion Hb >7 g/dL.
- Consider using Group O-negative blood early if haemorrhage is life-threatening.
- Uncrossmatched, group-compatible blood should be used until full crossmatch is confirmed by the blood bank.

Coagulation and blood products
- Severe coagulopathies may occur following small losses. Anticipate changes and measure coagulation regularly.

- Transfuse FFP and platelets as clinically indicated until coagulation screen available.
- Prolonged PT and PTT will correct with FFP transfusion.
- Falling fibrinogen levels (normally raised in pregnancy) will require cryoprecipitate transfusion.

Autotransfusion (cell salvage)
- Cell salvage techniques are used increasingly in obstetrics.
- Contamination with amniotic fluid does not appear to contraindicate cell salvage techniques.
- Likely to become a 'standard of care'.

Interventional radiology
- In situations where significant haemorrhage predicted (e.g. placenta accreta) consider prophylactic intra-arterial access that allows occlusion of the uterine arteries if required.
- Although unlikely to be helpful in acute massive haemorrhage, emergency interventional radiology may help in situations of persistent moderate haemorrhage.

Further reading

Boehlen, F., Morales, M.A., Fontana, P., Ricou, B., Irion, O., de Moerloose, P. (2004). Prolonged treatment of massive postpartum haemorrhage with recombinant factor VIIa: case report and review of the literature. *British Journal of Obstetrics and Gynaecology*, **111**, 284–7.

Esler, M.D., Douglas, M.J. (2003). Planning for hemorrhage. Steps an anesthesiologist can take to limit and treat hemorrhage in the obstetric patient. *Anesthesiology Clinics of North America*, **21**, 127–44.

Mousa, H.A., Alfirevic, Z. (2003). Treatment for primary postpartum haemorrhage. *Cochrane Database of Systematic Reviews*, **1**, CD003249. www.cochrane.org/reviews/en/ab003249.html

Su, L.L., Chong, Y.S., Samuel, M. (2007). Oxytocin agonists for preventing postpartum haemorrhage. *Cochrane Database of Systematic Reviews*, **3**, CD005457. www.cochrane.org/reviews/en/ab005457.html

:☠: Amniotic fluid embolus

Definition
- Severe reaction to entry of amniotic fluid into maternal circulation.

Presentation
- Diagnosis is by exclusion. Presents as respiratory failure with dyspnoea, hypoxaemia, hypotension, and circulatory collapse.
- Early phase of transient pulmonary hypertension and right heart failure is followed by left ventricular dysfunction.
- DIC is likely. Convulsions secondary to cerebral hypoxia.

Immediate management
- Mortality is high and prolonged CPR may be needed.
- Both increased pulmonary vascular resistance and left ventricular failure can occur.
- Coagulopathy may be prominent; order FFP and platelets along with blood.

Subsequent management
- A haematologist should be involved at an early stage.
- Appropriate radiological investigation (e.g. V/Q or spiral CT) to exclude pulmonary embolus.
- Echocardiogram to exclude specific cardiac lesions.
- 50% mortality, only 15% overall will survive without neurological impairment.

Investigations
- FBC, U&Es, coagulation, consider PAFC.

Risk factors
- Main period of risk is from the onset of labour until after delivery.
- Increased maternal age and parity.

Exclusions
- Hypovolaemia—obstetric examination to check for internal bleeding (intrauterine or extrauterine), will respond to adequate volume replacement, whereas with amniotic fluid embolus (AFE) there will be continuing circulatory depression after normal circulating volume is restored.
- Pulmonary embolus—history of risk factors; no coagulopathy.
- Eclampsia—recovery once convulsion is finished, possibly followed by hypertension. No pulmonary gas exchange problem in the absence of pulmonary aspiration.
- Local anaesthetic toxicity—temporal relationship to LA administration, prodromal symptoms, convulsions, prolonged cardiac depression, but no gas exchange impairment.
- Cardiac disease—variable presentation, echocardiogram ASAP.
- Anaphylaxis—temporal relationship to drug administration; bronchospasm, gas exchange impairment not marked; final diagnosis by serum tryptase assay.

Further reading
www.npeu.ox.ac.uk/ukoss/current-surveillance/amf

☉ Severe pre-eclampsia

Definition

Hypertension ≥160/110 mmHg and proteinuria ≥ +++ (≥300 mg/24 h).
May also include:
- Headache, visual disturbance, epigastric pain
- Hyperreflexia
- Platelet count <100 × 10⁹/L
- Abnormal LFTs

Presentation

Increased blood pressure after 24 weeks' gestation and/or proteinuria,
oedema, headache visual disturbances, and epigastric pain.

Immediate management: hypertension

First-line agent: labetalol

Oral therapy:
- Ensure no contraindications: exclude asthma.
- Oral therapy 200 mg stat dose.
- Repeat oral 200 mg dose if not controlled at 30 min.
- If BP not controlled 30 min after second dose or oral therapy is not
  tolerated, commence IV therapy.

Intravenous therapy
- Bolus of 50 mg.
- BP should be controlled within 5 min.
- Repeat at 5 min intervals to a maximum dose of 200 mg or until BP
  controlled.
- Commence labetalol infusion at 20 mg/h.
- Double infusion rate every 30 min to maximum 160 mg/h.

Second-line agent: nifedipine
- Indicated if labetalol fails or is contraindicated.
- 10 mg oral (not sublingual).
- Repeat after 30 min if BP not controlled.

Third-line agent: hydralazine
- 5 mg IV bolus.
- Repeat at 15 min.
- Infusion 5–15 mg/h.

Immediate management: prevention of eclampsia

Magnesium (see also pp308–9)
- Loading dose 4 g over 15 min.
- Infusion 1 g/h for 24 h minimum.
- Further 2 g bolus if eclamptic seizure occurs.
- NB In the event of magnesium overdose causing cardiorespiratory
  compromise, give 1 g calcium gluconate IV (10 mL of 10% solution).

Subsequent management
Team approach involving senior obstetrician, obstetric anaesthetist, and midwife.

Aims of treatment
- Stabilize *before* delivery—may take several hours.
- Control hypertension.
- Prevent eclampsia.
- Timely delivery of baby.

Fluid balance
- Fluid restrict—1 mL/kg/h background. Replace losses.
- Hourly fluid balance measurement. Tolerate oliguria.
- 'Fluid challenges' of more than 250 mL should only be given with CVP guidance.
- Central venous catheter placement should only be undertaken by experienced anaesthetist as the patient is awake, oedematous, and may have a coagulopathy. Consider ultrasound guidance or using peripherally introduced central catheter (PICC).

Anaesthetic management
Analgesia in labour
- Epidural analgesia indicated to prevent surges in blood pressure associated with pain of contractions.
- Epidural analgesia should not be used to treat hypertension.
- Uncorrected platelet count <50 × 10^9/L is a relative contraindication to regional anaesthesia; between 50 and 100 × 10^9/L, consult local protocol/consultant advice.
- Platelet function as well as platelet count may be depressed in pre-eclampsia.

Regional anaesthesia for Caesarean section
- Preferred to general anaesthesia.
- No clear advantage between single-shot spinal, combined spinal–epidural or epidural—choice should be made according to clinical situation.
- Traditionally, sudden hypotension was thought to be a major risk; this is now known to be considerably less common than previously thought.

General anaesthesia
- Call for senior help early.
- Patient frequently not fasted.
- Anaesthetic likely to interact with antihypertensive agents and magnesium.
- Airway oedema complicates intubation.
- Obtund pressor response to intubation and extubation (see Table 5.2)
- HDU monitoring postoperatively—airway oedema may worsen following extubation

Table 5.2 Methods of obtunding pressor response to intubation and/or extubation

Alfentanil	7.5–10 µg/kg
Magnesium sulphate	30 mg/kg
Esmolol	0.5 mg/kg
Labetalol	0.5 mg/kg
Lidocaine	1 mg/kg

Indications for ITU
Respiratory failure, renal failure, liver failure.

Investigations
- FBC, coagulation, U&Es, LFTs, urate
- Repeat 6-hourly

Risk factors
- Nulliparity
- New partner
- Afro-Caribbean race
- Underlying maternal condition (e.g. hypertension, renal disease, diabetes, obesity, antiphospholipid syndrome, cardiac disease)

Exclusions
- Pre-existing hypertension
- Renal or hepatic disease
- Acute fatty liver of pregnancy

Further reading
Ramanathan, J., Bennett, K. (2003). Pre-eclampsia: fluids, drugs, and anesthetic management. *Anesthesiology Clinics of North America*, **21**, 145–63.

Santos, A.C., Birnbach, D.J. (2003). Spinal anesthesia in the parturient with severe pre-eclampsia: time for reconsideration. *Anesthesia and Analgesia*, **97**, 621–2.

The Magpie Trial Collaboration Group (2002). Do women with pre-eclampsia, and their babies, benefit from magnesium sulphate? The Magpie Trial: a randomised placebo-controlled trial. *Lancet*, **359**, 1877–90.

www.rcog.org.uk/resources/Public/pdf/management_pre_eclampsia_mar06.pdf

☼ Eclampsia

Definition
Tonic–clonic seizure associated with pre-eclampsia.

Presentation
- Approximately 33% of seizures occur before labour, 33% during labour, and 33% in the puerperium.
- Seizures may occur over a week after delivery.

Immediate management
- Call for help.
- ABC.
- Left lateral recovery position.
- High flow oxygen—do not attempt to insert airway or hand ventilate.
- If undelivered, assess fetal condition once emergency situation over.
- Magnesium sulphate 4 g IV over 15 min followed by 1 g/h infusion.
- For recurrent seizures give further bolus of 2 g magnesium—consider measuring plasma levels.
- *Do not give diazepam for the first fit.*

NB Average length of first fit in eclampsia is 90 s. If seizure persists, consider diazepam, thiopental, or propofol once anaesthetist present. Consider other causes of fits, including intracranial haemorrhage.

Subsequent management
- Delivery should be undertaken when the mother's condition has stabilized.
- Control severe hypertension (>160/110 mmHg) with intravenous labetalol or hydralazine according to local protocol (see p156).
- Consideration should be given to the possibility that the fit was precipitated by an intracranial bleed—full neurological examination mandatory. Consider CT/MRI imaging.
- Mode of delivery is contentious.
- Consultant obstetrician and anaesthetist should be informed in all cases.
- If fetal distress severe and failing to respond to intrauterine resuscitation (see pp150–1), urgent delivery may be considered but may compromise maternal safety.

Investigations
FBC, coagulation, U&Es, LFTs, urate

Risk factors
- Pre-eclampsia
- Afro-Caribbean race

Exclusions
Epilepsy or other intracerebral events not associated with pre-eclampsia.

Further reading
Eclampsia Trial Collaborative Group (1995). Which anticonvulsant for women with eclampsia? Evidence from the Collaborative Eclampsia Trial. *Lancet*, **345**, 1455–63.

☼ Total spinal

Definition
Cardiorespiratory collapse caused by direct action of local anaesthetic on high cervical nerve roots and/or brainstem.

Presentation
- May vary from rapid maternal loss of consciousness and collapse to gradual rise of block, causing difficulty in breathing and/or respiratory failure before loss of consciousness.
- Tingling of hands and difficulty speaking are important warning signs of an ascending block (see pp246–7).
- Bradycardia and hypotension.
- Fetal bradycardia.

Immediate management
- ABC ... 100% O_2. Intubation will be required.
- Support blood pressure and circulation with incremental doses of ephedrine 6 mg, phenylephrine 25–50 µg, or adrenaline 5–10 µg.
- Deliver baby if appropriate (difficulty stabilizing mother or non-recovering fetal compromise).
- If ALS unsuccessful, baby should be delivered at 5 min.
- Once resuscitated, anaesthetic agents will be required to keep mother asleep while block resolves.

Subsequent management
- Block will often recede in under 1 h, but may persist for several hours.
- Persisting high block — transfer to ITU until extubated.

Investigations
Examine to exclude other causes of collapse. Assess fetus if undelivered.

Risk factors
- Accidental dural puncture (recognized and unrecognized).
- Accidental subdural placement of epidural catheter.
- Large or rapid epidural top-ups (e.g. for category 1 CS).
- Spinal injection with epidural *in situ*
- Epidural top-up after recent spinal injection.

Exclusions
Other causes of maternal collapse (e.g. pulmonary embolism, amniotic fluid embolus, cardiological, neurological).

Further reading
Yentis, S.M., Dob D.P. (2001). High regional block—the failed intubation of the new millennium? *International Journal of Obstetric Anaesthesia*, **10**, 159–61.

⊙ Accidental dural puncture

Definition
Accidental passage of an epidural needle through dura mater and arachnoid mater into the CSF.

Presentation
- Immediate—CSF through Tuohy needle or epidural catheter.
- Early—high block or total spinal (see pp160, 246–7).
- Late—postdural puncture headache.
- Rarely—epileptiform fit, subdural haematoma.
- Incidence 0.5–4%.

Immediate management

- Consider threading the epidural catheter into the CSF (see below) or re-site epidural a space above.
- Regardless of eventual positioning of epidural catheter, all further top-ups or infusions must be given by the anaesthetist.
- Accidental dural puncture no longer mandates instrumental delivery—second stage should be managed normally.
- Patient should be followed up closely after delivery.
- If CS becomes necessary, top-ups down the epidural catheter (regardless of eventual position) or de novo single-shot spinal both carry increased risk of high block or total spinal.

Postdural puncture headache (PDPH)
Features
- Incidence— >80% (16G Tuohy needle), 1% (25G pencil-point spinal needle).
- May occur up to 72 h following dural tap.
- Rarely occurs before 12 h.
- Postural—relieved by lying down.
- Worse with mobilization.
- Fronto-occipital headache.
- Neck stiffness common.
- Photophobia.
- Occasionally incapacitating.
- Transiently relieved by abdominal compression (diagnostic test).

Treatment
Early
- Bolus (20 mL) or infusion (1000 mL/8 h) of 0.9% saline down epidural catheter has been reported as being effective in some cases.
- 'Prophylactic' blood patch injected down epidural catheter before the headache occurs has been reported as effective, but headache more likely to re-occur when compared to 'delayed' blood patch. (NB Do not do this if catheter has been placed into CSF.)

Intermediate
- Keep patient well hydrated.
- Regular simple analgesics—paracetamol, NSAIDs, codeine.

- Caffeine may provide temporary relief. 50 mg tablets orally up to 1-hourly prn (max. 300 mg in 24 h).
- A number of other therapeutic agents, including ACTH and sumatriptan, have been tried, but results have been disappointing.

Epidural blood patch

- Considered the definitive treatment.
- Initially reported as over 90% effective, results now suggest that long-term success rate may be as low as 50%.
- Success improved by delaying until at least 24 h postdural tap, siting the patch at the same level as the tap or one level below, and injecting greater than 15 mL of autologous blood.

Investigations

Assess temperature and glucose content of fluid leaking through Tuohy needle or catheter. If warm and containing glucose, it is likely to be CSF.

Risk factors

- Moving target
- Increased BMI
- Inexperienced operator
- Rotating the Tuohy needle once in the epidural space
- ? Loss of resistance to air
- ? Sitting position

Exclusions

Other causes of headache—simple, meningitis, hypertension, subarachnoid haemorrhage.

Further reading

Reynolds, F. (1993). Dural puncture and headache. *British Medical Journal*, **306**, 874–6.

Sprigge, J.S., Harper, S.J. (2008). Accidental dural puncture and post dural puncture headache in obstetric anaesthesia: presentation and management: a 23-year survey in a district general hospital. *Anaesthesia*, **63**, 36–43.

Stride, P.C., Cooper, G.M. (1993). Dural taps revisited. A 20-year survey from Birmingham Maternity Hospital. *Anaesthesia*, **48**, 247–55.

Sudlow, C., Warlow, C. (2003). Epidural blood patching for preventing and treating post-dural puncture headache (Cochrane Review). *The Cochrane Library*, Issue 2. www.cochrane.org/reviews/en/ab001791.html

Turnbull, D.K., Shepherd, D.B. (2003). Post-dural puncture headache: pathogenesis, prevention and treatment. *British Journal of Anaesthesia*, **91**, 718–29.

☢ Category 1 Caesarean section

Urgency scale[1]

1. Immediate threat to life of woman or fetus.
2. Maternal or fetal compromise which is not immediately life-threatening.
3. Needing early delivery but no maternal or fetal compromise.
4. At a time to suit the patient and maternity team.

Presentation
- Usually for acute fetal compromise (see also 'Intrauterine Fetal Resuscitation', pp150–1).
- Commonest maternal indication is antepartum haemorrhage.

Preoperative preparation
- Rapid preoperative assessment—allergies, medication, past anaesthetics, general health, recent food or drink.
- Intravenous access if not already established. Start fast crystalloid infusion prehydration, or colloid/blood for hypovolaemia.
- Premedication—sodium citrate 0.3 M 30 mL PO. Intravenous metoclopramide 10 mg and ranitidine 50 mg may be given if there is time.
- Supine with left uterine displacement using a wedge or lateral table tilt. If there will be no delay in starting anaesthesia and surgery, this position may be used on arrival in the operating theatre. However, full left lateral position is associated with least aortocaval compression and should be used if there will be a delay.
- Preoxygenation should be started immediately on positioning on the operating table. Use high oxygen flow and tight mask fit.

Choice of anaesthesia
- General anaesthesia is the quickest to establish but is associated with more life-threatening maternal complications and early neonatal depression. The factors that must be identified rapidly to inform the choice of anaesthetic are: the urgency (communicate with surgeon), maternal preference (communicate with mother), and specific contraindications or difficulties (brief history as above plus preoperative examination of airway, body mass index, spine, and coagulation status). If regional anaesthetic is attempted, a time limit must be imposed and conversion to GA performed once this is exceeded.
- Management of the woman with an epidural *in situ* varies. Epidural anaesthesia is less reliable than spinal. Some units routinely top up the epidural once the decision for Caesarean section is made, whereas others attempt to insert a spinal wherever possible. A selective approach is outlined in Fig. 5.1. Spinal doses may have to be adjusted in the presence of an epidural (see 'Spinal after epidural', p166).

---

1 Lucas, D.N., Yentis, S.M., Kinsella, S.M., Holdcroft, A., May, A.E., Wee, M., Robinson, P.N. (2000). Urgency of caesarean section: a new classification. *Journal of the Royal Society of Medicine*, **93**, 346–50.

- The rate of GA conversion of regional anaesthesia in category 1 CS is significantly higher than in less urgent cases—be prepared!

General anaesthesia

(See also 'Rapid sequence induction', pp86–8; 'Failed intubation—obstetrics', p170.)

- Formal preoxygenation before GA involves breathing 100% oxygen from a well-fitting anaesthetic mask for 3 min. Preoxygenation with 4 vital capacity breaths is less effective at denitrogenation than 3 min tidal ventilation.
- Maintain 100% inspired oxygen until delivery if there is fetal compromise, increase inspired inhalation agent concentration to compensate for lack of N_2O.

Spinal

- In urgent cases, a 'rapid sequence spinal' may be appropriate (see below). After spinal insertion, the patient should be placed immediately supine with left lateral displacement.
- The addition of lipophilic opioid (25 µg fentanyl or 0.3 mg diamorphine) reduces discomfort or pain for a given level of sensory block, but the spinal should not be delayed if the drug cannot be rapidly obtained.

Rapid sequence spinal

- Deploy other staff for intravenous cannulation and monitoring— don't inject spinal until cannula secured
- Preoxygenate during attempt
- 'No touch' technique—gloves only; chlorhexidine on sterile swabs; use glove packet as sterile surface
- Local infiltration not mandatory
- **Add fentanyl 25 µg if time; if not consider increased dose of bupivacaine**
- Only one attempt at spinal unless obvious correction allows a second
- If necessary start surgery when block ≥ T10 and ascending—be prepared to convert to GA. Keep mother informed

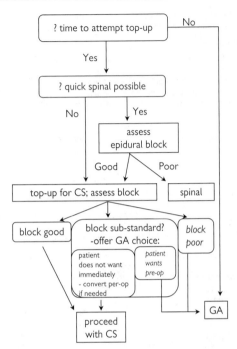

Fig. 5.1 Category 1 Caesarean section.

Spinal after epidural

- Sensory block level is higher for a particular spinal dose if administered after an epidural. This effect is greater with recent (<30 min) large-volume top-ups (volume effect) using concentrated local anaesthetic (addition-of-block effect). Dangerously high spinal blocks requiring respiratory support are more common after epidural (1:50) versus spinal alone (<1:4000). It is thought that this risk is greater if the epidural has been topped up recently. Many anaesthetists reduce the spinal dose by 20–40% if administering after a recent epidural 'Caesarean section' top up.

Epidural top-up

- Lidocaine is theoretically the quickest onset local anaesthetic available in the UK, though some favour bupivacaine/levobupivacaine.
- Possible adjuncts:
  - adrenaline 1 in 200 000 (100 µg per 20 mL of LA solution)
  - sodium bicarbonate 8.4% (2 mL per 20 mL of lidocaine, 0.2 mL per 20 mL of bupivacaine)
  - fentanyl 100 µg

- Some mixtures have been shown to speed onset time, but the preparation time must be offset against this.
- The safest practice is to give a slow fractionated top-up in the operating theatre with full monitoring. This may be too slow for category 1 Caesarean section. Consider starting the epidural top-up in the labour room and give the full top-up under close observation (see box).[1] If dural puncture has occurred or was suspected, do not top-up in the labour room.
- Have available:
  - free-running drip
  - vasopressors
  - oxygen supply and method to ventilate lungs
- Standard total volume for top-up is 20 mL. Consider reduction to 15 mL if the block is high or dense or the woman is of short stature.
- Top-up in left lateral position (right lateral if fetal heart rate problems on left).

Safety assessment (15 s)
- Is the epidural in (i.e. not leaking)?
- Is it spinal?—Has there been excessive motor block, recurrent hypotension?
- Is it intravenous?—poor block, need for frequent top-ups, symptoms of local anaesthetic toxicity.
- PERFORM ASPIRATION TEST.

Test dose (90 s)
- Give 3 mL; wait 30 s; assess change in block (e.g. any 'global' subjective change, cold sensation at S1, ankle dorsiflexion) indicating spinal placement.
- Give 3 mL; wait 60 s, assess symptoms (strange taste, tinnitus, sedation) indicating intravenous placement.

Main dose (90 s)
- Give remainder while observing for any changes as above.
- Stay with woman and maintain communication. Monitor pulse and BP. Be prepared to deal with high block.

Further reading
Yentis, S.M., Dob, D.P. (2001). High regional block—the failed intubation of the new millennium? *International Journal of Obstetric Anaesthesia*, **10**, 159–61.

1 Moore, P., Russell, I.F. (2004). Controversy: Epidural top-ups for category I/II emergency caesarean section should be given only in the operating theatre. *International Journal of Obstetric Anaesthesia*, **13**, 257–65.

① Problems during Caesarean section

Cardiovascular collapse before delivery
- Commonest with regional anaesthesia; consider IVC compression ± vasovagal syncope. Once a severe reaction is established, especially in the presence of a regional block, it may not resolve until delivery of the baby. If there is likely to be a delay use the full lateral position.
- Other causes include hypovolaemia, amniotic fluid embolus (see pp146–8), allergy to general anaesthetic drugs, high or misplaced regional anaesthetic, undiagnosed cardiac disease, pulmonary embolism.

Cardiovascular collapse after delivery
Undetected haemorrhage, amniotic fluid embolus (see p155), reaction to oxytocin, anaphylaxis to antibiotic.

Acute uterine relaxation (tocolysis)
- This may rarely be requested by the obstetrician where delivery is difficult.
- GTN IV is the drug of choice (50 µg boluses—double dose if effect is poor). Dilute 1 mg/mL solution 1 in 20 = 50 µg/mL. Other tocolytic agents either have too slow an onset or too protracted a duration. The use of general anaesthesia with inhalational agents to produce tocolysis is obsolete, although this effect may be utilized if GA is being used for other indications.

Haemorrhage—see pp152–4
Inhalational agents interfere with uterine contraction. If haemorrhage occurs during CS under general anaesthetic, consider switching to intravenous anaesthesia with propofol.

Nausea and vomiting
During Caesarean section with regional anaesthesia this is often related to a decrease in cardiac output and hypotension. Before delivery this usually responds to a vasopressor and optimizing position, whereas after delivery blood loss must be excluded.

Failed intubation—see pp68–73; 170–2

Endobronchial intubation—see pp92–3

Pre-eclampsia—see pp156–8

✪ **Failed intubation—obstetrics**

(See also 'Unanticipated difficult intubation', pp68–73)

Definition
Failure to intubate trachea during rapid sequence induction.

Presentation
- Induction of Caesarean section or any incidental operation in pregnancy requiring rapid sequence intubation.
- Incidence in obstetric practice, 1:250.

Immediate management
- Failed intubation drill—see Fig. 5.2 and pp68–73. (NB There are numerous variations in the literature, see 'Further reading', p172.)
- Avoid repeated attempts at intubation.
- DO NOT give a second dose of suxamethonium.
- Oxygenation of mother is priority.
- Mask and airway or LMA (release cricoid pressure during insertion).
- If failed intubation occurs, it is usually appropriate to wake the mother despite any perceived risk to the fetus, as the mother's life is the priority. Consider before starting the anaesthetic whether or not you would wake the mother if failed intubation were to occur.

Subsequent management
- Get senior anaesthetic help.
- Abandon the Caesarean section—the mother's life is the priority. Unless the un-intubated airway is difficult to maintain, turn on to left lateral side and allow to wake up.
- Consider a regional technique or an awake fibreoptic intubation.
- On rare occasions, when the airway is easy to maintain during a Category 1 Caesarean section, it may be appropriate to continue the GA using a facemask or LMA. Continue anaesthesia using drugs in the same way as with any spontaneously breathing patient—aspiration is unlikely, but maintain cricoid pressure if possible.
- If a well-positioned LMA is in place and intubation is necessary, consider fibreoptic intubation through it—a standard size 6.0 mm armoured ETT can be railroaded over an intubating fibreoptic bronchoscope through a size 3, 4, or 5 LMA, using 0.9% saline for lubrication. Leave the LMA in place.
- Alternative airway devices (e.g. iLMA, proseal LMA) may be considered if operator familiar, however this should not delay moving to surgical airway if required.

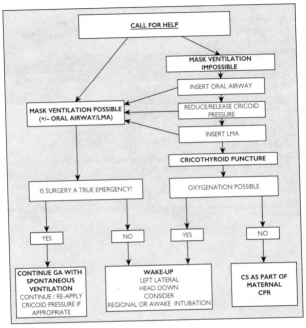

Fig. 5.2 Failed intubation drill—obstetrics.

Risk factors

- Anatomical:
  - full dentition
  - increased BMI
  - large breasts
  - tissue oedema (particularly in pre-eclampsia)
  - misplaced cricoid pressure
- Physiological:
  - reduced functional residual capacity and increased oxygen consumption results in rapid desaturation despite preoxygenation
  - increased intra-abdominal/intragastric pressure and reduced lower oesophageal sphincter tone result in reduced 'barrier pressure' increasing likelihood of aspiration
- Psychological:
  - urgency
  - highly stressful situation and environment

Special considerations

- Training and familiarity with appropriate equipment is important. Early identification of problems and thorough preoperative airway assessment may help.
- Rapid sequence induction: attention to detail—particularly preoxygenation.
- Failed intubation is a rare cause of maternal death but cases continue to occur.
- Regular failed intubation drills are essential.
- Exposure to anaesthetic simulators may be beneficial, though not universally available.

Further reading

Cooper, G. (2002). The drive for regional anaesthesia for elective caesarean section has gone too far. *International Journal of Obstetric Anaesthesia*, **11**, 289–95.

Hawthorne, L., Wilson, R., Lyons, G., Dresner, M. (1996). Failed intubation revisited: 17 year experience in a teaching maternity unit. *British Journal of Anaesthesia*, **76**, 680–4.

Morris, S. (2001). Management of difficult and failed intubation in obstetrics. *British Journal of Anaesthesia CEPD Reviews*, **1**, 117–21.

:O: Placenta praevia

Procedure	CS (occasionally vaginal delivery may be attempted if 'low grade' placenta praevia)
Time	<30 min if haemorrhage significant
Pain	***
Position	Supine
Blood loss	500 mL—possibly massive haemorrhage
Practical techniques	Regional (now more widespread) or GA, ETT

(See also 'Severe haemorrhage in obstetrics', pp152–4.)

Presentation
• Elective or emergency lower segment CS (LSCS).
• Diagnosis may already have been made antenatally.
• Painless revealed antepartum haemorrhage.

Classification
• Grade 1: Placenta in lower segment.
• Grade 2: Placenta reaches internal cervical os.
• Grade 3: Placenta partially covering internal cervical os.
• Grade 4: Placenta completely covering internal cervical os.

Anterior or posterior position.

'Major' = Grades 3 & 4
'Minor' = Grades 1 & 2

Causes of haemorrhage
• Premature antenatal partial separation of the placenta.
• Increased blood supply to lower segment at site of uterine incision.
• Placental site is in thin lower segment which is unable to contract effectively.
• Placenta accreta (5% if no previous LSCS, 25% if placental site overlies incision from one previous LSCS, 50% if placental site overlies incision from 2 or more previous LSCS).

Immediate management

- Two anaesthetists, 14G IV access with rapid infusion equipment, 4 units blood crossmatched and in theatre. (NB If significant antepartum haemorrhage, resuscitation and LSCS occur simultaneously—use O-negative or group-specific blood as appropriate).
- Administer blood and blood products early.
- Senior obstetrician must be present.
- Consider regional anaesthesia if cardiovascularly stable. Combined spinal–epidural preferable as operation may be prolonged.
- Consider intra-arterial and central venous monitoring, particularly if actively haemorrhaging or if increased risk of placenta accreta (e.g. anterior placenta praevia with previous LSCS scar).
- If GA required, use rapid sequence induction. Consider TIVA/TCI, as avoiding volatile anaesthetics may help uterine contraction.
- Oxytocin 5 IU slow IV for delivery of placenta followed by infusion of 30–40 IU over 4 h.
- Early recourse to ergometrine 500 µg IM, misoprostol 400–1000 µg PR/SL, or carboprost 250 µg IM or intramyometrial.

Subsequent management

- If intraoperative haemorrhage persists, surgeon should consider B-Lynch suture. Hysterectomy may be required.
- Cell salvage techniques are increasingly used in obstetrics and will become a standard of care.
- HDU monitoring following LSCS—increased chance of postpartum haemorrhage.

Special considerations

- USS, CT, and MRI have all been used to try to identify presence and severity of placenta accreta or percreta. None of them has proved highly predictive of intraoperative haemorrhage or outcome.
- Preoperative radiological placement of intrailiac balloon catheters has been reported as effective in a number of cases. However, this requires specialist skills and equipment in semi-elective/elective situations.
- Successful postoperative radiological embolization has been reported. Again, specialist skills and equipment are required.

Further reading

Parekh, N., Husaini, S.W., Russell, I.F. (2000). Caesarean section for placenta praevia: a retrospective study of anaesthetic management. *British Journal of Anaesthesia*, **84**, 725–30.

:O: **Retained placenta**

Procedure	EUA and manual removal of placenta
Time	1–3 h
Pain	Minimal
Position	Supine, lithotomy
Blood loss	500 mL—possibly massive haemorrhage
Practical techniques	Regional technique preferred if cardiovascularly stable. If GA required, rapid sequence induction mandatory

(See also 'Severe haemorrhage in obstetrics', pp152–4.)

Presentation

- Occurs in 0.5–1% of all deliveries.
- Usually immediately following delivery; but if only partial, may not be diagnosed for several days.
- Partially retained placenta may be diagnosed on examination of the rest of the placenta, or may be suspected if membranes appear 'ragged' or if persistent postpartum haemorrhage/uterine atony occurs.
- In any significant postpartum haemorrhage, EUA to exclude retained placenta must be considered.
- May be associated with minimal blood loss or with massive ongoing haemorrhage.

Exclusions

- Uterine atony without retained products of conception.
- Genital tract trauma.

Immediate management

- Intravenous access with 14G cannula.
- Fluid resuscitation if appropriate.
- G&S—crossmatch if blood loss if >500 mL and continuing.
- Consider oxytocin (5 IU slow IV), ergometrine (500 µg IM) to help deliver placenta.
- Catheterize and empty bladder.
- Transfer to theatre for EUA if placenta remains undelivered or if haemorrhage significant. Do not delay EUA to resuscitate patient. NB Even if haemorrhage minimal, do not delay transfer to theatre as sudden severe haemorrhage may occur at any time.
- Regional anaesthesia preferred—top up epidural if *in situ* or establish spinal anaesthesia. Block to T6 required.
- If regional technique contraindicated or cardiovascularly unstable, give GA with rapid sequence induction.

Subsequent management

- Give postoperative Syntocinon infusion for 4 h minimum.
- Consider further dose of ergometrine 500 µg IM, misoprostol 400–1000 µg PR/SL, or carboprost 250 µg IM or intramyometrial, if uterine atony persists despite evacuation of uterus.

- Consider central venous and intra-arterial monitoring if haemorrhage greater than 1000 mL.
- Consider HDU/ITU monitoring post-op.

Further reading

Broadbent, C.R., Russell, R. (1999). What height of block is needed for manual removal of placenta? *International Journal of Obstetric Anaesthesia*, **8**, 161–4.

Tandberg, A., Albrechtsen, S., Iversen, O.E. (1999). Manual removal of the placenta. Incidence and clinical significance. *Acta Obstetricia et Gynecologica Scandinavica*, **78**, 33–6.

✛ Ruptured ectopic pregnancy

Procedure	Laparoscopy/laparotomy
Time	1 h
Pain	***
Position	Supine
Blood loss	Possibly massive blood loss
Practical techniques	GA, ETT

Presentation
- Usually from 6 to 12 weeks of pregnancy.
- Sudden onset of left or right iliac fossa pain associated with a positive pregnancy test.
- May be associated with severe cardiovascular compromise or collapse.
- May be diagnosed by pelvic USS.

Immediate management
- 14G IV access (NB Even apparently 'stable' ectopics may suddenly decompensate).
- FBC, G&S—crossmatch 4 units if cardiovascularly compromised.
- Resuscitate and operate simultaneously.
- GA with rapid sequence induction once abdomen has been surgically prepared—GA may precipitate sudden cardiovascular collapse.
- GA may require modification if cardiovascularly compromised—consider ketamine.
- If cardiovascularly unstable, laparoscopy usually inappropriate.
- Consider intra-arterial and central venous monitoring.
- Consider HDU/ITU post-op. (NB Most patients with ruptured ectopics are young and fit and will recover rapidly so long as surgery is not delayed.)

Subsequent management
- Correct anaemia and coagulopathy
- PCA
- HDU/ITU until stable

Neurosurgery

Martin Smith and Katharine Hunt

☼ Raised intracranial pressure

Definition
Intracranial pressure (ICP) >25 mmHg.

Presentation
- ICP >25 mmHg measured by intraparenchymal microtransducer or external ventricular drain—the latter measures CSF pressure in lateral ventricles and this is the 'gold standard' for ICP measurement.
- Identification of abnormal ICP waveforms—these are often triggered by phasic cerebral vasodilatation in response to a fall in cerebral perfusion pressure (CPP), and terminated by rises in blood pressure.
  - plateau ('A') waves are paroxysmal rises to 50–100 mmHg (usually on a high baseline pressure) and last for several minutes (up to 20 min)
  - 'B' waves are shorter lived fluctuations lasting about a minute and peaking at 30–35 mmHg
  - abnormal ICP waveforms reflect reduced intracranial compliance
- Clinical signs of acute rises in ICP include deteriorating conscious level, sluggish or unequal pupil responses progressing to non-reactivity, hypertension and bradycardia, loss of consciousness, and death. Chronic rises in ICP cause pressure headache, vomiting, and papilloedema.

Immediate management
- Sedation and analgesia to control cerebral metabolic rate and minimize blood pressure surges.
- Mechanical ventilation to maintain PaO_2 >13.3 kPa (100 mmHg) and $PaCO_2$ 4.0–4.5 kPa (30–34 mmHg).
- Nurse in 20–30° head-up position with neck in neutral position and unobstructed neck veins.
- Maintain adequate cerebral perfusion pressure (>60 mmHg) but treat hypertension if mean BP >130 mmHg.
- Mannitol 20% (0.5 g/kg) or other osmotic agent such as hypertonic saline.

Subsequent management
- Maintain CPP >60 mmHg to ensure adequate cerebral perfusion (see 'Management of head injury', pp182–5) by volume resuscitation and inotropes/vasopressors.
- Treat blood pressure if above the upper limit of autoregulation (mean BP >130 mmHg) to minimize vasogenic brain swelling, using short-acting drugs such as labetalol or esmolol.
- Moderate hyperventilation to $PaCO_2$ 4.0–4.5 kPa (30–34 mmHg). Hyperventilation to $PaCO_2$ <4.0 kPa (30 mmHg) should only be undertaken with cerebral oxygenation monitoring guidance (e.g. jugular venous oximetry) since overzealous hyperventilation may worsen cerebral ischaemia by further reduction of critically low cerebral blood flow.
- Treat pyrexia.

- Consider induced moderate hypothermia (target temperature 34°C). Although this has not been shown to improve outcome in prospective randomized trials, modest reductions in temperature are effective in reducing ICP.
- Mannitol (0.5 g/kg), usually as a 20% solution or hypertonic saline.
- CSF drainage via a ventricular catheter is an efficient method of reducing ICP but is an invasive procedure and not without risk.
- Barbiturate infusion may be effective in intracranial hypertension refractory to other therapies.
- Decompressive craniectomy (removal of a bone flap) with enlargement of the dura (duraplasty) is a therapeutic option for intracranial hypertension refractory to conventional therapy.

Investigations

- ICP monitoring, invasive cardiovascular monitoring, regular ABGs, core temperature.
- Consider CT scan if acute rise in ICP.

Risk factors

- Head injury, intracranial haematoma
- Anoxic brain injury
- Intracranial infections

Special considerations

- Consider CT scanning following an acute rise in ICP to exclude a surgically remediable cause.
- There is no merit in persisting with therapies such as mannitol if they have no, or only a short-lasting, effect.

Further reading

Forsyth, R., Baxter, P., Elliott, T. (2001). Routine intracranial pressure monitoring in acute coma. *Cochrane Database System Review*, **3**, CD002043. http://www.cochrane.org/reviews/en/ab002043.html

Smith, M. (2008). Monitoring intracranial pressure in traumatic brain injury. *Anesthesia and Analgesia*, **106**, 240–8.

Stocchetti, N., Rossi, S., Buzzi, F., Mattioli, C., Paparella, A., Colombo, A. (1999). Intracranial hypertension in head injury: management and results. *Intensive Care Medicine*, **25**, 371–6.

⚙ Severe head injury

Definition

Severe traumatic head injury—GCS ≤8.

Presentation

- Clinical observation—unconscious patient following any trauma, clinically apparent head trauma, and obtunded conscious level.
- Radiology—cranial CT scan is the investigation of choice, skull X-ray is of little value if CT easily accessible.

Immediate management

- Oral endotracheal intubation under direct vision, with manual in-line immobilization of the cervical spine (association between cervical spine and head injury).
- IV induction agent to prevent rise in ICP secondary to laryngoscopy. Choice of agent not important, but appropriate dose should be chosen to avoid fluctuations in blood pressure (avoid ketamine due to hypertension and increases in CBF/ICP). Propofol is widely used.
- Rapid sequence induction using suxamethonium (1 mg/kg)—a full stomach or acute gastric dilatation must be assumed.
- Pass orogastric tube to decompress the stomach.
- Mechanical ventilation to maintain PaO_2 >13.3 kPa (100 mmHg) and $PaCO_2$ 4.5–5.0 kPa (34–38 mmHg).
- Maintain sedation and paralysis with short-acting agents (e.g. propofol, fentanyl, atracurium) to allow ventilation and prevent coughing.
- Fluid resuscitation with 0.9% saline or colloid to maintain mean BP >90 mmHg—if ICP monitored, aim for CPP >60 mmHg. Choice of fluid not as important as volume administered, but glucose-containing fluids and hypotonic solutions should be avoided.
- Inotropes may also be required to maintain BP at adequate levels, particularly to offset the hypotensive effects of sedative agents. Noradrenaline is the agent of first choice.
- Mannitol 20% (0.5 g/kg) or hypertonic saline may be used to reduce ICP pending definitive treatment—seek advice from neurosurgical centre.
- Urgent CT scan for patients at high risk of intracranial haematoma or postresuscitation GCS ≤ 8.

Subsequent management

- Detailed secondary survey and appropriate investigations to identify other injuries.
- Active bleeding and other life-threatening chest and abdominal injuries must be treated prior to definitive neurosurgical treatment, but it is sufficient to stabilize non-life-threatening injuries.
- Treat seizures with anticonvulsants—phenytoin 15 mg/kg loading dose.
- Discuss with neurosurgical unit (see p184).

The Glasgow coma scale (GCS)

	Score
Best motor response (observed in the upper limb)	
Obeys commands	6
Withdraws from painful stimuli	5
Localizes to painful stimuli	4
Flexes to painful stimuli	3
Extends to painful stimuli	2
No response	1
Best verbal response Orientated	
Orientated	5
Confused speech	4
Inappropriate words	3
Incomprehensible sounds	2
None	1
Eye-opening response Spontaneously	
Spontaneously	4
To speech	3
To pain	2
None	1

Indications for CT scanning after head injury

Indications for emergency CT scan

- GCS 12 or lower after resuscitation (i.e. eye opening only to pain or not conversing).
- Deteriorating conscious level (GCS falls by 2 points or more) or progressive focal neurological signs.

Indications for urgent CT scan

- Confusion or drowsiness (GCS 13 or 14) followed by failure to improve within 4h.
- Radiological or clinical evidence of a skull fracture, whatever the level of consciousness.
- New neurological signs which are not worsening.
- GCS 15 with no skull fracture but one of the following features:
  - severe and persistent headache
  - nausea and vomiting
  - irritability or altered behaviour
  - a single seizure

Investigations
- Check FBC, U&Es, ABGs, and crossmatch blood.
- Neurological examination—GCS and localizing signs and secondary survey
- Cranial CT scan

Risk factors
- Road traffic accident
- Assault
- Falls from significant height

Exclusions
- Alcohol or other drug intoxication
- Subarachnoid haemorrhage or other spontaneous intracranial haemorrhage
- Anoxic/hypoxic intracranial event

Paediatric implications
- The relatively large head size and weak neck muscles render the child's brain more susceptible to acceleration–deceleration injuries.
- In children under 2 years of age, brain swelling is accommodated by expansion of the skull and may be assessed by examination of the fontanelles and measurement of head circumference. Skull fractures are less common than in adults.
- Scalp lacerations and intracranial haematomas may result in hypotension because of the relatively large head size and small circulating blood volume.
- Surgically treatable intracranial haematomas occur less frequently than in adults (20–30% of paediatric head injuries compared to 50% in adults).
- Cerebral blood flow is higher in children than adults and this may offer some 'protection' against ischaemic damage.
- Neurological outcome is better for children than for adults with the same GCS after resuscitation.

Transfer
- Adequate resuscitation and stabilization prior to transfer.
- Appropriate emergency and monitoring equipment, drugs, intravascular access, and infusion devices should be available for the journey.
- Medical staff involved in transfer should have suitable training, skills, and experience in resuscitation and intensive care medicine and be accompanied by an appropriately trained assistant.
- Good communication between referring and receiving centre before and during transfer.
- Notes, prescription charts, observation charts, and CT scans should accompany the patient.

Further reading
Brain trauma foundation. (2007). The American Association of Neurological Surgeons. The Joint Section of Neurotrauma and Critical Care. *Journal of Neurotrauma*, S1–S106.

Ghajar, J. (2000). Traumatic brain injury. *Lancet*, **356**, 923–9.

Helmy, A., Vizcaychipi, M., Gupta, A. (2007). Traumatic brain injury: intensive care management. *British Journal of Anaesthesia*, **99**, 32–42.

Maas, A.I., Dearden, M., Servadei, F., Stocchetti, N., Unterberg, A. (2000). Current recommendations for neurotrauma. *Current Opinion in Critical Care*, **6**, 281–92.

Moppett I. (2007). Traumatic brain injury: assessment, resuscitation and early management. *British Journal of Anaesthesia* , **99**, 18–31.

NICE clinical guideline 56. Head injury: triage, assessment, investigation and early management of head injury in infants, children and adults. www.nice.org.uk/CG56

✪ Aneurysmal subarachnoid haemorrhage

Definition
Non-traumatic subarachnoid haemorrhage (SAH) is characterized by extravasation of blood into the CSF of the subarachnoid space. It occurs secondary to a ruptured intracranial aneurysm in 85% of cases.

Presentation
- Clinical observation—sudden onset headache (often described as 'worst imaginable' or 'like a hammer blow'), nausea, vomiting, photophobia, and neck stiffness. Focal neurological signs, including third or sixth cranial nerve palsies, motor deficits, or obtunded conscious level, may also be present. Catastrophic SAH presents as sudden loss of consciousness.
- Radiology—cranial CT demonstrates blood in the basal cisterns and throughout the CSF spaces.
- Lumbar puncture—should be carried out in patients with negative or equivocal CT. Typical findings include high CSF opening pressure, elevated red cell count and xanthochromia after 12 h.

Immediate management
- ABC ...
- Maintain systemic blood pressure in 'high normal' range prior to control of the aneurysm—maintains cerebral perfusion whilst minimizing risk of re-bleeding:
  - treat hypertension if systolic BP exceeds 160 mmHg in a previously normotensive patient
  - treat hypotension with intravenous fluids followed by vasopressors
- Oral endotracheal intubation and mechanical ventilation in unconscious patients or those with deteriorating conscious level:
  - maintain PaO_2 >13.3 kPa (100 mmHg) and $PaCO_2$ 4.5–5.0 kPa (34–38 mmHg).
- Urgent CT scan.
- Transfer to neuroscience unit.

Grades of SAH
- Several grading scales quantify the severity of SAH but that described by the World Federation of Neurological Surgeons (WFNS) is widely used:
- Grade 1:   GCS 15 and no motor deficit
- Grade 2:   GCS 14–13 and no motor deficit
- Grade 3:   GCS 14–13 with motor deficit
- Grade 4:   GCS 12–7 with or without motor deficit
- Grade 5:   GCS 6–3 with or without motor deficit

Subsequent management
- Nimodipine 60 mg PO 4-hourly.
- Regular neurological observations.
- Transfer to neurosurgical unit.

Investigations
- Check FBC, U&Es, ABGs, clotting, and crossmatch blood.
- Cranial CT scan.
- Lumbar puncture if CT-negative or equivocal.
- Four-vessel cerebral angiography to identify aneurysm and delineate vascular anatomy.

Risk factors
- 85% of cases of non-traumatic SAH are caused by ruptured intracranial aneurysm.
- Female sex.
- Afro-Caribbean and Japanese races.
- Hypertension.
- Alcohol intake >2 units/day.
- First-degree relative with SAH.

Exclusions
- Ischaemic or haemorrhagic stroke
- Migraine
- Tension headache

Further management
- Re-bleeding:
  - occurs in 7%
  - prevented by early protection of the ruptured aneurysm
  - endovascular intervention is now the treatment of choice for the majority of aneurysms
- Hydrocephalus
  - occurs in approx. 25% patients
  - treated by external ventricular drainage
- Vasospasm
  - can result in delayed ischaemic neurological deficit
  - most common cause of morbidity and mortality after re-bleeding
  - peaks at 4–10 days after the event
  - detected clinically by changes in conscious level or focal neurological deficits
  - confirmed by transcranial Doppler ultrasonography or cerebral angiography
  - triple-H therapy (hypervolaemia, hypertension and haemodilution) widely used to treat cerebral vasospasm after SAH
    - infusion of crystalloids and colloids (>3000 mL/24 h) to achieve daily positive fluid balance
    - maintain systemic BP using vasopressors/inotropes
  - balloon angioplasty and intra-arterial vasodilating agents may be applied in vasospasm resistant to triple-H therapy
- Systemic complications:
  - ECG changes and 'stunned' myocardial syndrome common in poor grade SAH
  - pulmonary oedema

- hyponatraemia—often secondary to SIADH (syndrome of inappropriate antidiuretic hormone secretion)
- fever and hyperglycaemia

Endovascular treatment of intracranial aneurysm

Procedures usually carried out in isolated areas of the hospital, at some distance from main theatre.

Complications include:

- Acute rupture of aneurysm
  - detected by:
    - visualization of extravasation of contrast media during angiography
    - abrupt rise in mean arterial pressure and change in heart rate
  - immediate management:
    - reduce systemic blood pressure with short acting hypotensive agent (e.g. labetalol) or by deepening anaesthesia to allow radiologist to gain control of bleeding
    - maintain $PaCO_2$ 4.5–5.0 kPa (34–38 mmHg)
    - consider reversal of heparin with protamine (1 mg for each 100 IU of heparin given)
    - consider mannitol (0.25–0.5 g/kg)
  - subsequent management:
    - urgent CT scan when bleeding controlled
    - alert main theatre (see below)
    - arrange transfer to an ICU post procedure
  - risk factors for intraprocedural aneurysmal rupture:
    - prolonged or anatomically difficult coiling
    - thin-walled aneurysm
    - anticoagulant and/or antiplatelet therapies
  - special considerations:
    - preferred treatment is packing of aneurysm with coils. Some patients may require emergency craniotomy to evacuate clot and clip the aneurysm
- Thromboembolism
  - consider administration of an antiplatelet agent such as abciximab
- Vasospasm
  - consider intra-arterial administration of vasodilators such as glyceryl trinitrate (GTN) or nimodipine via the angiographic catheter
  - Triple-H therapy post-procedure

Further reading

Smith, M. (2007). Intensive care management of patients with subarachnoid haemorrhage. *Current Opinion in Anaesthesiology*, **20**, 400–7.

Suarez, J., Tarr, R., Selman, W. (2006). Aneurysmal subarachnoid hemorrhage. *New England Journal of Medicine*, **354**, 387–96.

Varma, M. et al. (2007). Anaesthetic considerations for interventional neuroradiology. *British Journal of Anaesthesia* **99**, 75–85.

Wartenberg K.E., Mayer S.A. (2006). Medical complications after subarachnoid hemorrhage: new strategies for prevention and management. *Current Opinion in Critical Care*, **12**, 78–84.

Wilson, S., Hirsch, N., Appleby, I. (2005). Management of subarachnoid haemorrhage in a non-neurosurgical centre. *Anaesthesia*, **60**, 470–85.

:✪: **Spontaneous intracerebral haemorrhage**

Definition
Acute extravasation of blood into the brain parenchyma.

Presentation
- Clinical observation—rapid onset of focal neurological deficit, signs of raised ICP, decreased consciousness level. Severe intracerebral haemorrhage results in immediate unconsciousness. Acute hypertension (blood pressure >150/100 mmHg) occurs in >90% patients.
- Radiology—cranial CT scan allows estimation of volume of haematoma and differentiates between haemorrhagic and ischaemic stroke.
- Cerebral angiography—in young patients or those with no identified risk factors for intracerebral haemorrhage (ICH) and to exclude underlying vascular abnormality, such as arteriovenous malformation or cerebral aneurysm.

Immediate management
- ABC …
- Oral endotracheal intubation and mechanical ventilation in unconscious patients or those with deteriorating conscious level:
  - maintain PaO_2 >13.3 kPa (100 mmHg) and $PaCO_2$ 4.5–5.0 kPa (34–38 mmHg)
- Maintain systemic blood pressure within tight limits around premorbid BP—balancing risk of perihaematoma ischaemia against risk of haematoma expansion:
  - do not treat hypertension unless >180/105 mmHg
  - always maintain systolic BP >100 mmHg
- Consider mannitol (0.5 g/kg) or hypertonic saline if signs of raised ICP.
- Urgent CT scan.

Subsequent management
- Regular neurological observations.
- Reverse therapeutic anticoagulation:
  - vitamin K
  - fresh frozen plasma until normal coagulation indices are restored
- rFVIIa is not indicated—it reduces haematoma volume but does not reduce mortality or improve outcome.
- Treat hypertension:
  - consensus guidance recommends treatment only when systolic BP >180 mmHg
  - recent evidence suggests that reduction of systolic BP to 140 mmHg is associated with reduced haematoma expansion and no increase in cerebral ischaemic events, but further studies are required to determine if this is associated with improved outcome
- Seek neurosurgical advice for large ICH or deterioration in clinical status.

Investigations
- Check FBC, U&Es, ABGs, clotting, and crossmatch blood.
- Cranial CT scan.
- Angiography if no obvious risk factors for ICH or pattern of bleeding suggestive of underlying aneurysm/arteriovenous malformation.
- MRI if underlying lesion suspected (e.g. amyloid angiopathy, neoplasm).

Risk factors
- Warfarin therapy (5–10 fold increase in risk of ICH).
- High dose aspirin in the elderly.
- Hypertension—especially untreated.
- High alcohol intake.
- Cocaine abuse.
- Cerebral amyloid angiopathy.
- Arteriovenous malformation.

Exclusions
- Ischaemic stroke
- Subarachnoid haemorrhage—see p186

Further management
- Surgery:
  - evacuation of haematoma is controversial
  - cerebellar haemorrhage >3 cm should be evacuated because of risk of early deterioration
  - younger patients with lobar haemorrhage causing significant mass effect may also derive benefit from surgery
  - external ventricular drain for hydrocephalus
- Fever and glycaemic control.
- Thromboembolic prophylaxis.
- Seizures occur in 10% of patients and should be treated aggressively.
- Optimal time for resumption of anticoagulation therapy is unclear. Risks and benefits of withholding or restarting treatment should be assessed for each patient.

Further reading
Anderson, C., Huang, Y., Wang, J., *et al.* (2008). Intensive blood pressure reduction in acute cerebral haemorrhage trial (INTERACT): a randomised pilot trial. *Lancet Neurology*, **7**, 391–9.

Mayer, S., Rincon, F. (2005). Treatment of intracerebral haemorrhage. *Lancet Neurology*, **4**, 662–72.

Rincon, F., Mayer, S. (2004). Novel therapies for intracerebral hemorrhage. *Current Opinion in Critical Care*, **10**, 94–100.

① Sodium disturbances after brain injury

Definition

| Hyponatraemia | serum sodium <135 mmol/L (see also p302) |
| Hypernatraemia | serum sodium >145 mmol/L (see also p300) |

Presentation

- *Hyponatraemia*—lethargy, irritability, nausea and vomiting, headache, and muscle cramps/weakness in moderate hyponatraemia. Severe hyponatraemia (<120 mmol/L) presents with drowsiness, seizures, and unconsciousness.
- *Hypernatraemia*—thirst, lethargy, and irritability in moderate hypernatraemia. Severe hypernatraemia (>165 mmol/L) results in seizures and coma.

Immediate management

- Expectant and supportive treatment in asymptomatic patients—brain-injury related sodium disturbances are often transient and self-limiting.
- ABC ... in patients with decreased consciousness or those in coma.
- Prompt treatment of acute sodium disturbance in acute symptomatic patients to minimize risk of neurological complications and death.
- Gradual correction of sodium deficit (0.5 mmol/L/h or 8–10 mmol/L/day) to minimize neurological sequelae.
- Target treatment to the alleviation of symptoms rather than arbitrary serum sodium values.
- Correct associated water deficits.

Causes

- Hyponatraemia:
  - syndrome of inappropriate ADH secretion (SIADH)
  - cerebral salt-wasting syndrome (CSWS)
- Hypernatraemia:
  - cranial diabetes insipidus (DI)

Investigations

- Plasma sodium
- Plasma osmolality
- Urine sodium
- Urine osmolality
- Cranial CT scan

Risk factors

- Head injury (see p182)
- Subarachnoid haemorrhage (see p186)
- Iatrogenic
- Drugs:
  - diuretics
  - mannitol
- Water intoxication

Exclusions
- Inappropriate administration of hypotonic fluids.
- Inadequate water intake or excessive water loss.
- Hyperglycaemia.
- Adrenal insufficiency.
- Hypothyroidism.
- Renal failure.

Diagnosis
- SIADH:
  - serum Na$^+$ <135 mmol/L and osmolality <280 mOsm/kg—i.e. hypotonic hyponatraemia
  - urine osmolality > serum osmolality
  - urinary Na$^+$ concentration >18 mmol/L
  - normal thyroid, adrenal, and renal function
  - clinical euvolaemia
- CSWS:
  - low serum Na$^+$ concentration in association with normal or high serum osmolality
  - high or normal urine osmolality
  - high haematocrit and urea
  - biochemical criteria may be inconclusive—the key clinical diagnostic feature is the presence of volume depletion
- DI:
  - polyuria, polydipsia, and thirst in awake patients
  - high urine volume (>3000 mL/24 h)
  - serum Na$^+$ >145 mmol/L
  - serum osmolality >305 mOsm/kg
  - abnormally low urine osmolality (<350 mOsm/kg)

Specific management
- SIADH:
  - often self-limiting—treatment should be initiated if patient symptomatic or serum Na$^+$ significantly low or falling rapidly
  - fluid restriction (800–1000 mL/24 h)
  - 1.8% saline in acute symptomatic hyponatraemia–discontinue when serum Na$^+$ approx 125 mmol/L
  - pharmacological treatment if saline resuscitation fails and diagnosis certain—furosemide, demeclocycline (900–1200 mg/24 h; note this is higher than licensed dose) or ADH-receptor antagonists (e.g. conivaptan)
  - in general, do not increase serum Na$^+$ by more than 0.5 mmol/L/h or 8–10 mmol/L/day–over-rapid correction can lead to central pontine myelinolysis (see also p302)
- CSWS:
  - volume and saline resuscitation—initially with 0.9% saline
  - 1.8% saline in acute symptomatic hyponatraemia—discontinue when serum Na$^+$ approx 125 mmol/L
  - replace ongoing losses when normovolaemia and normonatraemia restored—0.9% saline IV or water and sodium tablets via NG tube
  - fludrocortisone (0.05–0.3 mg daily) in refractory CSWS
  - as with SIADH, avoid over-rapid correction of serum Na concentration (see also p302)

- DI:
  - key aims are replacement and retention of water and replacement of ADH
  - conscious patients are often able to increase their own water intake—may be sufficient treatment in self-limiting disease
  - 5% glucose IV or water via NG tube in unconscious patients
  - Desmopressin (100–200 µg intranasally or incremental doses of 0.4 µg IV) if urine output >250 mL/h
  - in general, do not reduce serum Na^+ quicker than 10 mmol/L/ day—over-rapid correction can result in pulmonary or cerebral oedema (see also p300)

Further reading

Diringer, M., Zazulia, A. (2006). Hyponatremia in neurologic patients: consequences and approaches to treatment. *Neurologist*, **12**, 117–26.

Lien, Y., Shapiro, J. (2007). Hyponatraemia: clinical diagnosis and management. *American Journal of Medicine*, **120**, 653–8.

Tisdall, M., Crocker, M., Watkiss, J., Smith, M. (2006). Disturbances of sodium in critically ill adult neurologic patients. *Journal of Neurosurgical Anesthesiology*, **18**, 57–63.

☣ Venous air embolism

(See also 'Air/gas embolism' pp62–3)

Definition

Entry of air into the pulmonary arterial circulation through open veins or sinuses.

Presentation

- Immediate fall in $ETCO_2$, fall in SpO_2.
- Rise in end-tidal nitrogen as air enters circulation. This is more specific than changes in $ETCO_2$ as it is not influenced by cardiovascular changes.
- Air entry noted by surgeon, detection of air bubbles with precordial ultrasonography or transoesophageal echocardiography.

Immediate management

- Inform surgeon.
- ABC … 100% O_2.
- Stop nitrous oxide (N_2O) if in use.
- Flood area with saline/cover wound with wet swabs.
- Raise venous pressure, elevate legs, compress neck veins (during cranial surgery), and occlude open ports on CVP lines.
- Attempt to aspirate air from CVP line.

Subsequent management

- Position patient in head-down, left lateral position to limit airflow to pulmonary circulation.
- Standard resuscitation if cardiovascular collapse ensues, initially with fluids, but with inotropes/vasopressors if necessary. NB Adrenaline may worsen arrhythmias precipitated by air embolism, therefore careful administration advisable.
- 8 mg dexamethasone IV followed by maintenance dosage may limit delayed cardiovascular and pulmonary sequelae, although clinical evidence for this is poor.

Investigations

- Capnography, ET nitrogen
- ABGs
- Precordial Doppler ultrasonography or transoesophageal echocardiography (if available)

Risk factors

- Presence of central venous catheters—particularly during insertion or removal.
- Surgery:
  - operative site above level of heart, creating negative hydrostatic pressure, e.g. posterior fossa surgery, ENT surgery
  - surgery involving lung parenchyma
  - cardiothoracic surgery

- iatrogenic introduction of air, CO_2, or other gases to systemic veins, e.g. laparoscopic, hysteroscopic, and arthroscopic surgery
  - obstetric surgery
- Blunt and penetrating chest trauma.
- Barotrauma:
  - IPPV, blast injuries

Exclusions

- Ongoing entrainment of air through venous catheters or open wounds:
  - ensure patient is head down and venous catheters are flushed prior to insertion
  - check lines are closed to air when not in use
  - flood open wounds with saline/cover with wet swabs
  - inform surgeon if during operative procedure

Special considerations

- Prevent venous air embolism in high-risk procedures by elevating central venous pressure—volume loading, compression of the lower limbs with bandages, 'G-suit', or medical anti-shock trousers.
- Do not use nitrous oxide in high-risk procedures—causes expansion of air bubbles.
- Closed chest compressions may give additional benefit by dissipating emboli into the pulmonary arterial tree.

Further reading

Domaingue, C.M. (2005). Anaesthesia for neurosurgery in the sitting position: a practical approach. *Anaesthesia and Intensive Care*, **33**(3), 323–31.

Gray, H., Smith, M. (2004). Anaesthesia for posterior fossa surgery. In *Handbook of Clinical Anaesthesia* (ed. B. Pollard), pp299–302. Churchill Livingstone, Edinburgh.

☢ Status epilepticus

(See also Fig. 6.1, 'Status epilepticus algorithm', p200)

Definition
- Continuous seizure activity lasting >30 min.
- Intermittent seizure activity lasting >30 min during which consciousness is not regained.

Presentation
Loss of consciousness, tonic–clonic muscle activity, tongue biting, and urinary incontinence.

Immediate management
- ABC ... 100% O_2.
- Check blood sugar and treat hypoglycaemia.
- Termination of seizures with IV lorazepam (0.1 mg/kg) or diazepam (0.1 mg/kg) as first-line therapy.
- Second-line therapy if seizures not terminated within 10 min
  - phenytoin 15–17 mg/kg by slow IV infusion (rate <50 mg/min), or fosphenytoin 22.5 mg/kg (equivalent to phenytoin 15 mg/kg) at a rate of up to 225 mg/min (equivalent to phenytoin 150 mg/min)
- Intubation and ventilation to maintain PaO_2 and $PaCO_2$ within normal range.
- Fluid resuscitation to maintain adequate systemic blood pressure and cerebral perfusion pressure.
- Inotropes may also be required, particularly if general anaesthesia is needed to control seizures.

Subsequent management
- Search for cause of seizures and treat underlying problem.
  - known epileptic ± recent change in anti-epileptic medication
  - alcohol withdrawal, drug overdose
  - CNS infection, intracranial pathology, e.g. stroke, subarachnoid haemorrhage
- Start propofol anaesthesia (under EEG control) for refractory status epilepticus if seizures not controlled after 30 min with second-line therapy.
- Ensure therapeutic levels of long-acting anticonvulsant drugs.
- Consider third-line therapy, e.g. phenobarbital 10 mg/kg by infusion (rate <100 mg/min; max 1g) or one of the newer anti-epileptic drugs such as levetiracetam or topiramate. Levetiracetam is now available as an IV preparation and is being widely used in the ICU setting because of rapid titration and ease of transition to maintenance therapy. There are limited data on its efficacy in status epilepticus.
- Management of complications—hyperthermia, rhabdomyolysis (screen for myoglobinuria and measure creatinine kinase), cardiac arrhythmias, pulmonary aspiration, and neurogenic pulmonary oedema.

Investigations
- ABGs, FBC and inflammatory markers, U&Es, blood glucose, thera-peutic drug levels
- EEG
- CT scan if intracranial lesion suspected

Risk factors
- Acute processes:
  - electrolyte imbalance, e.g. Na^+, Ca^{2+}, glucose
  - stroke, cerebral anoxic/hypoxic damage
  - CNS infection, e.g. encephalitis, meningitis
  - drug overdose/toxicity
  - sepsis syndrome
  - acute renal failure
- Chronic processes:
  - pre-existing epilepsy, poor compliance with therapy or recent change of anti-epileptic medication
  - alcoholism
  - brain tumour or other intracranial space-occupying lesion

Exclusions
- Rigors due to sepsis
- Myoclonic jerking
- Generalized dystonia
- Pseudostatus epilepticus, including seizures that are psychogenic in origin

Paediatric implications
- In children the most common cause of status epilepticus is fever/infec-tion.
- Drug efficacy is similar to that in adults, although children may tolerate more rapid IV administration.
- Drug doses are the same as for adult patients on a weight by weight basis, but the maximum dose of lorazepam should not exceed 4 mg/dose in children (compared with 8 mg/dose in adults).
- The adult treatment protocol is generally followed, although there is no evidence that this is applicable to children.

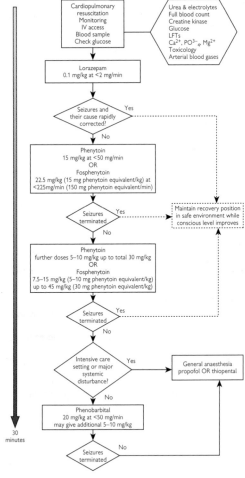

Fig. 6.1 Status epilepticus algorithm.

Special considerations

- General anaesthesia is the definitive treatment for refractory status epilepticus and should be undertaken in a specialist unit where continuous EEG monitoring is available to direct effective and rational therapy:
  - thiopental was previously the drug of choice, but the side-effect profile of high-dose barbiturate infusion severely limits its usefulness—a 250 mg bolus should be followed by an infusion of 2–4 mg/kg/h
  - propofol has potent anticonvulsant properties and is now widely used for the treatment of refractory status. An initial blus of 1 mg/kg is given over 5 min and repeated if seizure activity is not suppressed. A maintenance infusion should be adjusted to 2–10 mg/kg/h until the lowest rate of infusion to suppress epileptiform activity on the EEG is achieved
  - fosphenytoin is a pro-drug of phenytoin—fosphenytoin, 1.5 mg is equivalent to phenytoin 1 mg. Because fosphenytoin is water soluble it can be administered by IV infusion at three times the rate of phenytoin (up to 225 mg/min—equivalent to phenytoin 150 mg/min) and therapeutic concentrations are achieved in 10 min. Dosage is expressed in phenytoin equivalents (PE)
- Identify and treat systemic complications of status epilepticus or its treatment:
  - cerebral—hypoxia/anoxia, oedema, haemorrhage, venous thrombosis
  - cardiovascular—hypo/hypertension, arrhythmias, myocardial infarction, cardiogenic shock, cardiac arrest
  - respiratory—apnoea/hypopnoea, respiratory failure, aspiration pneumonia, pulmonary oedema
  - metabolic—dehydration, electrolyte disturbances (hyponatraemia, hyperkalaemia, hypoglycaemia), metabolic acidosis
  - other—acute renal failure, hepatic failure, acute pancreatitis, multiple organ dysfunction syndrome, DIC, rhabdomyolysis

Further reading

Chapman, M.G., Smith, M., Hirsch, N.P. (2001). Status epilepticus. *Anaesthesia*, **56**, 648–59.

Costello, D., Cole, A. (2007). Treatment of acute seizures and status epilepticus. *Journal of Intensive Care Medicine*, **22**, 319–47.

Penas, J., Molins, A., Puig, J. (2007). Status epilepticus: evidence and controversies. *Neurologist*, **65**, S62–S73.

Treiman, D.M. (1999). Convulsive status epilepticus. *Current Treatment Options in Neurology*, **1**, 359–69.

☼ Spinal shock

Definition
Interruption of sympathetic pathways in spinal cord injury.

Presentation
- Profound hypotension and reduced systemic vascular resistance in the acute phase of spinal cord injury. Often bradycardia due to interruption of cardiac sympathetic denervation.
- Impaired systolic function may manifest as congestive cardiac failure, particularly with fluid loading.
- Bladder and bowel atony are frequently present.

Immediate management
- ABC … 100% O_2.
- Place patient in Trendelenburg position.
- Large-bore IV cannula.
- *Careful* IV fluid boluses.
- Atropine—up to 3 mg in 0.3–0.6 mg increments for bradycardia.
- Consider vasopressors, e.g. noradrenaline, if patient remains hypotensive despite above treatment.

Subsequent management
- Insertion of central venous or pulmonary artery catheter/oesophageal Doppler to monitor responses in cardiac output and filling pressures to fluid challenges.
- Titration of vasopressors and inotropic agents to cardiac output and systemic vascular resistance.
- Nasogastric suctioning for gastric/bowel distension.
- Urinary catheterization for monitoring of fluid balance and bladder atony.

Investigations
FBC, U&E

Risk factors
- Most common in high thoracic or cervical cord injuries.
- Occurs in acute phase of spinal cord injury and progresses to autonomic dysreflexia within 4–6 weeks after injury.

Exclusions
- Exclude haemorrhagic shock as a cause of hypotension. Associated bradycardia is more indicative of neurogenic (spinal) shock.
- Anaphylaxis.
- Vascular volume assessment with CVP/pulmonary artery catheter or oesophageal Doppler monitoring may be helpful.

Special considerations

Hypotension should be treated aggressively with volume expansion and vasopressor/inotropic therapy to optimize spinal cord perfusion, thereby reducing the risks of 2° spinal cord injury.

Steroids and acute spinal cord injury

- Methylprednisolone may be administered to patients with an acute spinal cord injury within 3 h of the injury. Dose is 30 mg/kg bolus dose over 15 min, followed 45 min later by an infusion at 5.4 mg/kg/h for 23 h.
- While administration of methylprednisolone may not treat spinal shock, there is some evidence to suggest that it may produce some neurological improvement in incomplete spinal cord injury, although the potential side-effects of administration should also be considered.

Further reading

Stevens, R.D., Bhardwaj, Kirsch, J.R., Mirski, M.A. (2003). Critical care and perioperative management in traumatic spinal cord injury. *Journal of Neurosurgical Anesthesiology*, **15**, 215–29.

☼ Autonomic dysreflexia

Definition
Massive sympathetic discharge in patients with a spinal cord injury (SCI).

Presentation
- Condition characterized by massive autonomic discharge of the sympathetic chain, below the level of the spinal cord lesion, in response to certain stimuli.
- Severe hypertension (most common clinical feature), cardiac arrhythmias, headache, flushing, and sweating above the level of the lesion.
- Less common features—Horner's syndrome, nausea, anxiety.

Immediate management
- ABC ... 100% O_2.
- Place patient in upright position to produce fall in blood pressure.
- Loosen all tight clothing and shoes.
- Treat/stop any obvious precipitating stimuli (see below), including during general or local anaesthesia.
- Rapid-onset, short-acting vasodilators—nifedipine 10 mg capsule (contents) sublingually, glyceryl trinitrate (0.5–10 mg/h IV infusion, 0.3–1 mg sublingually prn, 5 mg in 24 h dermal patch), or phentolamine (2–10 mg IV prn).

Subsequent management
- Continue antihypertensive of choice in incremental doses until blood pressure is controlled.
- Consider long-term pharmacological therapies:
  - prazosin 1–20 mg PO daily
  - guanethidine 10–20 mg IM, repeated 3-hourly prn
  - calcium-channel blockers, clonidine, and hydralazine have also been recommended

Investigations
Clinical diagnosis

Risk factors
- Occurs from 3 weeks to 12 years after spinal cord injury.
- Most commonly seen in high spinal cord lesions—occurs in up to 60% of patients with cervical lesions and 20% in those with thoracic lesions. Rarely a problem with lesions below T10.
- Usually related to provoking stimuli such as bladder distension, blocked urinary catheter, faecal impaction, uterine contractions.

Exclusions
- Bladder distension
- Bowel distension
- Uterine contractions/labour
- Exclude other pathology—bone fractures, DVT/PE, phaeochromocytoma (rare)

Special considerations

- Episodes of autonomic dysreflexia may result in myocardial ischaemia, pulmonary oedema, cerebral haemorrhage, seizures, coma, and death. Severe hypertension should be treated promptly and these outcomes recognized, investigated, and treated as appropriate.
- Spinal anaesthesia obliterates autonomic dysreflexia, although numerous cases have been reported under general and epidural anaesthesia. In addition to short-acting antihypertensive therapy, increasing depth of anaesthesia may be effective in treating these cases.

Further reading

Bycroft, J., Shergill, I. S., Chung, E. A., Arya, N., Shah, P.J. (2005). Autonomic dysreflexia, a medical emergency. *Postgraduate Medical Journal*, **81**, 232–5.

Hambly, P.R., Martin, B. (1998). Anaesthesia for chronic spinal cord lesions. *Anaesthesia*, **53**, 273–89.

① Dystonic reactions

Definition
Severe, sustained muscular spasms or abnormal posturing.

Presentation
- Recent history of antipsychotic or antidepressant drug ingestion:
  - antipsychotics—phenothiazines (e.g. prochlorperazine), butyrophenones (e.g. haloperidol), thioxanthenes (e.g. flupentixol)
  - antiemetics—prochlorperazine, metoclopramide
  - antidepressants—selective serotonin reuptake inhibitors
  - in 90% of patients onset is within 4 days of start of medication.
- Characteristic muscle spasms:
  - oculogyric crisis—blepharospasm, upward/lateral deviation of eyes
  - torticollic crisis—spasm of neck muscles
  - buccolingual crisis—spasm of facial muscles and tongue, dysphagia, dysarthria
  - tortipelvic crisis—painful abdominal wall spasm
- Cessation of symptoms within 5–15 min of antimuscarinic administration.

Immediate management
- Assess and stabilize airway, consider 100% O_2.
- Reassure patient.
- IV access.
- Centrally acting antimuscarinic—benzatropine 1–2 mg IV or procyclidine 5–10 mg IV.
- Consider diazepam 5–10 mg IV in severe cases resistant to treatment with antimuscarinic agents.

Subsequent management
- If immediate management fails, consider another diagnosis.
- Discontinue trigger agent if possible.
- Consider longer term treatment with anticholinergic therapy:
  - procyclidine 5 mg PO tds or amantadine 100 mg od–tds

Investigations
U&Es, magnesium, calcium

Risk factors
- Recent treatment with triggering agents (see above)
- Male sex, teenagers/young adults
- Previous history of acute dystonia
- Cocaine abuse

Exclusions
- Tetanus, seizures/status epilepticus
- Metabolic disturbances, e.g. hypocalcaemia, hypomagnesaemia
- CVA
- Meningitis, particularly in young children

Special considerations
- Life-threatening dystonias may occur rarely.
- Severe stridor due to laryngospasm has been reported.

Further reading

Dressler, D., Benecke, R. (2005). Diagnosis and management of acute movement disorders. *Journal of Neurology*, **252**, 1299–306.

Van Harten, P.N., Hoek, H.W., Kahn, R.S. (1999). Acute dystonia induced by drug treatment. *British Medical Journal*, **319**, 623–6.

Thoracics

Adrian Pearce and Gerard Gould

☢ Intrathoracic tracheal/bronchial obstruction

(See also pp80–4)

Definition
Partial or complete obstruction of the tracheobronchial tree.

Presentation
- Dyspnoea, hypoxia, ineffective cough, weak voice, only a few words at a time, prefer to sit up (particularly to sleep).
- Narrowing visualized on CXR or CT, abnormal flow-volume loop.

Immediate management
- Make or consider diagnosis (often missed initially).
- 100% O_2.
- Consider Heliox (disadvantage is low FiO_2).
- Give dexamethasone 8 mg IV, then 4 mg 6–hourly.
- Arterial line and regular blood gases to check pH, $PaCO_2$.
- Move to HDU/ITU environment.
- CXR, preferably CT of airway and echocardiography.
- May need tracheal intubation in extremis—use small tube (5.0–6.0 mm) and make certain (with fibrescope) that tube tip is below level of obstruction. May be done awake with fibreoptic intubation and maintenance of spontaneous respiration, RSI with rigid bronchoscope or inhalational induction, depending on the clinical situation.
- Make plans for rigid bronchoscopy, debulking of tumour, or stenting.
- Carinal obstruction is difficult to overcome—try intubating one bronchus and surviving on one lung temporarily.
- If situation not critical, consider awake fibreoptic bronchoscopy to diagnose site and extent of problem and urgent radiotherapy to debulk malignancy.

Investigations
CXR, CT of airway, flow-volume loop, echocardiography

Risk factors
- Extrinsic or intrinsic narrowing, primary carcinoma of trachea/bronchus, lymphoma, carcinoma of oesophagus.
- Thymoma, retrosternal goitre, other mediastinal masses.
- Inflammatory conditions such as Wegener's granulomatosis.
- Problems likely if trachea narrowed by >50% on CT.
- May be associated pericardial effusion or cardiac involvement.

Exclusions
- Asthma
- Worsening of COPD

Subsequent management

- Rigid bronchoscopy under GA with Sanders injector.
- Surgeon can manipulate bronchoscope through obstruction or into bronchus.
- Tumour debulking by grabbing with forceps or laser.
- Stenting of narrowed airway under GA:
  - patient on X-ray lucent table
  - X-ray screening
  - wire placed through obstruction into distal bronchus
  - stent advanced over wire into bronchus, trachea, or both
- Lasering possible through flexible bronchoscope without GA.
- Consider radiotherapy, chemotherapy, or surgical removal of mass.
- Inflammatory tracheal narrowing requires tracheostomy followed by immunosuppression.

Special considerations

- Mediastinal masses are one cause of unexpected failed ventilation and intubation after induction of general anaesthesia.
- Anaesthetic plans to remove mediastinal masses might include cardiopulmonary bypass.

Further reading

Bechard, P., Letourneau, L., Lacasse, Y., Cote, D., Bussieres, J.S. (2004). Perioperative cardiorespiratory complications in adults with mediastinal mass. *Anesthesiology*, **100**, 826–34.

Conacher, I.D. (2003). Anaesthesia and tracheobronchial stenting for central airway obstruction. *British Journal of Anaesthesia*, **90**, 367–74.

Goh, M.H., Liu, X.Y., Goh, Y.S. (1999). Anterior mediastinal mass: an anaesthetic challenge. *Anaesthesia*, **54**, 670–82.

Hammer, G.B. (2004). Anaesthetic management for the child with a mediastinal mass. *Paediatric Anaesthesia*, **14**, 95–7.

☼ Inhaled foreign body

Definition
Foreign body (FB) in airway.

Presentation
- Immediate—inhalation episode may be witnessed, coughing, choking, stridor, cyanosis, respiratory distress, lateralizing clinical chest signs.
- Late—non-resolving collapse, consolidation, wheeze.
- 30% left bronchus, 60% right bronchus, 10% laryngotracheal.

Immediate management

- Encourage coughing and, if conscious:
  - *infant*—5 back blows, 5 chest thrusts, check airway, then repeat if necessary
  - *child*—5 back blows, 5 chest thrusts, check airway, 5 back blows, 5 abdominal thrusts (Heimlich manoeuvre), check airway, then repeat if necessary
  - *adult*—5 back blows, 5 abdominal thrusts (Heimlich manoeuvre), check airway, then repeat if necessary
- If unconscious, remove any visible obstruction, give two effective rescue breaths and commence chest compressions to relieve the obstruction.
- 100% O_2.
- Intubation and CPR in extremis (ETT may push FB distally, allowing ventilation).
- FB occasionally seen (and removed) at intubation.
- Consider trial of Heliox (if immediately available) for serious respiratory difficulties while transfer to theatre organized.
- Make diagnosis:
  - history and examination
  - CXR—FB visible or obstructive emphysema
  - if intubated, inspect airway with flexible fibrescope
  - may just be clinical suspicion
- Removal of FB by rigid bronchoscopy under GA: immediate transfer to theatre:
  - IV access, atropine 600mcg IV (or 20 mcg/kg for a child), standard monitoring (in compromised child may be obtained post induction)
  - O_2/sevoflurane or halothane induction, maintain SV
  - deep anaesthesia with inhalational agent (switch to O_2/halothane or isoflurane as sevoflurane wears off too rapidly)
  - lidocaine spray to cords and trachea (<3 mg/kg)
  - tape and pad eyes
  - insertion of rigid bronchoscope, connection to breathing system
  - maintain spontaneous respiration via breathing system attached to bronchoscope

- must avoid vocal cords closing when FB being removed (adequate anaesthesia or paralysis)
- consider dexamethasone 0.1 mg/kg IV
- procedure can be lengthy (i.e. hours) so remember IV fluids, keep patient warm and consider intubation at the end and transfer to ITU
- an alternative GA technique (particularly in adults) is rigid bronchoscopy under TIVA and muscle relaxation with ventilation by Sanders injector
- Retrieval possible in adults by flexible bronchoscopy under topical anaesthesia.

Subsequent management
- Mucosal inflammation secondary to organic material (particularly oily nuts) may take days to resolve.
- Antibiotics useful.

Investigations
CXR (inspiratory/expiratory views)

Risk factors
- Children under 3–5 years, lack of adult supervision, availability of nuts, seeds, beads
- Adults—dentures, senility, mental illness, intoxication

Exclusions
- Asthma, acute laryngotracheobronchitis
- Chest infection

Paediatric implications
- Common cause of accidental death in the home in children <6 years.
- 400 choking deaths/year in EU—food accounts for 85% choking deaths.

Special considerations
- May be more than one FB.
- FB may be organic or inorganic.
- Organic FBs liable to fragment at removal.
- Majority not visible on CXR.

Further reading
Farrell, P.T. (2004). Rigid bronchoscopy for foreign body removal: anaesthesia and ventilation. *Paediatric Anaesthesia*, **14**, 84–9.

Litman, R.S., Ponnuri, J., Trogan, I. (2000). Anesthesia for tracheal or bronchial foreign body removal in children: an analysis of ninety-four cases. *Anesthesia and Analgesia*, **91**, 1389–91.

Pinzoni, F., Boniotti, C., Molinaro, S.M., Baraldi, A., Berlucchi, M. (2007). Inhaled foreign bodies in pediatric patients: review of personal experience. *International Journal of Pediatric Otorhinolaryngology*, **71**, 1897–903

UK Resuscitation Council BLS Guidelines. www.resus.org.uk

☼ Tracheal injury or laceration

Definition
Loss of structural integrity of tracheobronchial tree.

Presentation
- Blunt trauma to cricoid region; beware disrupted larynx or cricotracheal discontinuity (high mortality):
  - superficial bruising, pain, stridor, respiratory embarrassment
  - surgical emphysema, vocal cord palsy
  - associated cervical spine trauma
  - associated oesophageal injury
- Tracheobronchial tears:
  - high tracheal tear due to penetrating injury
  - low tracheal tear due to crushing injury with closed glottis, double lumen tube, penetrating trauma (knife, gunshot)
  - surgical emphysema, hoarseness, cyanosis, respiratory embarrassment, bubbling or frothy blood in airway, pneumothorax, lung collapse
  - associated oesophageal, cardiac, aortic, or great vein injury

Immediate management
- 100% O_2.
- Maintain spontaneous respiration whenever possible—massive air leak may occur with IPPV.
- High index of suspicion—airway initially OK, then rapid deterioration.
- Cervical spine precautions.
- IV access essential, arterial line useful.
- Take Hb, crossmatch 4 units blood.
- CXR (pneumothorax, pneumomediastinum, collapse).
- Intercostal drain for pneumothorax.
- Consult with ENT or thoracic surgeons and plan joint care.
- May be possible to pass tracheal tube directly into trachea through penetrating injury of cervical trachea.
- Induction of general anaesthesia, muscle relaxation, intubation by direct laryngoscopy, and IPPV are all potentially hazardous.
- Intubation by direct laryngoscopy under GA may fail to intubate the distal trachea if there is laryngeal or tracheal disruption.
- Consider awake fibreoptic endoscopy and intubation (in theatre).
- Load a cuffed tube on intubating fibrescope.
- Use uncut small tube (6.0–7.0 mm) in case intubation of one bronchus required.
- Inspect airway fibreoptically using CCTV to allow surgeons a view of the whole airway.
- Fibre-endoscopy may be difficult (blood, oedema, laryngotracheal disruption.
- Attempt to pass scope and tube beyond any trauma, even down to intubation of an unaffected bronchus.

- Tracheostomy under LA (or directly into exposed trachea) may be required, particularly with blunt laryngeal trauma.
- Avoid IPPV until airway below tear has been isolated with cuffed tube.
- Repair of low tracheal tears may require median sternotomy or thoracotomy.

Subsequent management
- Exclude cervical spine trauma, treat accordingly if present.
- Look for oesophageal injury and treat.
- Fractured ribs, flail segment, pulmonary and cardiac contusion may be present in blunt trauma.

Investigations
CXR, flexible nasendoscopy

Risk factors
- Double-lumen tube insertion
- Blunt/penetrating injury to neck/chest
- Thermal injury

Special considerations
- Acute laryngotracheal injury in 0.5% of all trauma.
- 70–80% of patients with airway injury die before reaching hospital.
- Blunt thoracic trauma has higher mortality than penetrating trauma.
- 70% in-hospital mortality rate with severe tracheobronchial injury.
- 80% tears in blunt thoracic trauma are within 2.5 cm of carina.
- With cricoid cartilage fractures, 25% have recurrent laryngeal nerve palsy.
- Pulmonary vein laceration may allow left-sided air embolism, particularly with high airway pressure and low pulmonary venous pressure.
- Systemic air embolism indicated by haemoptysis, coronary and cerebral dysfunction, air in retinal vessels and in arterial sample.

Further reading
Fitzmaurice, B.G., Brodsky, J.B. (1999). Airway rupture from double-lumen tubes. *Journal of Cardiothoracic and Vascular Anesthesia*, **13**, 322–9.

Ho, A.M.-H., Ling, E. (1999). Systemic air embolism after lung trauma. *Anesthesiology*, **90**, 564–75.

Karmy-Jones, R., Wood, D.E. (2007) Traumatic injury to the trachea and bronchus. *Thoracic Surgical Clinics*, **17**, 35–46.

Naghibi, K., Hashemi, S.L., Sajedi, P. (2003). Anaesthetic management of tracheobronchial rupture following blunt chest trauma. *Acta Anaesthesiologica Scandinavica*, **47**, 901–3.

① Bronchopleural fistula (BPF)

Definition
Abnormal communication between bronchial tree and pleural cavity.

Presentation
- Cough, fever, dyspnoea, hypoxia, subcutaneous emphysema, CXR shows falling fluid level in postpneumonectomy space.
- Large air leak through intercostal drain.
- Severity of symptoms relates to the size of the fistula.

Immediate management
- Oxygen by mask.
- Antibiotics to treat infection secondary to soiling of lung.
- Prevent soiling of good lung. Sit patient up with affected side tilted down until unaffected lung is isolated.
- Insert chest drain (prior to induction) to drain any pus.
- Large air leak down chest drain may impair facemask ventilation.
- Isolate the unaffected lung by insertion of a DLT under FOB guidance.
- Use DLT which intubates the healthy bronchus.
- Clamp side of BPF.
- Suction frequently down tracheal lumen to remove pus.

Subsequent management
- Minimize airway pressures during IPPV using pressure-controlled ventilation (PCV).
- Attempt to extubate as soon as possible post-op.
- HDU/ITU post-op. as significant pre-op. morbidity and post-op. mortality.

Investigations
CXR, ABGs, check Hb, G&S

Risk factors
- Most frequent following lung resection, greatest incidence following pneumonectomy.
- Rupture of lung abscess, bronchus, bulla, cyst.
- Erosion of bronchus by carcinoma or chronic inflammation.

Exclusions
Bronchopneumonia—cough, fever, dyspnoea, hypoxia, ± haemoptysis.

Paediatric implications
- Smallest DLT available is 28 Fr, not suitable for children <30 kg.
- Bronchial blockers are available that pass through 3.5 mm ID ETT.
- Single-lumen ETT with 'built in' bronchial blocker available from 5.5 mm ID.

Special considerations

- Isolation and prevention of soiling of the unaffected lung is central to the anaesthetic management and can be achieved in a number of ways:
  - awake FOB-guided intubation with DLT
  - rapid IV induction and FOB-guided endobronchial intubation with DLT
  - inhalational induction and intubation with DLT with spontaneous ventilation (difficult to do)
  - single-lumen tube placed endobronchially (if pneumonectomy)
  - if unable to pass DLT, consider bronchial blocker, or endobronchial intubation with single-lumen tube under FOB guidance
- If DLT insertion unsuccessful or problematic in the presence of a *major* air leak, then consider the following:
  - intubate using uncut 6mm ETT. Guide ETT into intact main bronchus over FOB. Isolate and ventilate the 'good' lung
  - pass rigid bronchoscope and slide bougie or airway exchange catheter into intact bronchus. Railroad ETT into bronchus
  - attempt to control air leak by passing 'Arndt' bronchial blocker (guided by FOB) or Fogarty embolectomy catheter into the fistula. This will act as a holding measure.

Further reading

Hammer, G., Fitzmaurice, B., Brodsky, J. (1999). Methods for single lung ventilation in pediatric patients. *Anesthesia and Analgesia*, **89**, 1426–9.

Kozian, A., Schilling, T., Strang, C., Hachenberg, T. (2006). Anesthetic considerations in patients with previous thoracic surgery. *Current Opinions in Anaesthesiology*, **19**, 26–33.

⚙ **Hypoxia during one-lung ventilation (OLV)**

Definition

Oxygen saturation <90% during OLV.

Presentation

- Usually gradual decrease in SpO_2 following change from two-lung ventilation to one lung.
- Usually develops over 3–10 min, then gradually improves.

Immediate management

- Increase FiO_2 to 100%.
- Check DLT patency.
- Adjust tidal volume to 7–8 mL/kg or inflation pressure to 30 cmH$_2$O.
- Suction to the dependent lung to remove mucus, blood, or pus.
- Check the position of the DLT with fibrescope.
- Manual inflation of the dependent lung to assess compliance and to expand areas of collapse.
- Auscultate lower lung for added sounds.
- Ensure adequate cardiac output (for a given shunt fraction, a fall in cardiac output leads to lower arterial oxygen partial pressures).
- Re-inflate operative, non-dependent lung with 100% oxygen following discussion with the surgeon (particularly if saturations sustained at <85–90%).
- Insufflation of 1–2 L/min oxygen through catheter in tracheal limb.
- CPAP of 5–10 cmH$_2$O with 100% oxygen to the non-dependent lung is highly effective and may be acceptable to the surgeon.
- Try PEEP 5 cmH$_2$O to the dependent lung, but may be ineffective or worsen situation (by increasing PVR).
- Clamping the pulmonary artery will eliminate the shunt to the operative lung (consider during pneumonectomy).
- May need to revert to two-lung ventilation if hypoxia persists.

Subsequent management

- Surgery may need to continue with intermittent two-lung ventilation.
- Switching from inhalational to intravenous anaesthesia may help to preserve hypoxic pulmonary vasoconstriction—consider when all else fails, but beware of falling cardiac output during changeover.
- IV almitrine (4–12 µg/kg/min), a pulmonary vasoconstrictor, has been effective in small studies but is not available in the UK.
- Nitric oxide to the lower lung has usually little or no beneficial effect.

Investigations

ABGs, fibreoptic bronchoscopy

Risk factors

- Arterial oxygen tension always dips following institution of OLV, but O_2 saturation <90% occurs in only 5–10% patients.

- Young may be more susceptible than elderly.
- Best predictor is PaO_2 when ventilating both lungs.

Exclusions

- Malposition of DLT, malfunction of DLT or the bronchial cuff (cuff herniation).
- Soiling of the dependent lung with sputum, mucus or blood.
- Breathing circuit dysfunction:
  - kinks in the circuit
  - incorrect application of clamp to 'Y' connector
  - obstruction within the breathing circuit
- Bronchospasm, anaphylaxis.

Re-inflating the non-dependent lung

- Use 100% oxygen.
- Suction using catheter provided with the DLT to remove any blood or secretions before re-inflation.
- Re-inflate using high sustained CPAP (35–40 cmH$_2$O) to expand areas of atelectasis under direct surgical vision.
- May return to original two-lung ventilation settings (care if extensive lung resection).
- Maintain normocapnia.
- May need to return to OLV if complications occur, e.g. large air leak from operative lung.

Further reading

Eastwood, J., Mahajan, R. (2002). One-lung anaesthesia. *British Journal of Anaesthesia CEPD Reviews*, **2**, 83–7.

Guenoun, T., Journois, D., Silleran-Chassany, J., Frappier, J., D'Attellis, N., Salem, A., Safran, D. (2002). Prediction of arterial oxygen tension during one-lung ventilation: analysis of preoperative and intraoperative variables. *Journal of Cardiothoracic and Vascular Anaesthesia*, **16**, 199–203.

⊙ Sudden high airway pressure during one-lung ventilation

Definition
Peak airway pressure >30 cmH$_2$O on OLV with tidal volumes of 7–8 mL/kg.

Presentation
Airway pressure >30 cmH$_2$O during OLV with volume-controlled ventilation.

Immediate management
- 100% O$_2$ if SaO$_2$ <90%.
- Check delivered tidal volume only 7–8 mL/kg.
- Switch to manual ventilation to assess compliance and to exclude dynamic hyperinflation.
- Auscultate dependent lung for wheeze.
- Inspect DLT and connector for obvious kinks or obstruction to gas flow and ensure the DLT is at an appropriate distance at the teeth (see pp230–1).
- Check positioning of DLT with fibrescope, particularly in relation to RUL, and rule out cuff herniation.
- Ensure the clamp is applied to the appropriate limb of the 'Y' connector and the correct lumen is open to the atmosphere.
- Suction, using catheter provided with DLT, to remove particulate matter within the DLT.
- Treat bronchospasm appropriately.
- Ask the surgeon to evaluate the dependent lung space under direct vision.
- If the problem is serious, consider going to two-lung ventilation to regain control.
- Surgery may need to continue on two-lung ventilation (discuss with surgeon).

Subsequent management
- Continue high FiO$_2$ as required.
- Treat pneumothorax, bronchospasm, and suspected anaphylaxis appropriately.
- Always check position of DLT with fibrescope following any change in patient position or ventilatory dynamics.
- Pulmonary oedema treated by postoperative IPPV, CVP/PAP monitoring, diuretics, inotropes.

Investigations
Fibreoptic bronchoscopy

Risk factors
- The severity of underlying disease in the dependent lung will affect the peak airway pressure following institution of OLV.
- Surgical handling may displace tube.

Exclusions

- Malposition of DLT (especially right DLT).
- Obstruction within the DLT by sputum, blood.
- Clamp incorrectly applied to 'Y' connector.
- Dynamic hyperinflation—see pp224–5.
- Pneumothorax of the dependent lung—see p223.
- Bronchospasm in dependent lung.
- Anaphylaxis.
- Cardiogenic pulmonary oedema.

Special considerations

- Consider the use of pressure-controlled ventilation during one-lung anaesthesia to prevent exposure to high peak airway pressures.
- Airway pressures above $40\,cmH_2O$ have been associated with postpneumonectomy pulmonary oedema.
- In ARDS, consider ventilation strategies to limit tidal volume and accept hypercapnia.

Further reading

Klein, U., Karzai, W., Bloos, F. *et al.* (1998). Role of fibreoptic bronchoscopy in conjunction with the use of double-lumen tubes for thoracic anesthesia. *Anesthesiology*, **88**, 346–50.

Moloney, E.D., Griffiths, M.J.D. (2004). Protective ventilation of patients with acute respiratory distress syndrome. *British Journal of Anaesthesia*, **92**, 261–70.

☠ **Pneumothorax of dependent lung during one-lung ventilation**

Definition
Pneumothorax of ventilated 'good lung' during OLV.

Presentation
- Decreased SaO_2, BP, $ETCO_2$, increased P_{aw}, cyanosis, bradycardia.
- Decreased breath sounds on auscultation.

Immediate management
- Stop N_2O if used and increase FiO_2 to 100%.
- Ventilate both lungs gently to assess compliance and improve oxygenation.
- If during thoracotomy, ask surgeon to evaluate dependent pleural space and decompress tension pneumothorax without having to return patient supine.
- If during VATS, consider rapid needle decompression (2nd intercostal space mid-clavicular line (ICS MCL)).
- If tension:
  - turn patient supine
  - place chest drain

Subsequent management
- Formal chest drain insertion.
- CXR on table or in recovery/HDU.
- Insert arterial line if not *in situ*—check ABGs.
- Consider HDU post-op.
- Aim to return to spontaneous ventilation as soon as possible post-op.

Investigations
Clinical diagnosis, consider on-table CXR.

Risk factors
Incidence unknown, but risk is greater if bullous disease of non-operative side.

Exclusions
- Dynamic hyperinflation—see pp224–5
- Bronchospasm, anaphylaxis
- Obstruction to expiratory gas flow

Special considerations
Consider advisability of continuing with planned surgery (particularly major lung resection) if a critical stage not yet reached.

:✪: Dynamic hyperinflation (DHI)

Definition
Pulmonary gas trapping during IPPV in emphysema and bullous lung disease.

Presentation
- Increased P_{aw}, JVP/CVP, decreased BP and SaO_2, pulsus paradoxus, slow rising capnography trace.
- Expiratory gas flow continuing longer than time allowed for exhalation.
- Clinical improvement (i.e. increased SaO_2 and BP, decreased HR) following disconnection from the ventilator is pathognomonic of DHI or tension pneumothorax.

Immediate management
- Increase FiO_2 to 100%.
- Disconnect patient from ventilator and breathing circuit. This should lead to rapid improvement in clinical condition.
- Detect long expiration by listening at end of ETT.
- Stop N_2O and continue with air/oxygen mix.
- Limit minute ventilation, reduce V_t to 7–8 mL/kg.
- Accept hypercarbia—up to 8.5 kPa (64 mmHg).
- Switch to pressure-controlled (PC) ventilation and limit inspiratory pressure to <20 cmH$_2$O.
- Increase expiratory phase (I:E ratio 1:4).

Subsequent management
- Consider HDU post-op.
- Arterial line, monitor ABGs.
- Aim to return to spontaneous ventilation ASAP.
- Optimize bronchodilator therapy.

Investigations
Listen at the open end of the ETT for prolonged expiration.

Risk factors
- Dysfunctional airways as found in emphysema and bullous lung disease.
- Inappropriately large tidal volumes or high inflation pressures.

Exclusions
- Tension pneumothorax of dependent lung—see p222
- Distended giant bulla in dependent lung
- Malposition of DLT
- Bronchospasm—see pp54–6

Special considerations
There is no failsafe approach to IPPV in these patients. Techniques should aim at avoiding high inspiratory pressure (pressure-controlled ventilation) and prevent gas trapping.

Further reading

Conacher, I.D. (1997). Anaesthesia for the surgery of emphysema. *British Journal of Anaesthesia*, **79**, 530–8.

Conacher, I.D. (1998). Dynamic hyperinflation—the anaesthetist applying a tourniquet to the right side of the heart. *British Journal of Anaesthesia*, **81**, 116–17.

Ward, N.S., Dushay, K.M. (2008). Clinical concise review: mechanical ventilation of patients with chronic obstructive pulmonary disease. *Critical Care Medicine*, **36**, 1614–19.

✛ Cardiac herniation postpneumonectomy

Definition
Cardiac herniation following intrapericardial pneumonectomy.

Presentation
- 75% present in immediate postoperative period and all within 24 h.
- Usually dramatic symptoms/signs, but may occur with little initial disturbance:
  - right-sided—impaired venous return, distended neck veins, dusky face, and hypotension
  - left-sided—strangulation of the left ventricle with myocardial ischaemia, dysrhythmias, impaired left ventricular performance, profound hypotension.

Immediate management
- 100% oxygen by facemask.
- Intubate if patient collapsed.
- Turn patient so that non-operative lung is dependent.
- Alert surgeons.
- Keep chest drain (if present) clamped.
- Insert arterial line (if not present).
- Consider CVP line (if not present).
- Start inotropes as required.
- Urgent return to theatre for surgical correction.
- Induction in semi-lateral position, non-operative side dependent.
- Arterial monitoring during induction, sympathomimetics ready.
- Single-lumen tube.
- Pressure-controlled ventilation to limit pressure on bronchial stump.

Subsequent management
- Surgical repair of defect should prevent recurrence.
- LV dysfunction due to ischaemia, oedema, or infarction may persist.
- May require post-op IPPV and inotropes.

Investigations
CXR, ECG, echocardiography

Risk factors
Pneumonectomy when intrapericardial ligation of great vessels required, leaving pericardial defect.

Exclusions
- Myocardial ischaemia/infarction
- Primary arrhythmia
- Acute mediastinal shift
- Haemorrhage
- Cardiac tamponade
- Pulmonary embolism

Paediatric implications

Cardiac herniation can occur spontaneously through congenital pericardial defects.

Special considerations

- 100% mortality if unrecognized.
- 50% mortality when recognized and treated promptly.

Further reading

Chambers, N., Walton, S., Pearce, A. (2005). Cardiac herniation following pneumonectomy—an old complication revisited. *Anaesthesia and Intensive Care.* **33**. 403–9.

Self, R.J., Vaughan, R.S. (1999). Acute cardiac herniation after radical pleuropneumonectomy. *Anaesthesia*, **54**, 564–6.

Weinlander, C.M., Abel, M.D., Piehler, J.M. (1986). Spontaneous cardiac herniation after pneumonectomy. *Anesthesia and Analgesia*, **65**, 1085–8.

☠️ Major airway bleeding

Definition
Haemorrhage from tracheobronchial tree.

Presentation
- Acute haemoptysis
- Bleeding at bronchoscopy

Immediate management

- 100% O_2.
- Turn patient good lung up.
- Tracheal intubation and suction to remove blood and clots.
- Crossmatch 4 units and check haematocrit/Hb periodically.
- Consider DLT, particularly with known unilateral pathology or trauma.
- Rigid or flexible bronchoscopy in theatre.
- At rigid bronchoscopy (GA):
  - suction by surgeon under direct vision and wait
  - bronchial blocker (Fogarty catheter) into affected bronchus
- May need thoracotomy and, if so, insert DLT and arterial line—suction down DLT limb.
- Detect and correct any bleeding diathesis (FFP, platelets, cryoprecipitate).

Subsequent management
- Bleeding lesion may be treated by YAG laser via flexible bronchoscope.
- Pulmonary angiography (and possibly embolizing) helpful if lesion not amenable to bronchoscopy.
- Bleeding cavitating lesions (such as aspergillomas) will need pulmonary resection and possibly pneumonectomy. Need CVP and arterial monitoring, fluid warmer, and 6 units crossmatched.

Investigations
CXR, bronchoscopy

Risk factors
- Tracheobronchial tumour/trauma
- Biopsy at bronchoscopy
- Bleeding disorder
- Aspergilloma

☼ **Bleeding during mediastinoscopy**

Definition
Continued bleeding during mediastinoscopy.

Presentation
- Bleeding at mediastinoscopy—venous or arterial.
- May be serious injury to aortic arch vessels, especially brachiocephalic artery.

Immediate management
- Pack wound and wait 10 min.
- Observe heart rate and measure BP every 1–2.5 min.
- Set up 14G IV cannula in lower limb.
- Take blood, crossmatch 4 units (if not already done).
- Get equipment collected for arterial line, CVP, and blood warmer.
- Check NIBP (at least feel pulse) in both arms.
- If bleeding persists, prepare for thoracotomy or median sternotomy.
- Upper limb IV fluids may leak out if large vein opened, so *use lower limb access.*
- Site arterial line in best radial pulse, consider internal jugular CVP insertion.
- Keep single-lumen tracheal tube.
- Position patient appropriately.
- If OLV needed, use blocker or push single-lumen tube into bronchus.
- May need cardiopulmonary bypass (rare).

Subsequent management
- Consider likelihood of tracheal compression.
- Consider continued intubation post-op and transfer to ITU.

Investigations
FBC, coagulation, crossmatch 4 units

Risk factors
- Aberrant blood vessel in front of trachea
- Grossly abnormal mediastinal anatomy
- SVC obstruction

Special considerations
- Impaired cerebral blood flow possible if brachiocephalic artery damaged or compressed.
- Mediastinoscopy morbidity rate 1.5–3.0%, mortality 0.09%, haemorrhage 0.73%.

Further reading
Plummer, S., Hartley, M., Vaughan, R.S. (1998). Anaesthesia for telescopic procedures in the thorax. *British Journal of Anaesthesia*, **80**, 223–34.

Double-lumen tubes (DLT)

Indications for DLT
- Pulmonary surgery.
- Avoid contamination of lung secondary to infection, haemorrhage, bronchopulmonary lavage.
- Control distribution of ventilation if large air leaks or unilateral lung disease (e.g. giant bullae, lung cysts).

Double-lumen tubes
- Bronchocath single-use PVC:
  - 28–41 Fr, low-pressure, high-volume cuff
  - transparent with coloured endobronchial cuff for fibreoptic recognition
  - right-sided tubes have a slot for ventilation of RUL
- Robertshaw:
  - small, medium, or large, red-rubber, reusable
  - high-pressure, low-volume cuff

Pre-insertion checks
- What size?
  - use largest DLT that passes without difficulty through the glottis
  - 39–41 Fr Bronchocath (large or medium Robertshaw) for males, 35–37 Fr for females (medium or small Robertshaw)
- Which side?
  - left-sided DLT usually used. Easier to place and avoids problems with right upper lobe orifice (2.5 cm from carina)
  - will need right-sided DLT if surgery on left mainstem bronchus
- Cuffs and connectors:
  - check both bronchial and tracheal cuffs and connectors prior to insertion

Insertion of DLT
- Insert DLT initially with concavity facing anteriorly.
- Once tip is past the glottis, withdraw the stylet and rotate tube through 90° in direction of the bronchus to be intubated.
- To aid endobronchial intubation, rotate the patient's head to the side opposite the bronchus to be intubated.
- Advance the tube gently.
- Height determines depth of insertion.
- Usually 29 cm at the teeth in men, 27 cm in women.
- Depth increases by 1 cm for each 10 cm in height.
- Inflate the tracheal cuff and confirm ventilation of the lungs.
- Inflate bronchial cuff slowly (usually <3–4 mL air).

Checking position of DLT
- Clinical confirmation:
  - inflate tracheal cuff
  - check ventilation via bronchial lumen
  - clamp flow to tracheal lumen and open tracheal lumen to air

- inspect for correct unilateral chest movement (be aware of pre-op pathology) and confirm air entry to all lobes by auscultation
- check for leaks around the bronchial cuff
- inflate bronchial cuff slowly to abolish leak. If >4 mL air required, then DLT position incorrect, or incorrect size for the patient (care with cuff volume, bronchial rupture reported)
- check ventilation of contralateral lung by reconnecting tracheal limb and switching clamp to bronchial limb. Open bronchial lumen, and check selective ventilation by inspection and auscultation
- Fibreoptic confirmation:
  - 'gold standard' for checking placement of DLT
  - pass scope via tracheal lumen, visualize carina, and open main bronchus
  - superior surface of the bronchial cuff should be visible at the carina
  - ensure no bronchial cuff herniation into lower trachea
  - pass scope down endobronchial limb of right-sided DLT to check correct positioning of 'slit' opposite RUL orifice
  - scope can also be used to 'railroad' the DLT into the appropriate main bronchus if placement is difficult

Paediatric implications

- Smallest available DLT in this country is 28 Fr and is unsuitable for patients under 30 kg.
- Bronchial blockers are available that pass through 3.5 mm ID ETT.
- Single-lumen ETT with 'built in' bronchial blocker available from 5.5 mm ID.

Special considerations

- Position of DLT should always be checked following repositioning of patient or if difficulty with ventilation and oxygenation.
- Recommendations to avoid DLT-induced tracheobronchial injury are to inflate cuffs slowly, limit intra-cuff pressure to <30 cmH$_2$O, avoid N$_2$O, deflate endobronchial cuff when not needed, on turning patient, and repositioning the DLT.
- Olympus LF-DP fibrescope (external diameter 3.1 mm) goes down all DLTs. Standard intubating fibrescope (ED 4.0 mm) is a tight fit down 37 Fr and may not fit down 35 Fr.

Further reading

Campos, J.H. (2007). Which device should be considered the best for lung isolation: double-lumen tube versus bronchial blockers. *Current Opinion in Anaesthesiology*. **20**, 27–31

Klein, W., Karzai, W., Bloos, F. et al. (1998). The role of fibreoptic bronchoscopy in conjunction with the use of a double lumen tube for thoracic anaesthesia. *Anesthesiology*, **88**, 346–50.

⑦ Bronchial blockers (BB)

Definition
Balloon-tipped luminal catheters that occlude the operative bronchus.

Indications for use
Inability to place DLT, distorted anatomy, difficult intubation, tracheostomy, patient <30 kg, limited mouth opening, ITU patient already intubated, planned postoperative ventilation.

Function
Block main-stem bronchus or segmental bronchi to facilitate single lung ventilation or selective lobar blockade.

Types
- Wire-guided bronchial blocker (Arndt)
- Single-lumen ETT with enclosed bronchial blocker (Univent)
- Fogarty embolectomy catheter

'Arndt' wire-guided endobronchial blocker
- 7 Fr (use 7.0 mm ETT) or 9 Fr catheter (use at least 8.0 mm ETT)
- 65 or 78 cm in length
- Inner lumen 1.4 mm diameter
- Inner lumen contains flexible nylon wire, exits as a small flexible wire loop.
- Advantages:
  - passes through nasotracheal tube
  - use if tracheostomy *in situ*
  - can be used as selective lobar blocker
  - allows CPAP through inner channel
  - useful if anticipated or actual difficult intubation with DLT
  - guided directly into position with fibrescope
  - high-volume, low-pressure cuff
- Disadvantages:
  - difficult to pass if ETT <7.0 mm internal diameter
  - wire cannot be re-inserted once removed (repositioning difficult)
  - small suction channel (increased time to lung collapse when compared with DLT)
  - takes longer to place than DLT
- Placement:
  - passes through single-lumen ETT
  - attach 'Arndt multi port' adaptor and maintain ventilation
  - lubricate the distal part of the blocker
  - fully deflate balloon to prevent damage
  - insert blocker through port
  - insert FOB through port and place FOB through loop on the blocker
  - pass FOB into appropriate bronchus
  - slide blocker down over FOB into bronchus
  - advance far enough so that deflated cuff is within bronchus
  - withdraw FOB into trachea and check blocker position
  - inflate balloon (5–8 mL air for bronchial blockade)
  - once position confirmed with FOB, remove wire loop

- Complications:
  - malposition (reported as more frequent than with Univent)
  - prone to dislodgement when moving to lateral position
  - balloon shearing has been reported when withdrawn through multiport. Withdraw blocker along with multiport connector and not through unlocked blocker port

'Univent' endobronchial blocker
- Single-lumen tube, sizes from 3.5 to 9.0 mm ID.
- Tube incorporates a channel enclosing a moveable bronchial blocker.
- Advantages:
  - can block right, left, or any specific secondary bronchi
  - non-latex, small lumen for suctioning and oxygenation
- Disadvantages:
  - bronchial rupture reported, high-pressure, low-volume cuff
- Placement:
  - lubricate bronchial blocker
  - retract blocker into standard lumen of ETT
  - place tube in trachea and insert FOB
  - advance BB into appropriate bronchus under FOB vision
  - inflate cuff of blocker and listen for leaks
  - outer surface of cuff should be just below carina
  - end of Univent tube should be at least 1–2 cm above tracheal carina
- Complications:
  - failure to achieve lung separation (no seal, abnormal anatomy)
  - inclusion of blocker in stapling line (communication with surgeon!)
  - prolonged suctioning to facilitate lung collapse can cause pulmonary oedema (use low pressure for just a few seconds)
  - lung rupture has been reported (blind insertion)
  - malposition and displacement when turning patient

Fogarty embolectomy catheter
- Least commonly used, minimal literature to support use.
- 80 cm length, 0.5–10 mL air to achieve occlusion of bronchus.
- Passed down ETT or as a separate device external to ETT.
- Positioned in appropriate bronchus under vision with FOB or via rigid bronchoscope.
- Ideal position is with superior surface of cuff 10 mm distal to carina.
- Advantages:
  - can be passed through single-lumen ETT
  - used for selective lobar blockade
  - can be used with tracheostomy
  - can be used nasally
- Disadvantages:
  - high-pressure, low-volume cuff
  - vascular device, not designed for bronchial blockade
  - made of natural rubber latex
  - cannot suction or oxygenate
  - cannot be coupled with FOB placement

- Complications:
  - minimal use, so no complications reported, risk of airway rupture, but very soft catheter
  - inclusion in stapling line if used for selective lobar blockade

Further reading

Campos, J.H. (2003). An update on bronchial blockers during lung separation techniques in adults. *Anesthesia and Analgesia*, **97**, 1266–74.

Hammer, B., Fitzmaurice, B.G., Brodsky, J.B. (1999). Methods for single lung ventilation in pediatric patients. *Anesthesia and Analgesia*, **89**, 1426–9.

Regional anaesthesia

Matt Grayling

⊕ Local anaesthetic toxicity

Definition
Toxicity due to excessive local anaesthetic blood levels.

Presentation
- Light headedness, dizziness, drowsiness. Tingling around lips, fingers, or generalized. Metallic taste, tinnitus, blurred vision.
- Confusion, restlessness, incoherent speech, tremors or twitching, leading to full-blown convulsions with loss of consciousness and coma.
- Bradycardia, hypotension, cardiovascular collapse, and respiratory arrest.
- ECG changes (prolongation of QRS and PR interval, AV block and/or changes in T-wave amplitude)

Immediate management
- Discontinue injection.
- ABC ... 100% O_2.
- Intubate and ventilate if required to prevent hypoxic cardiovascular collapse. Hyperventilate may help by increasing pH in the presence of metabolic acidosis.
- CPR if pulseless—commence ALS protocol (see p5).
- Treat convulsions with midazolam (3–10 mg), diazepam (5–15 mg), lorazepam (0.1 mg/kg), propofol (20–60 mg) or thiopental (50–150 mg). Titrate against patient response.
- Consider cardiopulmonary bypass if available.
- Consider treatment with lipid emulsion.

Lipid emulsion therapy
- Give an intravenous bolus injection of Intralipid® 20% 1.5 mL/kg over 1 min (100 mL for a 70 kg patient).
- Start an intravenous infusion of Intralipid® 20% at 0.25 mL/kg/min (400 mL over 20 min for a 70 kg patient).
- Repeat initial bolus twice at 5 min intervals if an adequate circulation has not been restored.
- After 5 min, double the infusion rate if an adequate circulation has not been restored.
- Continue CPR and infusion until a stable adequate circulation has been restored.
- Propofol is NOT a suitable alternative to Intralipid® 20%.
- Mechanism thought to be through extraction of lipophilic local anaesthetics from aqueous plasma and tissues or by counteracting the LA inhibition of myocardial fatty acid oxidation.

Subsequent management
- Simple, short-lived toxicity—observe and then consider if surgery can proceed.
- Hypotension may be treated with small doses of vasopressors— ephedrine, phenylephrine, noradrenaline, or adrenaline.
- If cardiac arrest or complicated reaction has occurred, ICU admission.

- Cardiac problems usually occur after central nervous manifestations and include a reduction in myocardial contractility and conduction velocity, depression of the sinoatrial node leading to bradycardia, ventricular arrhythmias and cardiac asystole.
  - bradycardia should be treated with atropine
  - ventricular arrhythmia:
    — amiodarone may be used as a 150 mg IV bolus over 5 min
    — bretylium has been recommended, but is not always available
    — if due to adrenaline, will usually settle spontaneously, but may be treated with low doses of a beta-blocker

Investigations

- Heparin or EDTA plasma sample for local anaesthetic blood levels.
- If Intralipid® used, also collect blood in plain tube to measure plasma triglyceride concentrations.
- Report findings to National Patient Safety Agency (www.npsa.nhs.uk) and to www.lipidrescue.org

Risk factors

- Intravenous regional anaesthesia
- Large volumes/high concentrations of local anaesthetics
- Location of local anaesthetic injection (e.g. lumbar plexus/intercostal blocks higher risk)
- Failure to aspirate before and during injection
- Use of agent with narrow therapeutic window, e.g. bupivacaine vs. prilocaine

Exclusions

- Fainting—vasovagal episodes are common. If cerebral anoxia occurs, convulsions may result.
- 'Acute anxiety' reaction sometimes associated with adrenaline-containing solutions.
- Epilepsy.
- Allergic reaction to LA (rare) or other drugs administered.
- Anaphylaxis.

Paediatric implications

- Since most regional blocks are carried out in anaesthetized children, many of the early warning signs of toxicity are masked. CVS collapse may be the first sign.
- Ensure dose and concentration are appropriate for size.
- Small children are more prone to methaemoglobinaemia than adults.
- **Case reports of successful treatment with Intralipid® 20% are starting to appear.**

Special considerations

- Table 8.1 lists the maximum doses of some LAs.
- Incidence of significant local anaesthetic toxicity is between 10–20/10 000 for peripheral nerve blocks and 4/10 000 for epidurals.

- Bupivacaine binds to myocardial ion channels and may result in prolonged cardiac arrest. Resuscitation should include treatment of arrhythmias and should be continued for longer than normal (at least up to 1 h). Inotropes may be required.
- Lidocaine has been used to displace bupivacaine from myocardial binding sites but is also negatively inotropic.
- Bretylium (7 mg/kg) stabilizes the myocardium by exerting an LA effect and can be used in LA-induced arrhythmias.
- Allergic reactions to local anaesthetics are extremely rare. The ester groups are more prone to exhibit allergic reactions than amides because they are metabolized to para-aminobenzoic acid (PABA) which acts as a hapten. There is also a cross-sensitivity of ester-type of LAs with sulphonamides. Allergic reactions range from simple local irritation, rash or urticaria, to laryngeal oedema or anaphylaxis.

Table 8.1 Maximum local anaesthetic drug doses

Drug	Max. dose for infiltration (mg/kg)	Max. dose for plexus anaesthesia (mg/kg)
Lidocaine	4	5
Lidocaine with adrenaline	7	7
Bupivacaine	2	2
Bupivacaine with adrenaline	3	3
Prilocaine	6	7
Prilocaine with adrenaline/ Octapressin	8	8

Avoiding toxicity

- Maximum dose varies depending on site to be anaesthetized, vascularity of the tissues, individual tolerance, and anaesthetic technique.
- Aspiration during regional techniques should be gentle, as the side wall of a small blood vessel is easily sucked on to the needle/catheter.
- Epidurals:
  - use a test dose. When giving large volumes, give increments
  - gentle aspiration or allowing the catheter to hang below patient level for a few moments (observing for blood or clear fluid) is a sensible precaution
  - inadvertent intrathecal injection of 3 mL 0.5% bupivacaine or lidocaine will be quickly apparent clinically (paraesthesia and decreased sensation in lower limbs and buttocks, depression or absence of knee jerk reflexes in sedated patients)
  - use of adrenaline in the test dose may help to identify an intravascular injection. 3 mL of 1:200 000 (15 μg) adrenaline injected intravenously will cause an increase in heart rate of 20 bpm and systolic blood pressure of 15 mmHg. However, these changes are short-lived and can be missed unless ECG and frequent BP monitoring is employed
  - risk associated with subsequent 'top-ups': the incidence of catheter migration is estimated to be 1 in 255
- Levobupivacaine and ropivacaine are less toxic than bupivacaine. The higher toxicity of bupivacaine is related to the R-enantiomer which binds more firmly and is released more slowly from the myocardium. Although ropivacaine is less toxic than bupivacaine, in clinical practice, a higher concentration of ropivacaine is required.
- Toxicity from prilocaine is less likely because of its rapid metabolism (primarily by the liver). Methaemoglobinaemia may occur with high doses (>600 mg in an adult) and should be treated with methylthioninium chloride (methylene blue) (1–2 mg/kg).

Further reading

Guidelines for the management of severe local anaesthetic toxicity. www.aagbi.org/publications/guidelines/docs/latoxicity07.pdf

Veering, B.T. (2003). Complications and local anaesthetic toxicity in regional anaesthesia. *Current Opinion in Anaesthesiology*, **16**, 455–9.

! Epidural abscess

Definition

Abscess formation in the extradural space.

Presentation

- Classically four phases—spinal ache, root pain with or without paraesthesia, weakness, and paralysis at or below relevant nerve roots.
- Sphincter dysfunction.
- Pyrexia, general feeling of malaise, headache, neck stiffness or meningism, leading to full-blown meningitis.
- Possible evidence of skin infection with localized tenderness at site of recent needle puncture. However, some are haematologically seeded rather than tracking infections.

Immediate management

- Bloods for culture, FBC, C-reactive protein, coagulation screen.
- Document findings of a full neurological examination.
- Organize an urgent MRI scan and liaise with neurosurgical team.
- Monitor neurological function regularly to assess deterioration.

Subsequent management

- Neurosurgical opinion and usually exploration. Although there have been reports of successful conservative management, surgical decompression via laminectomy is the usual treatment of choice for patients with neurological deficit.
- Prolonged high-dose antibiotic therapy (including an anti-staphylococcal agent).
- Two successful reports on non-surgical drainage via fluoroscopically guided Tuohy needles have been described, involving irrigation of the abscess site with saline or antibiotics.
- Careful review of neurological loss/recovery.
- Likely outcomes—complete recovery (39%), residual neurological deficit (48%), death (13%). Poor outcome associated with increasing age (risk doubles with every decade of life), degree of thecal sac compression and duration of symptoms.
- Outcome worsened by delays in diagnosis and surgery. Adversely affected by the use of steroids.

Investigations

- Frequent neurological observations to assess trend
- FBC, serial C-reactive protein, coagulation screen, and blood cultures
- MRI scan

Risk factors

- Recent epidural or spinal.
- Time epidural catheter in situ (40% increased risk per day).
- General abdominal and thoracic surgery.
- Re-connection of separated filters and frequency of syringe/infusion changes.
- Diabetes mellitus (20–50% of cases), steroid therapy (worsens outcome), systemic and localized infection, HIV infection, pregnancy, alcoholism and cirrhosis.

- Malignancy, immune deficiency, degenerative joint disease.
- Intravenous drug abuse (10–40% of cases) and patients with indwelling vascular catheters.
- Can occur spontaneously (incidence 0.2–1.2 per 10000 hospital admissions).
- Sources of bloodborne infection including skin, infected indwelling catheters, respiratory tract, urinary tract, dental abscess, bacterial endocarditis, bacteraemia, or septicaemia. Direct spread may occur from osteomyelitis, psoas, paraspinal or retropharyngeal abscess, penetrating injury, or introduction of infection from the exterior by other means.
- Combined factors increase risk considerably.

Exclusions
- Profound but reversible blockade due to excessive LA dose or concentration.
- Epidural haematoma—see p242–3 (epidural abscess has a slower onset, 24–48 h vs. ≤24 h, and is associated with pyrexia and signs of sepsis).
- Malignancy has a much slower, insidious onset.

Special considerations
- The quoted incidence accompanying epidural catheterization in the obstetric population is between 1:2000 and 1: 505 000. These figures may be affected by case clusters or by under-reporting.
- Contrast-enhanced MRI has now superseded myelography as a means of confirming a clinical diagnosis of epidural abscess. Epidural abscesses that contain no gas are difficult to diagnose on MRI without contrast enhancement as pus gives a similar image to cerebrospinal fluid. Gadolinium–diethylenetriamine penta-acetic acid (Gd–DTPA) enhances actively inflamed tissue, delineating the abscess cavity more clearly.
- *Staphylococcus aureus* is consistently the most commonly isolated causative organism (50–90% of cases). MRSA is an increasingly prevalent organism and TB may be the causative organism in the immunocompromised.
- Permanent neurological damage is likely if surgery is delayed for more than 12 h.
- Often slow neurological recovery, despite surgical decompression of abscess, suggests that local pressure is not the only mechanism. Ischaemia due to leptomeningeal vessel thrombosis or spinal artery compression may be involved.
- Meticulous documentation is important.

Further reading
Grewal, S., Hocking, G., Wildsmith, J.A.W. (2006). Epidural abscesses. *British Journal of Anaesthesia*, **96**(3), 292–302.

Kindler, C.H., Seeberger, M.D., Staender, S.E. (1998). Epidural abscess complicating epidural anesthesia and analgesia. An analysis of the literature. *Acta Anaesthesiologica Scandinavica*, **42**, 614–20.

Mercer, M., McIndoe, A.K. (1998). Co-incidental diagnosis of an extradural abscess while siting an extradural catheter for postoperative analgesia. *British Journal of Anaesthesia*, **80**, 45–7.

National audit of major complications of central neuraxial block in the United Kingdom. www.roca.ac.uk/index.asp?pageID=717

Reihsaus, E., Waldbaur, H., Seeling, W. (2000). Spinal epidural abscess: a meta-analysis of 915 patients. *Neurosurgery Review*, **23**, 175–204.

ⓘ **Epidural haematoma**

Definition
Haematoma in the extradural space.

Presentation
- Unexpected neurological deficit following epidural and severe localized pain at the level of the haematoma. Neurological deficit may lag behind symptoms of pain (can be completely painless).
- Sensory/motor block at or below relevant nerve root distribution. Unilateral or bilateral.
- Spinal cord compression at the level of the epidural haematoma may produce urinary retention or incontinence, faecal incontinence, hemiplegia, or paraplegia.

Immediate management
- Discontinue infusion of local anaesthetic.
- Optimize systemic blood pressure, avoid hypotension.
- Document findings of an immediate, full neurological examination.
- Monitor neurological function regularly to assess any deterioration.
- Organize an urgent MRI scan and liaise with neurosurgical team.
- Restore normal coagulation.
- Surgical evacuation of the haematoma. For optimal results surgery should take place within 12 h of diagnosis. Surgery beyond this time has a worse outcome but neurological improvements can still be expected.

Subsequent management
Neurosurgical monitoring—meticulous documentation is important.

Investigations
- Frequent neurological observations to assess trend.
- FBC, C-reactive protein, coagulation screen, blood cultures.
- Arrange urgent MRI. If MRI is not available, CT myelography or conventional myelography may reveal a mass.

Risk factors
- Rarely, can occur spontaneously (incidence <1 in 150 000).
- Female, old age, history of gastrointestinal bleeding.
- Bleeding disorders or altered bleeding state (e.g. haemophilia, platelet deficiency, pre-eclampsia).
- Anticoagulation (e.g. warfarin, LMWH, heparin, etc.).
- Traumatic epidural or spinal technique.
- Spinal surgery.
- Removal or accidental displacement of extradural catheter shortly after VTE prophylaxis dose.
- Thrombolytic therapy—risks may exist for up to 10 days following the use of epidurals if a vessel was damaged during insertion or removal of the catheter.

Exclusions

- Epidural abscess—slower onset and associated with pyrexia and signs of sepsis (see pp240–1).
- Malignancy has a much slower, insidious onset.

Special considerations

- Use of minimal concentration of local anaesthetics reduces the incidence of unintended motor blockade and may allow earlier detection of neurological deficit.
- Concurrent use of several preparations (e.g. NSAIDs, clopidogrel, warfarin, LMWH) may increase the risk of haematoma without influencing clotting/platelet test results.
- Table 8.2 gives recommendations for central neuraxial blockade and anticoagulation.

Further reading

National audit of major complications of central neuraxial block in the United Kingdom. www.roca.ac.uk/index.asp?pageID=717

SreeHarsha, C.K. *et al.* (2006). Spontaneous complete recovery of paraplegia caused by epidural hematoma complicating epidural anesthesia: a case report and review of literature. *Spinal Cord*, **44**, 514–17.

Table 8.2 Recommendations for central neuraxial blockade and anticoagulation

Drug	Type	Recommendations	Notes
Thrombolytic therapy	rt-PA, streptokinase, etc.	Avoid administration for 10 days following block. Avoid block after thrombolysis therapy—time period unknown	Very high risk. Fibrinogen level *may* be useful indicator
Unfractionated heparin	Minidose SC	No contraindication to neuraxial block. If possible, delay dose until after block	Check platelet count after 4 days' therapy
	IV Intra-operative administration	Give heparin >1h after block. Do not remove catheter until 2–4h after dosage and repeat APTR	If bloody/traumatic tap, discuss need for heparin with surgeon
	Full IV anticoagulation (cardiac surgery)	Unknown risk if undertaken after neuraxial block	
LMWH	Pre-op. dose	Block more than 10–12h after dose	Anti-Xa levels not helpful
	High-dose treatment	Block more than 24h after last dose	
	2h before surgery (general surgery)	Avoid neuraxial block	
	Post-op. od dosing	First dose more than 6–8h post-op. Epidural catheter removed more than 10–12h after last dose and more than 2h before next dose	If bloody/traumatic tap, delay post-op. dose for 24h
	Post-op. bd dosing	Increased risk of haematoma. Give first dose more than 24h post-op. Remove catheter more than 2 h before *first* dose	
Warfarin	Long term	Stop 4–5 days pre-op. INR <1.5	Monitor INR
	Pre-op.	Check INR if first dose more than 24h pre-block, or more than one dose administered	No useful test of function

Drug	Type	Recommendations	Notes
Anti-platelets	NSAIDs	No increased risk	
	Clopidogrel	Stop for 7 days pre-block	
	Ticlopidine	Stop for 14 days pre-block	
	Abciximab	Stop for 24–48 h pre-block	Avoid for 28 days post-block
	Eptifibatide, tirofiban	Stop for 4–8 h pre-block	Avoid for 28 days post-block
Synthetic pentasaccharide	Fondaparinux (Arixtra®) 2.5 mg od	First dose more than 6 h post-op. Epidural catheter removed >36 h after last dose, and 12 h before next dose (omit one treatment)	

Source: Adapted from Second ASRA Consensus Conference on neuraxial anesthesia and anticoagulation (2003). *Regional Anesthesia and Pain Medicine*, **28**, 172–9.

⊕ Total spinal

(See also 'Total Spinal—Obstetrics', p160)

Definition

Blockade of all spinal nerves including CNS.

Presentation

- Profound onset of regional block within seconds to minutes following administration of local anaesthetic into the spinal, subdural, or epidural space.
- Tingling in fingers or hands warns of block to T1. Nauseated or faint due to severe fall in BP and/or bradycardia. Dilated pupils late sign when the brainstem becomes involved.
- Initial difficulty in breathing due to intercostal paralysis (T1–T12) may progress to gasping and respiratory arrest due to diaphragmatic paralysis (C3–C5). Inability to cough or difficulty in speaking or whispering suggests onset of phrenic nerve block.
- Initial tachycardia (from hypotension) followed by bradycardia (cardiac accelerator fibres T1–T4 or activation of the Bezold–Jarisch reflex). Other cardiac arrhythmias may occur.

Immediate management

- ABC … 100% oxygen. Reassure conscious patient that they are safe.
- Secure airway with ETT and ventilate as necessary. Unconscious patient will not need a GA. Conscious patient will need a GA or sedation as dictated by blood pressure.
- Raise legs to increase venous return (pillows/Trendelenburg).
- Monitor SpO_2, ECG, and BP.
- Establish large-bore intravenous infusion—infuse colloids or crystalloids 1000 mL stat. Repeat as necessary.
- Treat bradycardia with atropine 0.6–1 mg IV.
- Treat hypotension with IV vasopressors:
  - ephedrine 6–9 mg boluses
  - metaraminol 1–2 mg boluses
- Adrenaline 100 μg boluses—if not responding or imminent cardiac arrest.

Subsequent management

- If cardiovascular stability achieved, it is possible to proceed with urgent surgery.
- Patient may require ventilation for 2–4 h and block will regress from cranial to spinal. Sedation (propofol infusion ideal) when consciousness starts to return.
- Transfer to ICU post-op.
- Provide explanation to the patient afterwards.
- A total spinal during labour is not necessarily an indication for a CS—unless fetal distress occurs. After recovery, an assisted forceps delivery may be indicated. Hypotension should be managed appropriately.

Investigations
Clinical diagnosis

Risk factors
- 'Large' dose spinal anaesthesia—particularly in parturients, short, or obese patients
- Epidural anaesthesia without effective test dose or following dural tap
- Subdural catheter placement (may present with an unexpectedly high block, often with sacral sparing)
- Combined epidural/spinal anaesthesia
- Multiple attempts at siting epidural
- Caudal block
- Retrobulbar, interscalene, stellate ganglion block

Exclusions
- Vasovagal
- IV injection of LA may present as sudden loss of consciousness with or without convulsions and cardiovascular collapse.
- Anaphylaxis
- Hyperventilation may cause tingling in fingers in an anxious patient.
- Sensation of breathing difficulties occurs in spinals due to intercostal blockade.

Paediatric implications
- Same basic principles as in adults—although fluids may be more useful than vasopressors.
- Use appropriate needle size while doing caudal. Avoid cephalad advancement of needle further than absolutely necessary into caudal epidural space.

Special considerations
- Vasopressors are more effective than fluids to reverse hypotension, but both are required.
- Document incident in detail, since there is the possibility of medicolegal claim.
- Offer explanation and reassurance to the relatives and patient upon recovery. Write to GP with copy of letter to patient so details are understood.
- There should be no permanent sequelae if handled correctly. Total spinal was previously used as anaesthetic to reduce blood loss.

⊙ Intravenous regional anaesthesia: cuff deflation

Definition
Premature release of tourniquet during intravenous regional anaesthesia (IVRA), releasing large dose of local anaesthetic into the circulation.

Presentation
- Signs of LA toxicity—see pp236–8
- Cardiovascular collapse
- Convulsions

Immediate management
- Apply immediate proximal pressure to axilla (or groin if leg cuff).
- Re-inflate cuff to minimize amount of LA entering circulation.
- ABC ... 100% O_2.
- CPR if pulseless—commence ALS protocol (see p5).
- Cardiovascular support.
- Treat arrhythmias.
- Treat convulsions with midazolam (3–10 mg), diazepam (5–15 mg), or thiopental (50–150 mg).
- Consider the use of cardiopulmonary bypass if available.
- Consider lipid emulsion therapy (see p236).

Subsequent management
- Monitor vital signs (HR, BP, respiration).
- Neurological assessment.

Investigations
Clinical diagnosis

Risk factors
- Inappropriate or faulty equipment including gas supply. A double-cuff tourniquet should be used.
- Swapping cuff inflation to diminish tourniquet pain.
- Obese patient with large arm, very muscular arm, hypertensive patient.
- Complications are agent- and dose-dependent. Prilocaine is less toxic than bupivacaine and considerably safer. Lidocaine and ropivacaine have been investigated but have an inferior therapeutic index and/or offer no clinical benefits.

Exclusions
- Vasovagal.
- Epilepsy.
- True allergy to local anaesthetics or to any other drugs administered (reaction may be restricted distally to tourniquet)..
- Anaphylaxis (consider mast cell tryptase and/or skin testing).

Special considerations
- Always site a second cannula in contralateral limb before starting the procedure.
- Do not remove tourniquet for at least 20 min after injection of local anaesthetic.
- Monitor patients undergoing IVRA by talking to them.
- Never use bupivacaine for IVRA.

ⓘ Injection of adrenaline-containing local anaesthetic around digit

Definition
Inadvertent injection of adrenaline-containing solutions around end-arteries (e.g. digit, penis).

Presentation
- Error discovered on checking syringes.
- Pallor, blanching in affected digit, possibly pain and paraesthesia.

Immediate management
- Assess blood flow to the digit using pulse oximeter, capillary return, or blanching.
- Usually the effect is temporary, so observe over 30 min.
- Massage may help to disperse the solution.
- Injecting papaverine (40 mg in 20 mL saline; unlicensed use) into the affected area may relieve arterial spasm. Alternatively, use of 1 mL lidocaine 2% with 0.15 mg phentolamine has been described.
- Consider warming the affected area—it may hasten digit ischaemia, but may also relieve arterial spasm.
- Consider use of regional block technique (e.g. brachial plexus block) to increase blood flow.
- Do nothing (see below).

Subsequent management
If ischaemia remains severe after 30 min, refer for urgent vascular surgical review.

Investigations
Pulse oximetry of affected digit

Risk factors
- Concentration of adrenaline injected
- Volume injected
- Concurrent infection
- Use of mechanical tourniquets

Exclusions
Using a high volume of local anaesthetic for ring blocks can stop arterial blood flow due to a pressure effect. Massaging the area is usually effective.

Special considerations

The established tradition of avoiding adrenaline for extremity blocks is weakly supported by limited numbers of case reports involving unknown concentrations of adrenaline and other confounding variables (e.g. infection). No case reports of digital gangrene exist following the use of commercial lidocaine with adrenaline preparations, despite a number of case series and randomized controlled trials supporting its routine use. As always a balance of risk should be struck between the use of adrenaline in local anaesthetics and the potential advantages it may bring through the avoidance of mechanical tourniquets and prolonged analgesia.

Further reading

Denker, K. (2001) A comprehensive review of epinephrine in the finger: to do or not to do. *Plastic and Reconstructive Surgery*, **108**, 114–24.

Thomson, C.J. *et al.* (2006). Randomised double-blind comparison of duration of anaesthesia among three commonly used agents in digital nerve block. *Plastic and Reconstructive Surgery*, **118**, 429–32.

Wilhelmi, B.J. *et al.* (2001). Do not use epinephrine in digital blocks: myth or truth? *Plastic and Reconstructive Surgery*, **107**, 393–7.

ⓘ **Retrobulbar haemorrhage**

Definition
Bleeding behind the globe from puncture of vessels in the orbital cone usually following retrobulbar or peribulbar block.

Presentation
- Rapid onset of proptosis with a taut, immovable eye. Increase in intraocular pressure—may be high enough to be palpable (>26 mmHg).
- Pain, decreased visual acuity, and ophthalmoplegia.
- Blood may be visible in the subconjuctival space and eyelid.

Immediate management
- Withdraw needle.
- Main danger is retinal/optic nerve ischaemia due to retrobulbar pressure preventing blood flow through the central retinal artery.
- If haemorrhage is mild, then gentle external pressure for 20–30 min in sitting position may reduce bleeding. However, excessive pressure in the presence of raised intraocular pressure may further disrupt retinal artery circulation and worsen ischaemia.
- If haemorrhage is severe—discuss further management immediately with ophthalmic surgeon.
- Degree of haemorrhage is usually assessed clinically. A severe haemorrhage is indicated by:
  - globe that feels stony hard (compare with normal eye)
  - immobile globe due to severe proptosis
  - inability to close eyelid
  - pain
  - decreased blood flow in central retinal artery on fundoscopy (pale/white optic disc, white blood vessels)
- If circulatory compromise suspected, a lateral canthotomy is performed as a temporary measure to relieve pressure by increasing retrobulbar volume.

Subsequent management
- Formal decompression is carried out as an emergency under GA. Surgery within 2 h has an improved outcome.
- Acetazolamide (250–500 mg IV) or mannitol (0.5 g/kg) can be used to reduce intraocular pressure. Steroids may reduce inflammation and stabilize cell membranes against ischaemic damage.

Investigations
- Measure intraocular pressure using a tonometer (normal 10–21 mmHg).
- Record keeping is essential and all observations must be recorded.

Risk factors
- Use of sharp vs. blunt needles (sub-Tenon's block)
- Retrobulbar block/retrobulbar needle placement
- Long needles (>25 mm)
- Patients on anticoagulant (INR >2.0) or antiplatelet drugs
- Bleeding disorders (e.g. haemophilia, thrombocytopenia)
- Severe hypertension

Exclusions
- Accidental intraocular injection of local anaesthetic following inadvertent globe perforation—presents as severe, acute rise in intraocular pressure, associated with severe pain (see p254).
- Proptosis due to large volume of local anaesthetic agent.
- Allergic reaction to local anaesthetic.

ⓘ **Globe perforation**

Definition
Accidental perforation of the globe during administration of a local anaesthetic eye block.

Presentation
- Operator may feel sudden loss of resistance as the needle perforates globe, or notices marked globe deviation followed by sudden return to neutral gaze. If in doubt, ask patient to look right then left with needle *in situ*. May be single perforation (entry) or double perforation (entry and exit).
- Patient may experience sudden severe intraocular pain or sudden loss of vision.
- Poor red reflex (vitreous haemorrhage).
- 50% of cases of globe perforations go unrecognized at the time of their occurrence.

Immediate management
- Refer to surgeon for indirect ophthalmoscopy. Will look for puncture sites, retinal detachment, and vitreous haemorrhage.
- Surgery should be postponed.

Subsequent management
Management may be conservative, or may involve cryo/laser if vitreous haemorrhage, vitreous contraction, or retinal detachment occur.

Investigations
Urgent indirect ophthalmoscopy. 'B' scan (ultrasound) if dense cataract

Risk factors
- Abnormally shaped globe: long eye (myopic >26 mm axial length), enophthalmos, staphyloma.
- Previous extraocular surgery, e.g. for strabismus.
- Sharp needles vs. blunt needles. Sharp needles are more likely to perforate sclera but blunt needles that do perforate are likely to cause more intraocular trauma.
- Elevated, adducted gaze in an inferotemporal needle insertion increases the risk of optic nerve and macular damage.

Exclusions
Intraneural injection (optic nerve)

Further reading
Thind, G.S., Rubin, A.P. (2001). Local anaesthesia for eye surgery—no room for complacency. *British Journal of Anaesthesia*, **86**, 473–6.

Metabolic and endocrine

☣ Anaphylaxis

(See also 'Paediatric anaphylaxis', pp128–9)

Definition

Anaphylaxis is a severe, life-threatening, generalized or systemic hypersensitivity reaction.

Presentation

- There is a lack of consistent clinical manifestations and a wide range of possible presentations.
- Most common presentations include cardiovascular collapse (88%), erythema (48%), bronchospasm (40%), angioedema (24%), cutaneous rash (13%), and urticaria (8%).

Immediate management of anaphylaxis during anaesthesia.

- Stop any likely trigger agents including IV colloids, latex, and chlorhexidine. Maintain anaesthesia if necessary with an inhalational agent.
- Call for help and note the time.
- Maintain airway and give 100% oxygen.
- Exclude airway/breathing system obstruction. Intubate if necessary and ventilate with oxygen.
- If the patient is hypotensive, elevate the legs or tip the operating table head-down.
- If appropriate, start CPR immediately according to ALS Guidelines (see p5).
- Give adrenaline intravenously. An initial dose of 50 µg (0.5 mL of 1:10 000) is appropriate. Several doses may be required if there is hypotension or bronchospasm.
- If several doses of adrenaline are required, consider starting an adrenaline infusion IV. CVS instability may last several hours and 5% of cases relapse.
- Start rapid IV infusion with crystalloid. Adult patients may require 2–4 litres.

Subsequent management

- Give antihistamines (chlorphenamine 10 mg by slow IV injection).
- Give corticosteroids (200 mg hydrocortisone IV 6-hourly).
- If BP does not recover despite an adrenaline infusion consider adding in another vasopressor such as metaraminol.
- May need bronchodilators for persistent bronchospasm. Salbutamol 250 µg IV or 2.5–5 mg by nebulizer. Aminophylline 250 mg by slow IV injection (up to 5 mg/kg)—not if taking theophylline. Consider giving magnesium sulphate.
- Refer to ITU.
- Check for airway oedema by letting the cuff down prior to extubation and ensuring there is a leak.

Investigations

- Take three blood tests for mast cell-released tryptase, each 5–10 mL clotted blood:
  - as soon as feasible after resuscitation has started—do not delay resuscitation to take the sample
  - 1 h after the reaction
  - 24 h after the reaction or in convalescence. This is a measure of baseline tryptase levels
- Store sample at −20°C until it can be sent for measurement of serum tryptase.
- Elevated serum tryptase indicates the reaction was associated with mast cell degranulation, and rises after both anaphylactic and anaphylactoid reactions. A negative test does not completely exclude anaphylaxis.
- Plasma histamine rises during the first several minutes of a reaction and generally stays up briefly; measurement is impractical because it requires special collection and handling techniques. Whether measurement of urinary methylhistamine is useful in documenting anaphylaxis remains to be demonstrated.
- The patient should be referred to a regional allergy centre. With the referral send:
  - photocopies of anaesthetic chart
  - photocopies of drug chart
  - description of reaction and time of onset in relation to induction
  - a note of tests sent and their time
  - A standard referral form can be found on the AAGBI website under 'Suspected Anaphylactic Reactions Associated with Anaesthesia'.
- The allergist will perform skin-prick tests to GA drugs 4–6 weeks after the reaction. Specific IgE antibodies in the serum can be measured for suxamethonium.
- Suspected anaphylactic reactions associated with anaesthesia should be reported to the Commission on Human Medicines (CHM) and on a 'Yellow Card'.

Risk factors

- No valid predictor of anaphylaxis—history of previous exposure not necessary.
- Factors which increase severity include asthma, beta-adrenoceptor blockade, hypovolaemia, and neuraxial anaesthesia. These are associated with a reduced endogenous catecholamine response.

Exclusions

- Breathing circuit obstruction:
  - filter or catheter mount obstruction
  - kinked ETT
  - cuff herniation
  - endobronchial intubation/tube migration
- Check breathing system not at fault—disconnect breathing circuit distal to all connections/filters and ventilate directly with a self-inflating bag. If inflation pressure still feels high, the problem is due to airway/ETT obstruction or reduced compliance.
- Foreign body in the airway.
- Air embolus.

- Tension pneumothorax:
  - history of CVP line insertion or trauma
  - trachea not central
- Severe bronchospasm.
- Type IV allergy—localized cutaneous reaction to a substance. This is T-cell mediated and is not life-threatening. It occurs 6–48h after exposure. In the medical context it is generally an allergy to chemical accelerators used in the manufacture of both latex and synthetic gloves.

Paediatric implications

See pp128–9.

Special considerations

- UK Resuscitation Guidelines recommend the IM route for adrenaline administration as the best compromise between safety and speed of onset for most healthcare workers. IV adrenaline should only be given in specialist settings by those familiar with its use (e.g. anaesthetists), and if the patient is monitored and IV access is already available. It should not be given without continuous ECG monitoring because of the risk of precipitating dysrhythmias, especially in the presence of hypoxia and acidosis. SC adrenaline should be avoided because absorption time is extremely erratic.
- Latex anaphylaxis during anaesthesia presents in an atypical fashion. Most cases present 30–60min after induction. This coincides with either a delayed airborne exposure or with mucous membrane exposure at the beginning of the surgical procedure. Minimize risks by using a breathing circuit filter, non-latex gloves, and avoiding parenteral injection of latex corings from antibiotic bottles and IV-giving sets.
- 'Diprivan' TCI syringes are latex-free.

Further reading

Hepner, D.L., Castells, M.C. (2003). Anaphylaxis during the perioperative period. *Anesthesia and Analgesia*, **97**, 1381–95.

The Association of Anaesthetists of Great Britain and Ireland and British Society for Allergy and Clinical Immunology. (2008). Suspected anaphylactic reactions associated with anaesthesia. www.aagbi.org

UK Resuscitation Guidelines. www.resus.org.uk/pages/reaction.pdf

☤ Diabetic ketoacidosis

Definition
Acute, severe, uncontrolled diabetes characterized by hyperglycaemia, ketonaemia, and acidosis.

Presentation
- 2–3-day history of gradual deterioration, associated with polydipsia, polyuria, abdominal pain, nausea and vomiting, dehydration, and drowsiness.
- Triad of hyperglycaemia (blood glucose >10 mmol/L), ketonaemia (ketonuria—urinary ketones ≥3+), and acidaemia (pH <7.3).

Immediate management
- Assess ABC and conscious level.
- Calculate degree of dehydration and give 0.9% saline. Replace fluid deficit (average about 6 L) over 24 h. Give the average patient 1 L over 1 h followed by 1 L over 2 h, 1 L over 4 h, 1 L over 6 h, and then 8-hourly fluids. Be careful in elderly patients or those with cardiac dysfunction.
- Check serum potassium (K^+). If K^+ <3.3 mmol/L, withhold insulin and give 40 mmol K^+ over 1 h until K^+ level is ≥3.3 mmol/L. If K^+ ≥3.3 mmol/L start insulin infusion at 0.1 unit/kg/h). The actual amount of insulin given is less important than regular monitoring of the blood glucose, pH and K^+. If the blood glucose decreases by >5 mmol/h, then reduce insulin to 0.05 units/kg/h).
- If serum K^+ is 3.3–5.5 mmol/L, give 20 mmol K^+ in each litre of IV fluid, to keep level at 4–5 mmol/L. If serum K^+ ≥5.5 mmol/L, do not give potassium but check every 2 h.

Subsequent management
- Once glucose <11 mmol/L, switch to 5% glucose and 0.45% saline or 5% glucose depending on sodium levels.
- Prescribe insulin sliding scale.
- Measure glucose hourly.
- Investigate cause of diabetic ketoacidosis.
- Depending on severity of presentation, patient may require arterial line, CVP, and nasogastric tube.

Investigations
- To diagnose DKA—blood glucose, ABGs, dipstick urine
- To assess cause—FBC, U&Es, CRP, troponin I, cultures, MSU, ECG, and CXR

Risk factors
- Usually occurs with type I diabetes, but may occur with type II.
- Caused by infection, omission of/or inadequate insulin, medical illness (i.e. MI), or initial presentation of diabetes mellitus.

Exclusions

Severe metabolic acidosis in the absence of hyperglycaemia due to:

- Sepsis
- Renal failure
- Salicylate overdose
- Inborn errors of metabolism
- Alcoholic ketoacidosis
- Hyperosmolar non-ketotic coma (marked hyperglycaemia but no detectable ketoacidosis)

Paediatric implications

- See guidelines prepared for the British Society of Paediatric Endocrinology and Diabetes (web address in Further reading).
- Involve paediatricians early.

Special considerations

- The likelihood of intraoperative cardiac arrhythmias and hypotension is much reduced if the metabolic decompensation can be at least partially reversed prior to surgery. However, delaying surgery where the underlying condition will continue to exacerbate ketoacidosis is futile.
- Resuscitation should be continued perioperatively.
- If surgery necessary, hyperventilate to maintain respiratory compensation for metabolic acidosis—check ABGs.
- Sodium bicarbonate is virtually never indicated. A small percentage of patients who have diabetic ketoacidosis present with metabolic acidosis and a normal anion gap. Therefore, they have fewer ketones available for the regeneration of bicarbonate during insulin administration. Consider bicarbonate in this subset of patients or if pH <7.0 and compromised.

Hyperglycaemic, hyperosmolar, non-ketotic coma

- Only occurs in NIDDM.
- Patient is often old and presenting for the first time.
- Presents with a long history, marked dehydration, and a glucose >35 mmol/L.
- There is sufficient insulin to prevent lipolysis and ketogenesis, so no acidosis.
- Osmolality is >340 mOsm/kg.
- Treat as for DKA but give 0.45% saline if plasma Na^+ >150 mmol/L.
- Give insulin at 0.05 units/kg/h.

Risk of DVT is high and full heparin anticoagulation has been advised, despite inadequate clinical evidence for this. Heparin 5000 units SC is probably adequate if aggressive fluid replacement is instituted, but if thrombosis is suspected, full heparinization and radiological studies are warranted.

Further reading

BSPED recommended DKA guidelines (2001). http://www.bsped.org.uk/dka.htm

Chiasson J. Aris-Jilwan N. Belanger R. Bertrand S, Beauregard H. Ekoe J. Fournier H. Havrankova J. (2003) Diagnosis and treatment of diabetic ketoacidosis and the hyperglycemic hyperosmolar state. *Canadian Medical Association Journal*, **168**(7), 859–66.

Kian, K., Eiger, G. (2003). Anticoagulant therapy in hyperosmolar non-ketotic diabetic coma. *Diabetic Medicine*, **20**, 603.

☠ Malignant hyperthermia

Definition
Inherited disorder of skeletal muscle that can be triggered pharmacologically to produce a potentially fatal combination of hypermetabolism, muscle rigidity, and muscle breakdown.

Presentation
- Earliest indication is masseter muscle spasm following suxamethonium—defined as excess and prolonged jaw rigidity (2–4 min). NB Only 30% with masseter spasm as the sole sign go on to develop MH.
- Tachypnoea in the spontaneously breathing patient, or a rise in end-tidal CO_2 if mechanically ventilated, unexplained tachycardia, generalized muscle rigidity, progressing to hypoxaemia.
- Rise in body temperature is a later sign. Raised plasma CK and myoglobinuria occur even later. At this stage, hyperkalaemia, cardiac arrhythmias, and DIC are likely to develop.

Immediate management
- Discontinue volatile agents and give 100% oxygen.
- Call for help.
- Hyperventilate with high fresh gas flows and new breathing circuit (do not continue with circle).
- **Do not** switch to a system or machine that allows rebreathing, or limits hyperventilation.
- If intubation is required, **do not** use suxamethonium.
- Expedite surgery and maintain anaesthesia with intravenous drugs, e.g. propofol and opioid
- Give dantrolene—the only drug that is effective in limiting the accumulation of calcium ions within the muscle cell. Give intravenously in doses of 1 mg/kg up to 10 mg/kg until the tachycardia, rise in CO_2 production, and pyrexia start to subside. The average dose is 3 mg/kg. Warm solution to increase solubility and give through a blood administration set.

Subsequent management
- Commence active cooling by infusing cold IV solutions, applying ice to the axilla/groins, applying a cooling blanket. Avoid peripheral vasoconstriction which will prevent heat loss. Cold-flush nasogastric tube or urinary catheter.
- Take regular blood gas and electrolyte measurements. Acidosis and hyperkalaemia should be anticipated and treated using bicarbonate and insulin with glucose.
- Measure clotting and creatine kinase (peaks at 12–24 h after episode).
- Limit renal tubular damage from myoglobin by maintaining a diuresis of at least 2 mL/kg/h preferably with alkalinized urine (0.2–0.5 g/kg mannitol ± 1 mL/kg 8.4% sodium bicarbonate when $PaCO_2$ is within normal limits).

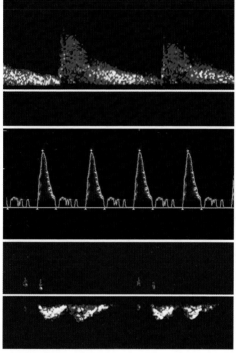

Plate 1 Typical CardioQ® waveforms.

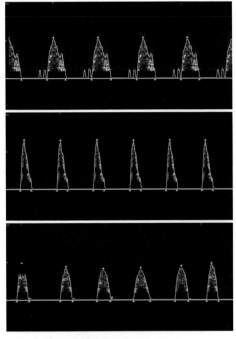

Plate 1 (cont.) Typical CardioQ® waveforms.

- Treat coagulopathies and arrhythmias as usual. Do not use calcium-channel blocking drugs, which in combination with dantrolene can produce marked cardiac depression.
- Transfer to ITU.
- After crisis, give dantrolene 1 mg/kg every 4–6 h for 24 h.

Investigations
- ABGs, U&Es, CK, FBC, and clotting
- Muscle biopsy for *in vitro* contracture testing (see below)

Risk factors
- Family history.
- May occur despite previously uneventful anaesthetics.
- History of unexpected death of relative during anaesthetic (50% risk of being MH).
- 1:10 000–1:15 000 patients.

Exclusions
- Inadequate anaesthesia/analgesia.
- Infection/sepsis—sepsis may present with tachycardia and pyrexia, with a metabolic acidosis which requires respiratory compensation; whereas MH presents with tachycardia, hypertension, and a mixed respiratory and metabolic acidosis. Both may cause a reduction in PaO_2 and subsequently SaO_2.
- Tourniquet ischaemia can cause tachycardia, hypertension and in children in particular, a rise in core temperature. End-tidal CO_2 will rise briefly when tourniquet is released, but then symptoms settle.
- Anaphylaxis. Check blood pressure—usually decreased in anaphylaxis.
- Phaeochromocytoma.
- Thyroid storm.

Paediatric implications
In children <20 kg, give dantrolene in doses of 1 mg/kg up to 10 mg/kg as required.

Special considerations
Confirmation of diagnosis
- MH is confirmed by *in vitro* contracture testing (IVCT) using a muscle biopsy from the vastus medialis taken under regional anaesthesia. The tissue is exposed to halothane and caffeine and the tension measured.
- MH is an inherited disorder so once a case is confirmed, further family members are investigated. DNA analysis can aid diagnosis but cannot be used in isolation.

Anaesthesia for susceptible patients

- Avoid trigger agents (Table 9.1).
- Use regional anaesthesia where appropriate.
- For general anaesthesia, prepare the anaesthetic machine by removing vaporizers and flushing the machine and ventilator with 100% oxygen at maximum flows for 20–30 min. Use a new breathing circuit. Prophylactic dantrolene is not needed. It has side-effects of nausea and vomiting, muscle weakness, and prolongation of non-depolarizing muscle relaxants.
- Monitor closely for signs of MH.
- Can be discharged 4 h after surgery if no problems.

Table 9.1 Trigger and safe agents in MH

Trigger agents for MH	Safe agents to use in MH
Suxamethonium	Nitrous oxide
All volatile agents	IV anaesthetic agents including ketamine
	Benzodiazepines
	Non-depolarizing neuromuscular blocking drugs
	Local anaesthetics
	Opioids
	Neostigmine
	Atropine
	Glycopyrronium
	Metoclopramide
	Droperidol

Further reading

Halsall, P.J. (2006). Malignant hyperthermia. In *Oxford Handbook of Anaesthesia*, Second Edition (ed. K.G. Allman, I.H. Wilson), pp. 260–5, 894–5. Oxford University Press, Oxford.

Hopkins, P.M. (2000). Malignant hyperthermia: advances in clinical management and diagnosis. *British Journal of Anaesthesia*, **85**, 118–28.

Malignant Hyperthermia (2003). CEPD reviews. *British Journal of Anaesthesia*, **3**, 1.

Rosenberg, H. (2007) Malignant hyperthermia. *Orphanet Journal of Rare Diseases*, **2**, 21.

⊙ **Porphyric crisis**

Definition

The porphyrias are a group of inherited or acquired enzymatic defects of haem synthesis.

Presentation

- Autonomic neuropathy—acute abdominal pain (lasts days), vomiting, constipation, hypertension, tachycardia, fever, and postural hypotension.
- CNS changes—confusion, hysteria, depression, convulsions. Peripheral neuropathy: motor > sensory.
- Red/purple urine—Hyponatraemia secondary to inappropriate secretion of ADH.

Immediate management

- Withdraw possible precipitating factors.
- Rehydrate with IV fluids.
- Aim is to decrease haem synthesis and the production of porphyrin precursors. High doses of glucose (400 g/day) can inhibit haem synthesis and are useful in treating attacks. If possible, give carbohydrate loading orally or via nasogastric. If not, give 10% glucose IV.
- Give propranolol for hypertension and tachycardia.

Subsequent management

- Treat any underlying infection. Treat pain with any opioid apart from pentazocine. Treat nausea with prochlorperazine. Avoid metoclopramide. Treat seizures with diazepam, propofol, or magnesium sulphate. Avoid barbiturates and phenytoin.
- For severe attacks, particularly those with neurological symptoms, treat with haem arginate (3 mg/kg IV once daily for 4 days). This provides negative feedback to the haem synthetic pathway and shuts down production of porphyrins and precursors. It can lead to intense thrombophlebitis so should be given through a central line.
- Refer to ITU.

Investigations

- U&Es, urinary porphobilinogen, and 5-aminolaevulinic acid
- A raised urine porphobilinogen is pathognomic of the acute attack

Risk factors

- Maintain a high index of suspicion in first-degree relatives of those with porphyria presenting with the features expressed above.
- Only acute porphyrias can precipitate a crisis—acute intermittent porphyria, variegate porphyria, hereditary coproporphyria, and plumboporphyria (very rare).
- Precipitating factors for a crisis may be drugs, dehydration, fasting, stress, infection, fluctuations in hormone levels during menstruation/pregnancy, alcohol.
- Patients are at greatest risk on first presentation since an abdominal emergency may be simulated.

Exclusions

- Acute abdomen—appendicitis, diverticulitis, biliary problems, pyelonephritis.
- Acute neurology, predominantly motor, can mimic Guillain–Barré syndrome.
- Manic–depressive illness.

Paediatric implications

Acute crises usually occur from puberty to 40 years of age, but porphyrinogenic drugs should be avoided in all children with a family history.

Special considerations

Anaesthetic drugs considered safe to use in a porphyric crisis

- Provided appropriate precautions are taken, most patients with acute porphyria can tolerate surgery and GA.
- It is difficult to be precise about which drugs definitely cause a porphyric crisis, since crises can also be triggered by infection or stress (Table 9.2).
- For further details on safe drugs to use in a porphyric crisis, see the Further reading list for the University of Queensland, Department of Medicine website..
- In certain cases, regional anaesthesia may be preferred to general anaesthesia, in which case bupivacaine is the LA of choice. In the presence of any peripheral neuropathy, detailed preoperative examination and documentation are essential.
- Remember, the onset of a porphyric crisis may be delayed for 5 days after exposure to a porphyrinogenic drug.

Further reading

James, M.F.M., Hift, R.J. (2000). Porphyrias. *British Journal of Anaesthesia*, **85**, 143–53.

Jenson, N.F., Fiddler, D.S., Streioe, V. (1995). Anaesthetic considerations in porphyria. *Anesthesia and Analgesia*, **80**, 591–9.

University of Queensland Department of Medicine website: *www.uq.edu.au/porphyria*

Table 9.2 Safety of drugs in porphyria

	Definitely unsafe	Probably safe	Controversial
Induction agents	Barbiturates, etomidate	Propofol	Ketamine
Inhalational agents	Enflurane	Nitrous oxide, ether, cyclopropane	Halothane, isoflurane, sevoflurane, desflurane
Neuromuscular blocking agents	Alcuronium	Suxamethonium, tubocurarine, gallamine, vecuronium	Pancuronium, atracurium, rocuronium, mivacurium
Neuromuscular reversal agents		Atropine, glycopyrronium, neostigmine	
Analgesics	Pentazocine	Alfentanil, aspirin, buprenorphine, codeine, fentanyl, paracetamol, pethidine, morphine, naloxone	Diclofenac, ketorolac, sufentanil
Local anaesthetics	Mepivacaine, ropivacaine	Bupivacaine, prilocaine, procaine	Cocaine, lidocaine
Sedatives	Chlordiazepoxide, nitrazepam	Lorazepam, midazolam, temazepam, chlorpromazine, chloral hydrate	Diazepam
Anti-emetics and H_2-antagonists	Cimetidine, metoclopramide	Droperidol, phenothiazines	Ondansetron, ranitidine
CVS drugs	Hydralazine, nifedipine, phenoxybenzamine	Adrenaline, α-agonists, β-agonists, β-blockers, magnesium, phentolamine, procainamide	Diltiazem, sodium nitroprusside, verapamil
Others	Aminophylline, oral contraceptive pill, phenytoin, sulphonamides		Steroids

:☼: Thyrotoxic storm

Definition

Life-threatening exacerbation of hyperthyroid state with evidence of decompensation in one or more organ systems. Mortality 20–30%.

Presentation

- Usually 6–24 h after surgery. Hyperpyrexia—temperature $\geq 41°C$, sweating. CNS dysfunction including agitation, delirium, and coma. May present as renal failure secondary to rhabdomyolysis
- CVS signs:
  - sinus tachycardia >140 bpm
  - atrial fibrillation or ventricular arrhythmias
  - hyper- then hypotension
  - congestive cardiac failure (25%)
- GI symptoms:
  - nausea and vomiting
  - diarrhoea
  - hepatocellular dysfunction with jaundice

Immediate management

- ABC … 100% oxygen.
- Rehydrate with IV saline and glucose, due to large insensible losses and depletion of hepatic glycogen stores. Heart failure may occur, particularly in the elderly.
- Treat hyperpyrexia with tepid sponging and paracetamol. **Do not** use NSAIDs or aspirin as these displace thyroid hormone from serum binding sites.
- To treat hyperadrenergic state give propranolol (1 mg increments IV up to 10 mg) with CVS monitoring (may precipitate CCF). Aim to decrease pulse rate to <90 bpm. Or give esmolol (loading dose 250–500 µg/kg followed by continuous infusion of 50–100 µg/kg per minute). Alternatively, use the antiadrenergic agent reserpine intramuscularly 2.5–5.0 mg qds (unlicensed).
- Give hydrocortisone (200 mg IV qds) to treat adrenal insufficiency and to decrease T_4 release and conversion to T_3 at very high levels.
- Dantrolene has been used with effect in treating thyroid crisis. High circulating T_4 has an effect on calcium flux across the sarcoplasmic reticulum and dantrolene may inhibit this pathological mechanism.

Subsequent management

- Give propylthiouracil (1 g loading dose via NG tube followed by 200–300 mg qds). This inhibits thyroid hormone release and also decreases the peripheral conversion of T_4 to T_3.
- Following blockade with propylthiouracil, give sodium iodide (500 mg tds IV), or potassium iodide (5 drops qds via NG) or Aqueous Iodine Oral Solution (Lugol's iodine) (5–10 drops qds via nasogastric). Iodine can exacerbate release of thyroid hormone if given without prior propylthiouracil.
- Transfer to ITU post-op.

Investigations
- T_3, free T_4, and TSH (but levels correlate poorly with severity)
- U&Es—hypercalcaemia, hypokalaemia (50%), and hypermagnesaemia

Risk factors
- Precipitating factors include intercurrent illness (especially infection), trauma, surgery, uncontrolled DM, labour, and pre-eclampsia/eclampsia.
- A crisis is precipitated intraoperatively due to excessive palpation of the gland, incomplete preparation, and inadequate doses of beta-blockers preoperatively.

Exclusions
- Malignant hyperthermia—do not get mixed metabolic and respiratory acidosis in thyrotoxic storm and no raised CK.
- Phaeochromocytoma—would not expect pyrexia in phaeochromocytoma.
- Infection, sepsis.

Special considerations
- It is important to establish an adequate depth of anaesthesia to avoid exaggerated sympathetic nervous system responses.
- Reversal of muscle relaxants should include glycopyrronium instead of atropine.
- Treat any intraoperative hypotension with a direct-acting vasopressor, such as phenylephrine.
- Non-cardioselective beta-blockers are more effective (e.g. propranolol). β_1-Adrenergic blockade treats the symptoms of tachycardia, but β_2-adrenergic blockade prevents peripheral conversion of T_4 to T_3.

Further reading
Bennett, M.H., Wainwright, A.P. (1989). Acute thyroid crisis on induction of anaesthesia. *Anaesthesia*, **44**, 28–30.

Farling, P.A. (2000). Thyroid disease. *British Journal of Anaesthesia*, **85**, 15–28.

:✚: Undiagnosed phaeochromocytoma

Definition
A functionally active catecholamine tumour of chromaffin cells typically found in the adrenal medulla (90%).

Presentation
- Sustained or paroxysmal hypertension, arrhythmias, MI.
- Most likely to occur during induction of anaesthesia/endotracheal intubation, or tumour manipulation.
- History of severe headache, anxiety, palpitations, tremor, weakness, chest pain, faintness, paraesthesia, drenching perspiration, facial pallor, anxiety, and tremor.

Immediate management
- Stop all noxious stimuli immediately, administer opioids and deepen inhalational anaesthesia to at least 2 MAC.
- Give phentolamine (1–2 mg increments IV up to 20 mg) to control hypertension. Titrate according to blood pressure. This is a competitive α_1- and α_2-blocker with a half-life of 10–15 min.
- Alternatively/additionally, give magnesium sulphate, which inhibits catecholamine release, exerts a direct vasodilator effect, and reduces alpha-receptor sensitivity. Give 5 g (20 mmol) loading dose then 2 g/h (8 mmol/h) to achieve a therapeutic level of 1.5 mmol/L. Beware of giving further muscle relaxation after magnesium.
- Establish arterial line monitoring while establishing BP control.
- If HR >100 bpm or >1:4 VEs after alpha-blockade, give labetalol—predominantly β-blocker (5–10 mg increments IV).
- Abandon surgery, but expedite if already commenced. Do not attempt to remove phaeochromocytoma at this stage.
- Consider sodium nitroprusside. Initial infusion 0.5–1.5 µg/kg per min. Titrate to BP with mean dose of 3–5 µg/kg/min.
- Control further tachyarrhythmias with esmolol (1.5 mg/kg bolus IV).

Subsequent management
- Transfer to ITU. Maintain magnesium (2 g/h), or sodium nitroprusside, until established on phenoxybenzamine or doxazosin orally.
- 24-hour urine collection for free catecholamines.
- Do not rebook for theatre until patient is stabilized with alpha-blockers (phenoxybenzamine up to 30 mg twice daily or doxazosin up to 16 mg daily).

Investigations

- 24-h collection for urinary catecholamines, vanillylmandelic acid, and metanephrine.
- Serial ECGs, CK-MB, troponin, and echocardiogram for evidence of acute and chronic heart damage.

Risk factors

Can be associated with other syndromes:

- MEN type-2 syndrome (phaeochromocytoma, medullary thyroid carcinoma, hyperparathyroidism)
- MEN type-3 syndrome (phaeochromocytoma, medullary thyroid carcinoma, mucosal ganglioneuromas, Marfinoid habitus)
- Von Hippel–Lindau disease (phaeochromocytoma, retinal angiomas, hemangioblastoma of CNS, renal and pancreatic cysts, renal cell carcinoma)
- Neurofibromatosis

Exclusions

- Inadequate anaesthesia/analgesia
- Uncontrolled hypertensive disease during stimulating surgery or when in pain postoperatively
- Pre-eclampsia
- Raised intracranial pressure
- Cocaine/amphetamine abuse
- Thyroid storm—fever sweating, and tachycardia dominate
- Malignant hyperthermia—get mixed respiratory and metabolic acidosis

Paediatric implications

- Phaeochromocytomas are more often multifocal and extra-adrenal in children when compared to adults.

Special considerations

- Perioperative undiagnosed phaeochromocytoma carries a 50% mortality.
- Excess catecholamine secretion results in vascular contraction and a relatively low intravascular volume. α-Blockers cause a fall in peripheral resistance, mainly by a reduction in arteriolar tone. β-Blockers can then be used to counteract the resulting tachycardia. β-Blockade should never be instituted until α-blockade is fully established, as unopposed α–stimulation may lead to severe hypertension and fulminant congestive cardiac failure. Labetalol is not suitable as a solo therapy despite being both an α- and β-blocker. When given IV it is seven times more potent at β-adrenoceptors than α-adrenoceptors; following oral administration the relative potencies are 3 to 1.

Further reading

Prys-Roberts, C. (2000). Phaeochromocytoma—recent progress in its management. *British Journal of Anaesthesia*, **85**, 44–57.

☼ Addisonian crisis

Definition
Primary adrenal insufficiency secondary to autoimmune adrenalitis or infectious adrenalitis (TB, AIDS, and fungal infections).

Presentation
- Severe hypotension or hypovolaemic shock, usually refractory to fluids and vasopressors.
- Acute abdominal pain, vomiting, and hyper- or hypothermia. May be misdiagnosed as having an acute abdomen.
- Mild hyponatraemia, hyperkalaemia, hypoglycaemia, and mildly elevated urea may be present.
- Addison's disease is typified by weakness, fatigue, and excess pigmentation.
- In patients with type-I diabetes, deterioration of glycaemic control with recurrent hypoglycaemia can be the presenting sign of adrenal insufficiency.

Immediate management
- ABC … 100% oxygen.
- IV fluids: colloids to restore blood volume, saline 0.9% to replace Na^+ deficit and glucose for hypoglycaemia.
- Hydrocortisone 200 mg stat followed by 100 mg qds.
- Inotropes/vasopressors as required. May be resistant in the absence of cortisol replacement.

Subsequent management
- Need to treat primary cause or precipitating factor. Give antibiotics as clinically indicated.
- Refer to ITU.

Investigations
- U&Es and glucose.
- Baseline cortisol and ACTH prior to administration of hydrocortisone. Short Tetracosactide (Synacthen®) test—no response.
- Take blood, urine, and sputum for culture.
- ECG to exclude MI.

Risk factors
- Usually occurs in someone with Addison's disease, or one who is on long-term steroids but has forgotten to take their medication. Precipitating factors include:
  - surgery
  - trauma
  - cessation of steroid therapy
  - sepsis
  - coagulopathy
  - acute illness
  - burns

- In autoimmune polyendocrine syndrome type 2, onset of autoimmune hyperthyroidism can precipitate adrenal crisis due to enhanced cortisol clearance.

Exclusions
- Acute abdomen
- Septic shock

Paediatric implications
- In children, acute adrenal insufficiency often presents as hypoglycaemic seizures.
- Give hydrocortisone initially 2–4 mg/kg IV.

Further reading
Oelkers, W. (1996). Adrenal insufficiency. *New England Journal of Medicine*, **335**, 1206–11.

:O: Disseminated intravascular coagulation (DIC)

Definition
A serious medical condition that develops when the normal balance between bleeding and clotting is disturbed.

Presentation
- Presents with symptoms relating to underlying disease process.
- DIC can also present with bleeding (64%) or symptoms related to thrombotic complications, i.e. renal dysfunction (25%), hepatic dysfunction (19%), respiratory dysfunction (dyspnoea and cough), shock, and altered consciousness (2%).

Immediate management
- Treat underlying disease.
- Routine replacement of platelet and coagulation factors not indicated in acute DIC unless ongoing bleeding is present or invasive procedures planned. However, most clinicians give platelets if count falls below 20 ×10^9/L.
- When there is significant DIC-associated bleeding and fibrinogen levels <100 mg/dL, give FFP. FFP contains all the coagulation factors and inhibitors deficient during active DIC and lacks traces of activated coagulation factors which may exacerbate the coagulation disorder. It is therefore better to use FFP than cryoprecipitate which may contain some of the activated coagulation factors.

Subsequent management
- Consult a haematologist.

Anticoagulants
The use of anticoagulants in the treatment of DIC remains controversial:
- Antithrombin has been used in patients with sepsis and DIC. However the beneficial effect is not conclusive.
- Activated protein C (APC) concentrates have been found to improve survival over that of heparin in the treatment of DIC.

Other agents
- Recombinant factor VIIa (rFVIIa) may be used in patients with severe bleeding unresponsive to other treatment options.

Investigations
- Diagnosis made from the clinical picture and coagulation tests.
- Check platelet count, fibrin-related markers (D-dimer and fibrin degradation products), fibrinogen, PT and APTT.
- The International Society on Thrombosis and Haemostasis developed a simple scoring system (Table 9.3). A score of 5 or more indicates overt DIC; a score of less than 5 does not rule out DIC but may indicate non-overt DIC.

Table 9.3 Scoring system for DIC

Score	0	1	2	3
Platelet count	>100	<100	<50	
Elevated fibrin marker	No elevation		Moderate increase	Strong increase
Prolongation of PT (s)	<3	>3, <6	>6	
Fibrinogen level (g/L)	>1	<1		

Risk factors

DIC can be caused by:

- Infections (Gram-positive and -negative bacteria, viruses, fungi, and protozoa)
- Malignancy (acute myelocytic leukaemias)
- Obstetrics conditions (placental abruption, amniotic fluid embolism, acute fatty liver of pregnancy, eclampsia, retained dead fetus syndrome)
- Trauma
- Burns
- Snake envenomation
- Blood transfusion
- Acute hepatic failure

Exclusions

- Consumptive coagulopathies, e.g. trauma and major surgery.
- Severe liver disease may result in markedly reduced production of coagulation factors and inhibitors.
- Thrombotic thrombocytopenic purpura.
- Idiopathic thrombocytopenic purpura and heparin-induced thrombocytopenia are both also associated with low platelets with thrombus formation, but do not have the consumptive coagulopathy of DIC which causes APTT and PT to be elevated.

Paediatric implications

- 10–15 mL/kg FFP will increase coagulation factors by 10–20% in ongoing consumption.

Further reading

Franchini, M., Lippi, G., Manzato, F. (2006). Recent acquisitions in the pathophysiology, diagnosis and treatment of disseminated intravascular coagulation. *Thrombosis Journal*, **4**, 4.

:✪: Hypoglycaemia

Definition
- Blood glucose <3.3 mmol/L (normal 3.5–5.5 mmol/L).
- Clinical signs more pronounced <2.5 mmol/L.

Presentation
- Early:
  - shaking
  - pins and needles
  - palpitations
  - slurred speech, headache, double vision
  - hunger
- Intermediate to late:
  - altered behaviour, poor concentration
  - restlessness, sweating
  - fits
  - coma

Immediate management

Conscious patient
- 4 glucose tablets, 3 spoonfuls of sugar (15 g glucose) in warm water, or any high-sugar drink, e.g. Lucozade®.
- Check blood sugar after 10 min, if clinical symptoms remain repeat glucose tablets/sugar drink.
- Glucogel® may be more readily available.
- Once symptoms have resolved, a high-fibre snack or carbohydrate meal should be eaten if the next meal is not due within 1 h. Continue with normal regime.

Unconscious patient
- Establish IV access.
- Give glucose IV—50 mL 20% glucose, otherwise 25 mL 50% glucose (highly irritant, if given peripherally the cannula must be flushed with saline afterwards).
- Repeat if little or no resolution of symptoms after 10 min.
- If no IV access, give glucagon 1 mg IM/SC (lasts 5–10 min)—can also be given IV.
- In cases of insulin or oral hypoglycaemic agents' overdose, start an infusion of 5 or 10% glucose—aim for maintenance of normoglycaemia.
- Consider long-acting carbohydrates once patient is conscious.

Subsequent management
- Give longer acting carbohydrate or glucose infusion if blood sugar remains unstable.
- Liaise with diabetic team to improve blood sugar control.
- Monitor blood sugars closely for 24 h, rebound hypo/hyperglycaemia may occur.
- Investigate cause if not obvious (e.g. incorrect insulin dosage).

Investigations
Blood glucose

Risk factors
- Insulin or oral hypoglycaemic overdose—generally accidental
- Insufficient oral intake—delayed meals, excess activity
- Medical conditions—insulinoma, hypopituitarism, acute liver failure
- Postoperative—pancreatectomy, gastric surgery
- Extremes of age
- Pregnancy
- Alcohol excess
- Severe sepsis, quinine therapy

Exclusions
Any patient with an altered conscious level or CVS instability should have their blood sugar checked, as many conditions can mimic hypoglycaemia:
- excess alcohol intake
- drug overdose
- epilepsy and cerebral irritation of any cause
- sepsis
- cardiogenic shock

Paediatric implications
- Different age groups present differently.
- Children can develop nocturnal hypoglycaemia despite good diabetic control, therefore consider hypoglycaemia in children found collapsed in bed.
- Infants <1 year can develop hypoglycaemia with fasting.
- Neonates:
  - brisk reflexes, lethargy, coma
  - poor feeding
  - hypothermia
  - apnoeas/respiratory distress
  - bradycardia
- Infants/children:
  - sweating
  - hunger/poor appetite
  - anxiety/confusion/bad behaviour/seizures/coma
  - respiratory distress
  - cardiovascular instability
- Treatment:
  - If awake, encourage oral intake of simple carbohydrates, e.g. sugary drinks, milk.
  - If reduced conscious level:
    - 2.5 mL/kg of glucose 10% IV
    - repeat as necessary and infuse to maintain blood sugar >2.5 mol/L
    - glucagon 500 µg IM/SC/IV (1 mg if >25 kg)

Special considerations
- Severe and prolonged hypoglycaemia may result in cerebral oedema. Intensive care and organ support may be required.
- 50% glucose can be highly irritant to blood vessels; therefore care should be taken at time of injection. Avoid use in children due to small vessel size.
- Glucagon is relatively ineffective in liver failure and after alcohol ingestion.
- Ongoing hypoglycaemia in the presence of liver disease may be a marker of acute liver failure.
- Hypoglycaemic attacks in previously well-controlled, insulin-dependent diabetics may indicate secondary pathology, e.g. Addison's disease.
- Patient information and follow-up is vital. Liaise with local diabetic services.
- If the patient is not a known diabetic, investigate other causes.
- In cases of a hypoglycaemic agent overdose , rebound hypoglycaemia can occur after initial treatment, therefore consider transfer to HDU and initiate treatment with 10% glucose.
- NB: Blood glucose range on ABGs is lower than recorded on BM stix.

Further reading
Watkins, P.J. (2003). ABC of Diabetes. BMJ Books, London.

☼: Acute liver failure

Definition

- Encephalopathy and jaundice in individuals with no pre-existing liver disease. Defined according to the speed of onset of encephalopathy:
  - hyperacute: <7 days
  - acute: 7– 28 days
  - subacute: >28 days to 12 weeks

Presentation

- Depends on the underlying cause:
  - non-specific symptoms; nausea, vomiting, abdominal pain
  - jaundice
- Bleeding—deranged INR.
- Cardiovascular instability—patients usually have a high cardiac output with vasodilatation.
- Encephalopathy—grading is essential for management:
  - Grade I—Slow mental function, rousable, altered mood
  - Grade II—Inappropriate behaviour, drowsy but able to talk
  - Grade III—Drowsy, can be agitated or aggressive
  - Grade IV—Coma, may respond to painful stimulus

Immediate management

- Depends on degree of encephalopathy—treatment is supportive initially, i.e. fluids, antibiotics, monitor urine output.
- Grade III/IV encephalopathic patients should be transferred to ITU. Renal support (haemodialysis) nearly always required.
- Do not correct INR unless bleeding as this is used as a marker of hepatic impairment
- In those with paracetamol overdose or where there is a possibility of paracetamol overdose N-acetylcysteine (NAC) should be administered.

Subsequent management

- All patients with encephalopathy should be referred to a specialist liver unit.
- Paracetamol overdose—administer NAC at earliest opportunity (also consider in those whose history is unclear and if overdose is more than 24h previously). Loading dose 150mg/kg followed by an infusion (see *BNF*).
- CVS—many patients require large volumes of fluid and should have CVP monitored. Acute liver failure results in a high cardiac output, vasodilated state, hence inotropes and vasoconstrictors are often required.
- RS—patients with Grade III/IV encephalopathy should be intubated and ventilated to ensure airway protection and control of carbon dioxide in the presence of raised ICP.

- CNS—ICP is elevated in those with encephalopathy. Signs of raised ICP are late and as such ICP monitoring can be useful— ICP monitoring devices should be placed with caution due to concurrent coagulopathy. To reduce ICP consider head-up position, avoid tight ETT ties and practise minimal intervention care. If ICP remains high (>25 mmHg for >10 min) consider mannitol (0.5 g/kg). Maintain a high normal serum sodium (145–150 mmol/L) to help reduce cerebral oedema.
- Metabolic—renal failure is common especially in those with hyperacute liver failure. Haemodialysis/haemofiltration are frequently required and allow some control of the continuing metabolic acidosis. Use lactate-free buffer solutions. Hypocalcaemia and hypoglycaemia can occur. Where hypoglycaemia is a problem an infusion of 10% glucose should be administered centrally and titrated according to blood glucose.
- Coagulation—patients should be crossmatched due to the risk of spontaneous haemorrhage. However FFP should not be used to correct the INR unless bleeding occurs. The INR is used as a measure of hepatic synthetic function and as such reflects severity of disease. Thrombocytopenia also occurs.

Investigations
- To diagnose the cause and assess ongoing status:
  - viral serology
  - FBC, U&Es, LFTs (bilirubin, AST, ALT)
  - clotting—INR is used as an indicator of disease severity
  - monitor blood glucose
  - image hepatic vasculature (ultrasound)
  - send for immunology, microbiology (urine, sputum, blood for MC&S) and toxicology—including paracetamol levels

Risk factors
- A thorough history is vital as the cause has implications for management, severity and outcome.
- Infection—ask about recent travel and social history (sexual partners, recreational drug usage, recent tattoos).
- Drugs, e.g. paracetamol overdose (still the commonest cause in the UK), MAOIs, carbamazepine, isoniazid, Ectasy, phenytoin.
- Toxins—mycose phylloides (mushrooms), herbal remedies.
- Vascular anomalies—Budd–Chiari syndrome, ischaemic hepatitis.
- Other—non-A non-B hepatitis, acute fatty liver of pregnancy, lymphoma.

Special considerations
- Antibiotic prophylaxis should be considered early. Patients are prone to fungal infections.
- Early involvement of a specialist liver unit is important for advice and decision making with regard to transplantation.
- Despite advances in managing these patients, there is still a high mortality and morbidity associated with acute liver failure. Those with sub-acute liver failure tend to have the worst prognosis.

Criteria for consideration of liver transplantation in acute liver failure

Paracetamol overdose
- Arterial pH <7.3 (or 7.25 if NAC given)

or
- Prothrombin time >100 s   **and**
- Creatinine >300 µmol/L   **and**
- Grade III/IV encephalopathy

Non–paracetamol
- Prothrombin time >100 s
- **or** three of the following:
- Age <10 or >40 years
- Jaundice >7 days prior to encephalopathy
- Prothrombin time >50 s
- Bilirubin >300 µmol/L
- Aetiology—non-A, non-B hepatitis, drug-induced hepatitis

Further reading

Gagan, K. Sood. (2008). Acute Liver Failure eMedicine. www.emedicine.com/Med/topic990.htm

Lai, W.K., Murphy, N. (2004). *Management of Acute Liver Failure. Continuing Education in Anaesthesia, Critical Care & Pain (CEACCP)*, Vol. 4, Number 2. Oxford University Press, Oxford.

:✪: Sickle cell crisis

Definition
Acute, painful, and life-threatening occlusion of blood vessels by sickle cells. Often accompanied by haemolysis.

Presentation
- Signs of tissue infarction due to reduced blood flow and poor tissue oxygenation. Occlusion of vessels can occur at any site in the body:
  - RS—'acute chest syndrome'—hypoxia, dyspnoea, haemoptysis, chest pain. Long-term respiratory failure with pulmonary hypertension
  - CNS—CVA, blindness, subarachnoid haemorrhages
  - haematological—acute drop in haemoglobin levels, bone marrow failure resulting in neutropenia. Sequestration of cells in the spleen causes thrombocytopenia and increased sickling in the presence of a crisis
  - skeletal and soft tissue—bone pain; disruption of growth plates, leading to gross limb deformities; osteomyelitis and cutaneous ulceration due to skin infarcts
  - abdominal—renal impairment, priapism, haematuria, ileus, jaundice, gallstones, ascending cholangitis/empyema of gallbladder, liver failure
- Evidence of multi-organ involvement due to recurrent episodes of vaso-occlusion.

Immediate management
- Supportive initially, the aim is to break the cycle of sickling. Establish IV access, admit to a specialist ward or HDU, give oxygen and keep warm.
- Analgesia—follow the WHO pain ladder. In addition to NSAIDs and paracetamol, consider:
  - Entonox until IV access achieved
  - morphine 0.1 mg/kg (IV or SC) every 20 min until pain controlled (monitor for respiratory depression), then give 0.05–0.1 mg/kg every 2–4 h
  - PCAs should be prescribed according to local protocols
- Monitor patients every 20 min until pain is controlled, and then at least every 2 h.
- Oxygen and anti-emetics should also be prescribed.
- Fluids—rehydrate, alternating 0.9% saline and 5% glucose with 20 mmol/L KCl, aim to administer 4 L/24 h.
- Oxygen—35% oxygen via facemask:
  - PaO_2 <7.5 kPa (56 mmHg) on oxygen—ventilate on ITU. Exchange transfusion may be indicated in patients with respiratory failure unresponsive to treatment. Discuss with haematology.
  - $PaCO_2$ >6.7 kPa (50 mmHg)—ventilate as likely to worsen.

Subsequent management
- Antibiotics—not routinely indicated unless proven infection.
- Blood transfusion—indicated when Hb <5 g/dL (or decrease of >2 g/dL) and clinical crisis.
  Transfuse to Hb >10 g/dL but <12 g/dL. Aim for HbA >70%. Limitation of blood transfusions reduces the risk of long-term complications.
- Exchange transfusion is at times indicated for major surgery, but specialist advice must be sought from a consultant haematologist.

Investigations
- FBC—including reticulocyte count (see sickle cells, sideroblasts, and Howell–Jolly bodies). 'Sickledex' test—induces sickling in susceptible red blood cells. Hb electrophoresis—to differentiate between homozygous (sickle cell disease) and heterozygous (sickle cell trait).
- G&S, U&Es, LFT, CXR, ABGs, AXR, amylase, CT/MRI.
- Blood, sputum, urine, stool cultures.

Risk factors
- Patients with sickle cell disease after 6 months of age.
- Sickle cell crisis is extremely rare in those with sickle cell trait.
- Hypoxaemia and acidosis.
- Infection of any cause.
- Cold, hypotension, pain, and dehydration.

Paediatric implications
- On admission, prescribe oral, or PR medication: paracetamol (PO: 20 mg/kg/dose 6-hourly), and NSAIDs—diclofenac (1 mg/kg 8–12 hourly) or ibuprofen (5–10 mg/kg 4–6 hourly).
  Apply tetracaine gel.
- If no improvement or deterioration, give morphine 0.05–0.08 mg/kg and repeat at 5-min intervals up to 0.4 mg/kg. Consider prescribing a PCA for those deemed competent.
- Causes failure to thrive.

Special considerations
- Chronic low haemoglobin levels are normal in those with sickle cell disease. Normal Hb is approx. 6–9 g/dL, therefore a low Hb is not in itself an indication for transfusion or cancellation of elective surgery.
- Patients with sickle cell disease have often had multiple admissions, many insist on pethidine for analgesia. If pethidine is used in high doses, then also prescribe carbamazepine 100 mg tds to reduce the side-effects of norpethidine accumulation.
- Many patients have renal impairment therefore use NSAIDs and renally excreted drugs with caution.
- Avoid use of tourniquets, bandages, etc. as they can promote further occlusion of vessels.
- Caution is needed when considering regional techniques for localized pain. Many patients are started on heparin in view of the vaso-occlusive nature of this disease, hence regional techniques are relatively contraindicated.
- Sickle cell crisis is rare in those with sickle cell trait only—consider a different cause for their pain.

Anaesthetizing a patient with sickle-cell disease

- Active management pre-, intra-, and postoperatively of known precipitants—such as dehydration, infection, acidosis, hypothermia, and pain—reduces the likelihood of a sickle crisis developing.
- Fasting times should be kept to a minimum.
- IV fluids should ideally be established the night before theatre.
- Patients should be first on the list.
- Liaise with haematology (preferably the patient's physician) with regard to blood transfusion requirements. Some patients may require exchange transfusion prior to major surgery.
- Preoxygenate and keep inspired oxygen >40% (correct end-tidal volatile concentration appropriately).
- Core temperature measurement—aim for normothermia using warmed IV fluids, Bair Hugger®, ambient theatre temperature control, etc.
- Regional techniques for pain relief should be considered (NB Patients may be receiving anticoagulation for previous crises and may therefore be unsuitable under normal criteria).
- Use of tourniquets has been described in patients with sickle cell disease, but may increase the risk of crisis. Limbs must be exsanguinated fully as sickling can occur locally in vessels.
- Ideally, nurse in a unit experienced at caring for patients with sickle cell disease.
- Postoperative oxygen must be prescribed—ideally for 72 h after surgery.
- Continue with intravenous fluids until patients are receiving free fluids orally.
- Tailor analgesia to the patient's needs—they may require higher than normal doses of analgesics, especially opioids.
- Inform Outreach/Acute Pain Team.

Further reading

Allman, K., Wilson, I. (2006). *Oxford Handbook of Anaesthesia*, (2nd edn), pp. 200–2. Oxford University Press, Oxford.

Claster, S. (2003) Clinical review; managing sickle cell disease. *British Medical Journal*, **327**, 1151–5.

Lucas, S.B., Mason, D.G., Mason, M., Weyman, D. (2008). *A Sickle Crisis: A report of the National Confidential Enquiry into Patient Outcome and Death*. National Confidential Enquiry into Patient Outcome and Death, London.

Rees, D.C., Olujohungbe, A.D., Parker, N.E. *et al.* (2003). Guidelines for the management of the acute painful crisis in sickle cell disease. *British Journal of Haematology*, **120**, 744–52.

Stoddart, P., Lauder, G. (2004). *Problems in Anaesthesia—Paediatric Anaesthesia*. Taylor and Francis, London.

Vijay, V., Cavenagh, J.D., Yate, P. (1998). The anaesthetist's role in acute sickle cell crisis. *British Journal of Anaesthesia*, **80**, 820–8.

⚠ TURP syndrome

(See also 'Hyponatraemia', pp302–3)

Definition
Excess absorption of irrigation fluid during transurethral resection of prostate (TURP).

Presentation

Early
- CVS—bradycardia, hypertension
- GI—nausea and vomiting, abdominal distension
- CNS—anxiety/confusion, headache, dizziness, slow waking after GA.

Late
- CVS—hypotension, angina, cardiac failure
- RS—dyspnoea, tachypnoea, cyanosis (pulmonary failure)
- CNS—twitching, visual disturbance (transient blindness due to glycine), seizures, coma
- GU—renal tubular necrosis, reduced urine output

Immediate management

- ABC ... 100% oxygen.
- Stop irrigation fluid infusion and operation as soon as possible, and insert urinary catheter.
- Take blood for serum sodium levels and haemoglobin—check regularly.
- Give diuretics, e.g. furosemide 20 mg (consider use when operating time exceeds 60 min).

Subsequent management for severe/late TURP syndrome

- Neurological symptoms indicate increasing severity of TURP syndrome.
- Admit all patients with neurological manifestations to ITU as there is a risk of cerebral oedema and respiratory failure.
- Establish invasive monitoring—CVP and arterial line early in severe cases.
- Consider hypertonic saline—to calculate volume of 3% hypertonic saline required:
  - (1) calculate total body water:

    TBW = 0.6 × weight (kg) (e.g. 70-kg man, TBW = 42 L)
  - (2) calculate volume needed to raise serum sodium by 1 mmol/L:

    2 × TBW/1000 = mL of 3% saline (e.g. 2 × 42 = 84 mL of 3% saline
  - (3) calculate need over 24 h and titrate according to serum sodium levels
- Aim to correct serum sodium to 120–125 mmol/L (*should not increase by more than 12 mmol in 24 h*).
- Respiratory and cardiovascular support may be required. Watch for convulsions and consider ICP monitoring.

- Metabolic acidosis can occur, which requires renal support, i.e. haemofiltration.

Investigations
Serum sodium levels

Risk factors
- Related to speed of absorption of irrigation fluid. Generally, absorption is approximately 1–2 L of irrigation per 40 min of operating.
- Large prostate (>45 g).
- Prolonged operation time >90 min.
- Hypotonic fluids given IV intraoperatively.
- Volume of irrigation >30 L.
- Inexperienced surgeon.
- Height of irrigation fluid bag >60 cm above the patient.
- Comorbidities, e.g. liver disease, genitourinary stones, UTI.

Exclusions
Congestive cardiac failure

Special considerations
- Elderly population with myocardial impairment may be more symptomatic due to fluid shifts.
- Regional techniques are thought to reduce the incidence of TURP syndrome:
  - conscious level of the patient can be monitored throughout operation and hence early signs can be identified
  - less absorption of irrigation fluid due to reduced venous pressure in the prostatic bed
- Clinical signs are absent in those under general anaesthesia—watch for unexplained tachycardia and hypertension. If concerned check serum sodium.
- Tracer substances—some centres advocate adding ethanol 10% to irrigation fluid and measuring blood level (>0.6 mg/mL indicative of >2 L absorption).

Further reading
Allman, K.G., Wilson, I.H. (2006). *Oxford Handbook of Anaesthesia*, (2nd edn), pp. 570–1. Oxford University Press, Oxford.

Chambers, A. (2002). Transurethral resection syndrome—It does not have to be a mystery. *AORN (Association of Operating Room Nurses)*, **75**, 155–78.

☼ Hypothermia

Definition

Core temperature   <35°C
- mild   32–35°C
- moderate   28–32°C
- severe   <28°C

Presentation

Varies according to temperature:
- <35°C:
  - apathy
  - confusion and disorientation
  - incoordination
  - shivering
- <32°C:
  - metabolic acidosis and hyperkalaemia
  - hypovolaemia
  - coagulopathy
  - dilated pupils
  - arrhythmias and reduced cardiac output
- <28°C:
  - unconsciousness
  - unresponsive EEG (at 18°C)
  - cardiac dysrhythmias/cardiac arrest, VF and vasoconstriction
  - ECG—J waves
  - diuresis—but loss of concentrating ability of the kidney
  - apnoea
- <15°C:
  - asystole

Immediate management

- ABC ... 100% oxygen.
- Active resuscitation, according to ALS guidelines (p5). Drugs and defibrillation may be ineffective below 30°C. Use active and passive re-warming methods.
- Warming may reveal hypovolaemia.
- Aim to correct hypothermia as quickly as it developed, although this maybe difficult. If time frame is uncertain, aim to increase temperature by 1°C/h.
- Modify immediate management according to clinical situation.

Postoperative hypothermia

Ideally—prevention using warming blankets, warmed fluids, and HME filters on breathing circuits reduces the chance of post-op. hypothermia. If it does develop:
- warm patient using warming blankets
- maintain ambient temperature >21°C
- warm IV fluids and all irrigation fluids

- transfer the patient to recovery, as generally higher ambient temperature than in theatres
- admit to ITU post-op. and warm up slowly prior to waking and weaning

Emergency surgery patient

- ABC … 100% O_2 (warmed to 40–42°C and humidified).
- Passive re-warming:
  - remove wet clothes and dry patient
  - turn up ambient temperature
- Active re-warming:
  - radiant heaters
  - heating blankets and warming mattresses
  - warmed IV fluids—consider using a rapid transfusion system (e.g. Level-1®) if large transfusions are required
- Humidify inspired gases.
- Central access and invasive BP monitoring are mandatory (NB Caution with line insertion, as possible coagulopathy).
- Blood gases—interpret uncorrected (for temperature) arterial blood gases as they are easier to understand and can be used for trend analysis during re-warming.
- Consider warmed fluid for irrigation of body cavities while in theatre.
- Aim to warm to 32–34°C as hyperthermia can be detrimental—hypothermia is thought to be neuroprotective.
- Consider the need for postoperative intensive care early.

Cold immersion/submersion (see also pp122–3)

Immersion—head above water. Patients suffer hypothermia and cardiovascular instability.

Submersion—head below water. Patients develop asphyxiation and hypoxia.
- Both groups are at risk of traumatic injuries.
- Manage cardiac arrest and re-warming as above.
- Vomiting is often seen in submersion victims. If the patient is conscious, place in the recovery position. Unconscious patients require definitive airway control, therefore intubate and ventilate. Decompress the stomach by inserting a large-bore NG tube.
- Submersion victims suffer a multisystem insult and, as such, require Intensive Care support. Both submersion and immersion patients should be invasively monitored if they arrive unconscious.

Resuscitation in the hypothermic patient

- ABC … 100% oxygen, intubate and ventilate, oesophageal temperature probe. Initiate passive and active re-warming.
- Follow ALS protocols, adjusted for hypothermia.
- With a continued fall in core temperature, bradycardia, atrial fibrillation, ventricular fibrillation, and finally asystole develop.
- Hypothermia renders the myocardium unresponsive to drugs, defibrillation, and pacemakers; consider withholding drugs until the patient's temperature is above 30°C. Below this temperature three DC shocks can be tried, but if there is no response then no further shocks should be given until the core temperature is above 30°C.

- At 30°C give drugs required, but at twice the time interval and the lowest recommended dose; resume normal drug protocols from ALS as the patient's temperature approaches normothermia.
- Death cannot be confirmed until profound hypothermia is excluded, i.e. the patient has been re-warmed and there is no cardiac output, or attempts at re-warming have failed. Check for a central pulse for at least 1 min with ECG monitoring, and look for signs of life before withdrawing support.
- If the patient has other life-threatening injuries, or is completely frozen, active resuscitation should probably not be started.
- Chest wall stiffness occurs in hypothermia, which can make chest compressions and ventilation difficult—aim to see the chest move with ventilation, and for 4-cm depression with cardiac massage.
- Central access is vital due to peripheral vasoconstriction (poor access, poor flow, and drug accumulation in vessels with sluggish flow).
- In specialist centres, cardiopulmonary bypass can be used to actively re-warm patients. If this is not available, standard venovenous haemofiltration can be used, and the replacement fluid warmed. The return line from the filter can also be insulated to prevent passive heat loss. Percutaneous bypass lines reduce haemorrhage. In all cases, beware of coagulopathy.
- Active warming causes progressive venous dilatation, therefore large volumes of fluids are likely to be required.
- Regular blood gas and electrolytes/clotting checks:
  - intra-/extracellular electrolyte shifts can develop rapidly, causing hyperkalaemia
  - DIC can also occur, due to failure of the clotting cascade (loss of homeostasis with cold)
  - hypoglycaemia can develop, requiring glucose-containing fluids

Subsequent management
- Most patients require intensive care as multi-organ failure can develop several days after the hypothermic episode. Watch for neurological sequelae.
- Watch limbs, especially digits, for signs of frostbite—amputation may be required.
- Treat infections early.
- Pancreatitis can develop, but may be masked in the initial stages.
- Exclude underlying metabolic disorder, e.g. hypothyroidism, diabetes mellitus.

Investigations
- Core temperature, e.g. oesophageal, rectal, or tympanic (axillary temperature 1°C less than core).
- Thyroid function tests should be considered in patients after successful resuscitation, as undiagnosed hypothyroidism can potentiate hypothermia, especially in the elderly.

Risk factors

- Extremes of age—elderly and infants can become hypothermic very easily.
- Prolonged exposure/near-drowning.
- Impaired conscious level.
- Trauma victims, including those with head injuries.
- Drug overdose—especially antidepressants.
- Endocrine—hypoglycaemia, hypothyroidism.
- Perioperatively—anaesthesia and surgical exposure promote heat loss from the body.

Exclusions

- Hypothyroid
- Diabetes mellitus

Paediatric implications

Survival from severe prolonged hypothermia in children is much greater than that for adults. A long (>1 h) resuscitation time may be required to regain a cardiac output in the hypothermic child.

Special considerations

- Hypothermia occurs all year round and bears no relation to the ambient temperature.
- Hypothermia can be neuroprotective, but hypothermia with comorbidities is a poor indicator of outcome.
- Neuroprotective hypothermia is now recommended for post out-of-hospital cardiac arrest patients.

Further reading

Kirkbridge, D.A., Buggy, D.J. (2003). Thermoregulation and perioperative hypothermia. *British Journal of Anaesthesia CEPD Reviews*, **3**(1), 24–8.

NICE (2008). *Perioperative Hypothermia (inadvertent)*. NICE Clinical Guideline No.65 (April).

ⓘ **Hyperkalaemia**

Definition

Normal serum potassium   3.5–5.5 mmol/L
- mild   5.5–6.0 mmol/L
- moderate   6.1–7.0 mmol/L
- severe   >7.0 mmol/L

Presentation

- Incidental laboratory finding. Acidotic, dehydrated patient ± renal impairment. Nausea, vomiting and diarrhoea.
- Effects on skeletal muscle:
  - generalized fatigue, weakness, paraesthesia, paralysis
- Effects on cardiac muscle:
  - ECG changes progressing through peaked T waves, prolonged PR interval, widened QRS, loss of P wave, loss of R-wave amplitude, sine wave pattern and asystole
  - ECG changes are potentiated by low calcium, low sodium, and acidosis

Immediate management

- Cardiac monitor, IV access.
- Calcium stabilizes the myocardium by increasing the threshold potential.
- If hyperkalaemia severe, or ECG changes are present, give calcium chloride (3–5 mL of 10% over 2 min) or calcium gluconate (10 mL of 10% over 2 min).
- Insulin 10 units in 50 mL 50% glucose IV over 30–60 min.
- If acidotic, give sodium bicarbonate (50 mmol).
- β-Agonist: salbutamol, 5 mg nebulizer (beware tachycardia).

Subsequent management

- Re-check K^+ level frequently.
- Ion-exchange resin—calcium resonium 15 g PO or 30 g PR 8-hourly.
- If initial management fails, will need dialysis or haemofiltration.
- Do not consider elective surgery.
- For life-threatening surgery, first treat hyperkalaemia. Avoid suxamethonium.
- Ascertain and treat cause of hyperkalaemia.

Investigations

U&Es, Ca^{2+}, ABGs, ECG

Risk factors

- Increased intake:
  - ingestion of foods high in K+ (e.g. bananas), or potassium supplements
  - rapid blood transfusion

- Intercompartmental shift:
  - trauma, including crush injuries with rhabdomyolysis, burns
  - suxamethonium (particularly burns and spinal injuries)
  - malignant hyperthermia
  - acidosis
- Decreased excretion:
  - acute or chronic renal failure
  - adrenocortical insufficiency
- Medications—potassium-sparing diuretics, NSAIDs, beta-blockers, digoxin.

Exclusions

Pseudohyperkalaemia (*in vitro* lysis of cells) occurs most commonly during blood-taking due to tourniquet being too tight, or blood left sitting too long. Also occurs in severe thrombocytosis (platelets >1000 × 10^9/L) or severe leukocytosis (WBC >70 × 10^9/L).

Paediatric implications

- Calcium chloride 0.2 mL/kg of 10% solution IV over 5 min, not to exceed 5 mL.
- Calcium gluconate 1 mL/kg of 10% solution IV over 3–5 min, not to exceed 10 mL.
- Glucose (25%) 0.5 g/kg (2 mL/kg) with insulin (0.1 unit/kg) IV over 30 min.

Special considerations

- Do not give Hartmann's or suxamethonium.
- Avoid hypothermia and acidosis. Control ventilation to prevent respiratory acidosis.
- Monitor neuromuscular blockade during anaesthesia. Effects may be accentuated.
- If a rapid assessment of K^+ is required, check a venous sample with blood gas analyser on ITU.

Further reading

Vaughan, R.S. (1991). Potassium in the perioperative period. *British Journal of Anaesthesia*, **67**, 194–200.

① **Hypokalaemia**

Definition

Normal serum potassium 3.5–5.5 mmol/L
- mild   3.0–3.5 mmol/L
- moderate   2.5–3.0 mmol/L
- severe   <2.5 mmol/L

Presentation

- Incidental laboratory finding. Palpitations, muscular weakness, abdominal cramping, nausea and vomiting, arrhythmias, polyuria, respiratory failure, and ECG changes.
- ECG may show small or inverted T waves, prominent U waves (after T wave), prolonged PR interval, and depressed ST segment.

Immediate management

- ABC ... including cardiac monitor and IV access.
- For severe hypokalaemia with cardiac arrhythmias, give KCl at 20 mmol/h via a central line, with cardiac monitoring, and in a high-dependency environment.
- If moderate hypokalaemia, use 40 mmol K^+ in 1-litre bag and infuse peripherally. Consider oral K^+ supplements, but may not be appropriate in perioperative setting. Sando K® two tablets four times a day = 96 mmol K^+.
- Withhold loop or thiazide diuretics.

Subsequent management

- Check K^+ level every 1–2 h initially.
- Ascertain cause of hypokalaemia.
- Decision to proceed to surgery depends on urgency of surgery, rate of onset of hypokalaemia, and comorbidity. Chronic hypokalaemia is less significant than that of acute onset.
- Switch any diuretics to potassium-sparing diuretics (e.g. spironolactone or amiloride).

Investigations

- U&Es, creatinine, Mg^{2+}, Ca^{2+}, PO_4^{3-}, and glucose. ECG. Consider ABGs to check for alkalosis.

Risk factors

- Decreased intake:
  - iatrogenic—No K^+ added to IV fluids
  - malnutrition
- Renal losses:
  - renal tubular acidosis
  - hyperaldosteronism
  - leukaemia
  - magnesium depletion

- GI losses:
  - diarrhoea
  - enemas or laxative use
  - vomiting or nasogastric suctioning
  - intestinal fistula, villous adenoma of rectum
  - pyloric stenosis
- Intercompartmental shift:
  - insulin
  - alkalosis
  - hypothermia
- Drug side-effects:
  - diuretics (most common)
  - steroids
- Beta-adrenergic agonists

Exclusions

- Cushing's syndrome
- Conn's syndrome—suspect if hypertensive, hypokalaemic alkalosis in someone not taking diuretics
- Hypomagnesaemia
- Hypocalcaemia

Paediatric implications

- Dose of KCl is 0.5 mmol/kg over 1 h.

Special considerations

- Potassium depletion sufficient to cause a 0.3 mmol/L drop in serum potassium requires a loss of about 100 mmol of K+ from total body store.
- If bicarbonate is raised, then loss is probably longstanding with low intracellular potassium, and will take days to replace.
- Patients should receive no more than 20 mmol/h potassium, to avoid potential deleterious effects on the cardiac conduction system.
- High concentrations of potassium are damaging to the small peripheral veins, so peripheral infusion of K+ should always be diluted (max. 40 mmol/L). In theatre/ITU/HDU it is easier to give more concentrated solutions of KCl through a central line, to avoid fluid overload.
- Aim for K+ of 4.0 mmol/L in a digitalized patient, since hypokalaemia increases the risk of digoxin toxicity. Aim for a K+ of 4.0–5.0 mmol/L if cardiac arrhythmias are present.
- Always use readymade KCl infusions on safety grounds. If 'Strong' KCl ampoules are used, these should be stored carefully to avoid the risk of inadvertent IV injection.
- Resistant hypokalaemia—check magnesium and correct if low.

Further reading

Wong, K.C., Schafer, P.G., Schultz, J.R. (1993). Hypokalaemia and anaesthetic implications. *Anesthesia and Analgesia*, **77**, 1238–60.

ⓘ **Hypernatraemia**

Definition

Normal serum sodium 135–145 mmol/L
- mild   145–150 mmol/L
- moderate   151–160 mmol/L
- severe   >160 mmol/L—high mortality

Presentation

- Depends on the cause—fluid status of patient is important (see below). CNS disturbance likely when >155 mmol/L.
- Hypovolaemic—*low total body sodium, excess water loss*:
  - diarrhoea and vomiting, open wounds (urinary Na^+ <10 mmol/L)
  - osmotic diuresis, e.g. following mannitol (urinary Na^+ >20 mmol/L)
  - ACTH insufficiency
- Euvolaemic—*normal total body sodium*:
  - insufficient water intake or excessive loss
  - diabetes insipidus
  - urine osmolality very high, reflecting intact ADH axis but urinary sodium variable
- Hypervolaemic—*increased total body sodium, with excess water*:
  - iatrogenic—sodium bicarbonate or hypertonic saline administration (urinary Na^+ >20 mmol/L)
  - Cushing's syndrome
  - hyperaldosteronism—serum sodium rarely very high

Immediate management

- Depends on cause, but correction of sodium should take at least 48 h.
- Hypovolaemic hypernatraemia:
  - isotonic fluid resuscitation to correct hypovolaemia
  - thereafter 0.45% saline or 5% glucose to correct water deficit
- Euvolaemic hypernatraemia:
  - give water to correct deficit—encourage oral intake, 0.45% saline or 5% glucose IV
  - monitor serum sodium to avoid water intoxification
  - diabetes insipidus—replace urinary losses and give desmopressin 1–4 µg/day IV/SC/IM
- Hypervolaemic hypernatraemia:
  - stop administration of high sodium infusions—use 5% glucose
  - consider furosemide (20 mg initially) or dialysis with low sodium dialysate

Subsequent management

- Monitor potassium and calcium. Reduce sodium intake.
- Investigate most likely cause and treat appropriately.

Investigations

U&Es, urinary sodium levels, serum osmolality, urine osmolality

Risk factors
- Very old and very young—limited water intake
- Altered conscious level—dehydration
- Uncontrolled diabetes mellitus
- Treatment with osmotic diuretics, e.g. mannitol
- Hypertonic saline infusions
- Sampling error—'drip arm'

Exclusions
- Sampling error.
- Acute liver failure—serum sodium should be maintained >145 mmol/L to increase osmolality and control ICP.

Paediatric implications
- Dehydration:
  - diarrhoea and vomiting
  - renal impairment resulting in loss of urinary concentrating ability
- Salt poisoning:
  - accidental excessive intake, e.g. incorrect diet in infants
  - Munchausen's by proxy—purposeful administration of salt

Special considerations
- Rapid correction of hypernatraemia can induce cerebral oedema.
- Acute hypernatraemia can be corrected over hours rather than days—aim for a decrease of 1 mmol/L/hour. In this group the risk of rapid correction causing cerebral oedema is reduced.

Further reading

Coulthard, M., Haycock, G. (2003). Distinguishing between salt poisoning and hypernatraemic dehydration in children. *British Medical Journal*, **326**, 157–60.

Kumar, S., Beri, T. (1998). Electrolyte quintet: Sodium. *Lancet*, **352**, 220–8.

Reynolds, R.M., Padfield, P.L., Seckl, J.R. (2006) Disorders of sodium balance. *British Medical Journal*, **332**, 702–5.

⊙ Hyponatraemia

(See also 'TURP syndrome', pp290–1)

Definition

Normal serum sodium 135–145 mmol/L
- mild   125–134 mmol/L
- moderate   120–124 mmol/L
- severe   <120 mmol/L

Presentation

- Important to differentiate between acute and chronic hyponatraemia.
- Depends on fluid status of patient, but commonly nausea and vomiting, headache and weakness, ataxia, psychiatric disturbance, cerebral oedema.

Immediate management

Management depends on the rate of onset and the patient's symptoms.

Symptomatic hyponatraemia (usually rapid onset)

e.g. TURP/hysteroscopy syndrome, induced hyponatraemia, SIADH
- Give 0.9% saline.
- Aim for rise of sodium of 5–10 mmol/L per 24 h.
- Watch for resolution of cerebral irritation.
- Avoid rapid correction as sudden rise in osmolality (serum sodium rise of >0.5 mmol/L/h) may result in central pontine myelinolysis, which can be fatal.
- Hypertonic saline should only be used in extreme cases.
- In cases of fluid excess or cerebral oedema, use 100–500 mL of 20% mannitol or furosemide (20 mg) to promote fluid excretion.

SIADH requires specific investigations and treatment. Discuss management with endocrinologist.

Asymptomatic hyponatraemia

- Fluid-restrict to 1 L/day.
- Monitor potassium and magnesium concentrations, as they can alter dramatically.

Chronic hyponatraemia

- Treat the cause.
- Fluid-restrict to 1 L/day.
- Aim to correct sodium by 12 mmol/L/day.
- Give IV 0.9% saline as maintenance.
- Consider furosemide in the presence of water overload.

Subsequent management

Watch for other electrolyte disturbance and treat accordingly. Treat specific cause.

Investigations

U&Es, urinary sodium levels, serum osmolality, urine osmolality

Risk factors

- Sampling error—'drip arm'.
- Very old and young—excess water administration.
- Diuretics, especially thiazides, e.g. bendroflumethiazide.
- Medical conditions—pancreatitis, cardiac and hepatic failure, renal disease, pneumonia, SIADH.
- Inappropriate fluid administration:
  - excess infusion of hypotonic fluids post-op. (increased ADH secretion due to anaesthesia, pain, etc.)
  - glycine absorption during TURP/hysteroscopy
- Falsely low readings—hyperglycaemia (reduces Na^+ by 1.5 mmol/L per 3.5 mmol/L rise in plasma glucose), and hyperlipidaemia. Define osmolar gap: measure serum osmolality and compare with calculated $[2 \times (Na + K)] + Urea + Glucose$.

Exclusions

Sampling error, hyperglycaemia, hyperlipidaemia.

Special considerations

- *Hypovolaemic*—*deficiency of total body water and sodium:* Loss of body fluid stimulates secretion of ADH, thus conserving body water. However, subsequent administration of hypotonic fluid exacerbates problem.
- Renal (urinary Na^+ >20 mmol/L): diuretics, diabetic ketoacidosis, Addison's disease (raised K^+, urea, and creatinine).
- Extrarenal (urinary Na^+ <20 mmol/L): gastrointestinal (vomiting and diarrhoea), third space loss (pancreatitis, burns).
- *Euvolaemic (more common)*—*slight increase in total body sodium but little or no oedema:* urinary sodium is generally >20 mmol/L, serum osmolality <270 mOsmol/kg and urinary osmolality >100 mOsmol/kg:
  - stress response, e.g. post surgery, inappropriate ADH secretion, glucocorticoid deficiency, hypothyroidism, HIV
- *Hypervolaemic*—*raised total sodium but total body water raised further:* generalized oedema is present due to water overload:
  - cardiac and hepatic failure (urinary Na^+ <20 mmol/L). Marker of poor prognosis
  - renal failure (urinary Na^+ >20 mmol/L)
  - measure urinary sodium for an idea as to cause
- Acute correction of hyponatraemia can induce cerebral oedema and central demyelination.
- If condition is chronic, correct more slowly.
- Symptomatic patients must be treated immediately (which may be intraoperatively) and may require Intensive Care support.
- Surgery should not be delayed in those with chronic or asymptomatic cases of hyponatraemia, but if Na^+ <120 mmol/L, proceed cautiously so as not to exacerbate the situation.
- Emergency cases may require surgery despite low serum Na^+.
- Consult with endocrinologists for advice.

Further reading

Ackrill, P., France, M. (2002). Common electrolyte problems. *Clinical Medicine JPCPL*, **2**, 205–8.

Kumar, S., Beri, T. (1998). Electrolyte quintet: Sodium. *Lancet*, **352**, 220–8.

Reynolds, R.M., Padfield, P.L., Seckl, J.R. (2006). Disorders of sodium balance. *British Medical Journal*, **332**, 702–5.

⚠ Hypercalcaemia

Definition
Normal serum calcium 2.2–2.5 mmol/L (ionized 0.9–1.1 mmol/L)
- mild   2.6–3.0 mmol/L
- moderate   3.0–3.4 mmol/L
- severe   >3.4 mmol/L

Presentation
- 'Bones, stones, abdominal groans, and psychiatric moans'.
- CVS—dehydration secondary to polyuria, raised BP, bradycardia, dysrhythmias, abnormal P–R and short Q–T interval.
- GI/GU—nausea and vomiting, abdominal pain, peptic ulceration, constipation, kidney stones and renal failure, pancreatitis.
- CNS—psychiatric disturbance, coma, hyperreflexia, tongue fasciculations.

Immediate management
- ABC ... 100% O_2.
- Rehydrate with IV fluids (0.9% saline)—consider loop diuretics to avoid fluid overload.
- Ca^{2+} >3.4 mmol/L: give disodium pamidronate 60 mg in 1 L 0.9% saline IV over 4h. Can take 48 hours to work.
- If possible, with severe hypercalcaemia (Ca^{2+} >3.4 mmol/L) postpone all elective surgery.
- If patient symptomatic consider haemodialysis.
- Malignant disease may warrant surgery in the face of moderate hypercalcaemia (risk/benefit ratio).

Subsequent management
- Measure serum PTH levels.
- Aim to decrease serum calcium by 0.5 mmol/L over 1 or 2 days.
- Bisphosphonates, e.g. disodium pamidronate (60 mg in 1 L 0.9% saline IV over 4h); sodium clodronate (300 mg/day for 7–10 days); etidronate sodium (7.5 mg/kg/day over 4h for 3 days).
- In renal failure-induced hypercalcaemia—haemodialysis with low-calcium dialysate.
- Glucocorticoids are effective in malignancy and granulomatous disease, where gastrointestinal absorption of calcium is inhibited, e.g. prednisolone up to 60 mg/day.
- Calcitonin increases calcium excretion and inhibits bone resorption—causes moderate and transient decrease therefore little benefit acutely, but give 4 units/kg IM/SC 6–12-hourly.
- Phosphate therapy: oral phosphate 3g/day (causes diarrhoea).
  IV phosphate must be administered slowly (<9 mmol/12 h). Phosphate increases calcium uptake into bone, reduces calcium absorption from GIT, and inhibits bone breakdown. Can be administered to children.
- Consult endocrinologist for expert advice.
- Treat the underlying cause. Investigate if there are clinical features of associated conditions, e.g. cachexia, bone pain with malignancy.

Investigations
- FBC, U&Es, phosphate, albumin, CXR, ECG, PTH levels, amylase
- Associated low K^+ and Mg^{2+} if on diuretics

Risk factors
- Hyperparathyroidism/thyrotoxicosis/phaeochromocytoma.
- Malignancy—often clinically evident, e.g. squamous-cell lung tumour, metastatic breast cancer, myeloma.
- Renal disease— chronic failure and post-transplantation.
- Drugs—thiazide diuretics, lithium, theophylline toxicity.
- Granulomatous disease—sarcoid, TB.
- Hypophosphataemia (<1.4 mmol/L).
- Sampling error—tourniquets used when sample taken.
- Rare—vitamin overdose, excess calcium antacids, milk–alkali syndrome, familial conditions.

Special considerations
- Ionized calcium is physiologically active, therefore measure in preference to total serum calcium. Changes in serum albumin cause changes in total calcium levels, but do not alter the unbound fraction. To calculate the corrected calcium level (mmol/L) deduct 0.1 mmol/L for every 4 g albumin above 40 g/L.
- Hypercalcaemia can cause pancreatitis, therefore check serum amylase regularly. (NB Hypocalcaemia occurs in pancreatitis).
- Anaesthetic agents potentiate the risk of serious arrhythmia in the presence of hypercalcaemia.

Further reading
Bushinsky, D.A., Monk, R.D. (1998). Electrolyte quintet: Calcium. *Lancet*, **352**, 306–11.

Khan, M.M., Desborough, J.P. (2003). Calcium homeostasis. *The Royal College of Anaesthetists Bulletin*, **18**, 883–6.

ⓘ Hypocalcaemia

Definition
Normal serum calcium 2.1–2.6 mmol/L (ionized 0.9–1.1 mmol/L)
- Hypocalcaemia <2.1 mmol/L (ionized calcium <0.9 mmol/L)

Presentation
- CVS—cardiac arrhythmias, prolonged P–R interval, reduced contractility causing reduced cardiac output, hypotension, heart failure.
- CNS—carpopedal spasm, muscle cramps, tetany, convulsions. Chvostek's (facial twitch seen on tapping the facial nerve) and Trousseau's (metacarpophalangeal joints and thumb flexion with hyper-extended fingers on occlusion of the brachial artery) signs are pathognomonic of hypocalcaemia.

Immediate management
- ABC … 100% O_2.
- Calcium intravenous injection:
  - calcium chloride (10% 5–10 mL) over 10 min
  - calcium gluconate (10% 10–20 mL)—has to be metabolized by the liver to become active, therefore less effective in the acute setting
- If required, start calcium infusion, e.g. 10% calcium chloride at 5–10 mL/h.
- Support CVS with inotropes if necessary.

Subsequent management
- Biochemical investigations to establish and treat cause.
- Chronic hypocalcaemia can be treated with oral calcium carbonate and vitamin D supplements. In those with hypoparathyroidism, some vitamin D supplements are inactive, therefore use alfacalcidol or calcitriol.

Investigations
- FBC, U&Es, amylase, serum creatine kinase, serum PTH, urine myoglobin
- CXR

Risk factors
- Transfusion of blood products, clotting factors—administration of a large quantity of blood products containing citrate can cause an acute reduction in ionized calcium.
- Alkalosis, e.g. hyperventilation—reduces ionized calcium.
- Chronic renal failure—reduced vitamin D activity.
- Calcium channel blockers overdose.
- Post parathyroidectomy—hypo- and pseudohypoparathyroidism.
- Acute pancreatitis.
- Septic shock.
- Rhabdomyolysis.
- Vitamin D deficiency—poor diet, low UV light exposure.

- Hypomagnesaemia—exacerbates low calcium.
- Transient—secondary to drug administration, e.g. protamine, glucagon, or heparin.

Special considerations

- Bolus administration of calcium can cause a transient but dramatic increase in blood pressure and should be administered over 5–10 min, with full monitoring.
- Ideally, calcium should be administered centrally as it can cause vasoconstriction and tissue ischaemia at the injection site. If not possible, administer calcium gluconate (in preference) into a fast-running IVI.
- To calculate the corrected calcium level (mmol/L) add 0.1 mmol/L for every 4 g albumin below 40 g/L.

Further reading

Bushinsky, D.A., Monk, R.D. (1998). Electrolyte quintet: Calcium. *Lancet*, **352**, 306–11.

Cooper, M., Gittoes, N. (2008). Clinical review: Diagnosis and management of hypocalcaemia. *British Medical Journal*, **336**, 1298–303.

Khan, M.M., Desborough, J.P. (2003). Calcium homeostasis. *The Royal College of Anaesthetists Bulletin*, **18**, 883–6.

⏺ Hypermagnesaemia

Definition

Normal serum Mg^{2+} levels 0.7–1.0 mmol/L (1.8–3.0 mg/dL)

- Hypermagnesaemia—serum level >1.1 mmol/L
- ITU and obstetrics—aim for magnesium level >2.0 mmol/L

Presentation (Table 9.4)

Table 9.4 Serum magnesium levels

Physiological range	0.7–1.0 mmol/L
Therapeutic range	1.25–2.5 mmol/L
Knee jerks abolished	3.3–5.5 mmol/L
Respiratory arrest risk	5.0–7.5 mmol/L
Cardiac arrest risk	>15.0 mmol/L

- CVS—vasodilatation and hypotension (worse with volatile agents and/or narcotics), bradycardia, prolonged PR interval, wide QRS, cardiac arrest.
- RS—bronchodilatation and respiratory depression.
- CNS—sedation, coma, weakness. Reduced acetylcholine at the neuro-muscular junction causes potentiation of muscle relaxants. Loss of deep tendon reflexes and facial paraesthesiae.
- Metabolic—bone mineralization.
- Coagulopathy—clotting may be impaired.

Immediate management

- Calcium chloride 10% 5–10 mL over 10 min and repeat if necessary.
- Enhance excretion with IV fluids and forced diuresis, e.g. with furose-mide 20 mg initially, repeat according to response.
- If life-threatening complications ± renal failure—dialysis with Mg^{2+}-free dialysate.

Subsequent management

Biochemical investigations to find possible cause.

Investigations

- Monitor serum Mg^{2+} levels
- U&Es, creatinine clearance, T_4/TSH, endocrine/hormone screen

Risk factors

- Excessive intake—rare if normal renal function:
  - iatrogenic—excessive administration
  - antacids
  - purgatives—anorexia nervosa
- Renal failure—especially with dialysis as patients take Mg^{2+} supplements.
- Hypocalcaemia and hyperkalaemia (exacerbate the complications of hypermagnesaemia).

- Adrenocortical insufficiency, hypothyroidism.
- Depression—especially with lithium ingestion.

Special considerations

- 1 g magnesium sulphate = 4 mmol Mg^{2+}.
- Treatment of severe asthma—aim for Mg^{2+} >1 mmol/L.
- Treatment of pregnancy-induced hypertension and eclampsia—aim for serum Mg^{2+} of 2–4 mmol/L.
- Lower dose of muscle relaxants may be required—Mg^{2+} decreases twitch response without train-of-four fade.
- Caution in patients with myasthenia gravis or muscular dystrophy (avoid Mg^{2+} administration in these groups).
- Hypotension with GA.
- Phaeochromocytoma—administration of magnesium can improve cardiovascular stability intraoperatively, due to blocking of calcium channels. Effective at serum concentrations exceeding 1.5 mmol/L.

Further reading

Watson, V.F., Vaughan, R.S. (2001). Magnesium and the anaesthetist. *British Journal of Anaesthesia CEPD Reviews*, **1**(1), 16–20.

Weisinger, J.R., Bellorin-Font, E. (1998). Electrolyte quintet: Magnesium and phosphorus. *Lancet*, **352**, 391–6.

⊙ Hypomagnesaemia

Definition
Normal serum Mg^{2+} levels 0.7–1.0 mmol/L (1.8–3.0 mg/dL)
- Hypomagnesaemia <0.6 mmol/L (ionized)

Presentation
- CVS—hypertension with angina due to coronary artery spasm, increased risk of digoxin toxicity, dysrhythmias (VT/VF, torsade de pointes, SVT, AF), ECG changes (increased PR/wide QRS/inverted T-waves).
- CNS—abnormal nerve conduction (myoclonus, stridor, cramps), convulsions, coma.
- Psychiatric changes—anxiety, depression, confusion, psychosis, Wernicke's encephalopathy.
- Metabolic—hypokalaemia, hyperinsulinaemia.
- Bone—(chronic signs) osteoporosis and osteomalacia.

Immediate management
- Acute management (dysrhythmias or acute severe resistant asthma): magnesium sulphate 2 g (8 mmol magnesium) IV in 5% glucose or saline over 15 min. Torsades de pointes— 2 g magnesium sulphate over 1–2 min. Continue an infusion 12.5–25 g (50–100 mmol) over 24 h.
- PIH/eclampsia: magnesium sulphate loading dose 4 g (16 mmol) in 5% glucose or saline over 10–20 min IV. Maintenance infusion 1 g/h (4 mmol/h). Continue for 24 h following last convulsion. If convulsions recur, give 2–4 g (8–16 mmol) over 5 min. Aim for plasma concentration of 2–4 mmol/L.

Subsequent management
- Aim to maintain serum magnesium >0.8 mmol/L.
- Maintenance dose: 2.5–5 g/day (10–20 mmol/day).

Investigations
Serum Mg^{2+} levels

Risk factors
- Decreased intake:
  - poor diet
  - elderly
  - chronic alcohol abuse
  - excessive administration of IV fluids
  - TPN with inadequate magnesium
- Intensive Care patients—multifactorial
- Decreased absorption:
  - pancreatic insufficiency—pancreatitis
  - short bowel syndrome—after small bowel resection

- Excessive renal losses:
  - drugs—loop diuretics, digoxin, gentamicin, ethanol, ciclosporin, amphotericin
  - renal disease—diuretic phase of ATN, interstitial nephritis, excessive diuresis
  - hyperaldosteronism
- Non-renal losses:
  - GI tract—diarrhoea/prolonged NG suctioning/drainage
  - primary hyperparathyroidism
  - diabetic ketoacidosis with insulin administration
- Massive blood transfusion

Special considerations

- 1 g magnesium sulphate = 4 mmol Mg^{2+}.
- Administration of magnesium can lead to a profound reduction in blood pressure and cardiac output. Care must be exercised in patients who are hypotensive or who have cardiovascular instability.
- Dysrhythmias occurring on ITU, in the presence of likely hypomagnesaemia, should be treated with a loading dose of magnesium as described above.
- Hypomagnesaemia is common after cardiopulmonary bypass and is associated with malignant arrhythmias.
- Pregnancy-induced hypertension and eclampsia—adequate magnesium levels have been shown to reduce intracerebral vascular spasm and decreased resistance in the internal and middle cerebral arteries, thus reducing the incidence of convulsions.
- Low Mg^{2+} increases the risk of stridor/bronchoconstriction at induction of anaesthesia and intubation of the trachea.
- Convulsions—magnesium has been used as a second-line treatment for status epilepticus.
- Asthma—magnesium therapy is used to treat bronchospasm unresponsive to standard treatment. Aim to keep serum Mg^{2+} >1.0 mmol/L.

Further reading

Watson, V.F., Vaughan, R.S. (2001). Magnesium and the anaesthetist. *British Journal of Anaesthesia CEPD Reviews*, **1**(1), 16–20.

Weisinger, J.R., Bellorin-Font, E. (1998). Electrolyte quintet: Magnesium and phosphorus. *Lancet*, **352**, 391–6.

Recovery problems

Richard Riley

⊙ Chest pain

Definition
Discomfort experienced anywhere in the thorax.

Presentation
Patient reports pain, or may appear dyspnoeic, distressed, pale, clammy, and may become hypotensive.

Immediate threats to life
Myocardial infarction (MI), pulmonary embolism, tension pneumothorax, aortic dissection.

Other important diagnoses
Myocarditis, pericarditis, pneumonia, pancreatitis, peptic ulcer disease, chole-cystitis, oesophageal spasm, musculoskeletal pain.

Immediate management
- ABC … 100% O_2.
- Establish continuous ECG, NIBP, SpO_2 monitoring.
- Call for senior assistance if patient looks unwell.
- Maintain SpO_2 >94% with high-flow O_2, non-rebreathing mask, CPAP, or intubation.
- Examine chest for symmetrical movement, tracheal position, altered percussion resonance, reduced breath sounds.
- Check 12-lead ECG—new focal ST- and T-wave changes suggests evolving myocardial ischaemia. Tachycardia, new RBBB and S_1QT_3 changes should raise suspicion of PE. Pericarditis and myocarditis and cardiomyopathies often have widespread ST changes across multiple coronary territories. Arrange for an urgent CXR, erect if possible. Pneumothorax and mediastinal widening can easily be missed if the patient is lying supine. A CXR with relatively clear lung fields in a hypoxic patient should raise the suspicion of PE.
- Maintain blood pressure and heart rate within the patient's normal range.
- Analgesics (usually diamorphine 1–5 mg IV, fentanyl 25–100 µg IV).

Subsequent management
- Disposition and ongoing care will be stratified according to the most likely diagnosis. Most patients will require admission to CCU/HDU/ICU.
- Consider arterial line, central venous access, ± Swan–Ganz catheter.
- **Acute coronary syndromes (ACS)**—see pp318–20
- **Pneumothorax**—acutely decompensated patient with clinical diagnosis of tension pneumothorax should receive urgent decompression by placing a 2–inch (50 mm) 14-gauge IV cannula in the 2nd intercostal space at the mid-clavicular line followed by the insertion of chest drain and underwater seal (see pp448–50).

- **Pulmonary embolism (PE)**—clinically presents as a shunt (significant hypoxia despite high oxygen flows) in a patient with a relatively clear CXR. Massive PE (patient shocked) has a high mortality rate (20–30%) and usually warrants mechanical reperfusion strategies (percutaneous or surgical embolectomy) because thrombolysis is contraindicated (see pp30–2). Submassive PE (PE with RV dysfunction but no shock) has a mortality rate of 4–5%. Reperfusion strategies are controversial in these patients and the potential harm almost certainly outweighs the benefit in postoperative patients. Discuss with the surgical team about an IVC filter and early systemic anticoagulation as soon as it is safe to do so. Normotensive PE patients with a normal RV have a low mortality (1%) and should be considered for early systemic anticoagulation ± IVC filter.
- **Aortic dissection**—is uncommon and more often seen in elderly or hypertensive patients, but may occur in younger patients with connective tissue disorders (Marfan's syndrome). Severe chest and/or back pain, new neurological deficits, unequal blood pressures in the upper limbs and/or cardiac tamponade. The erect CXR may reveal a widened mediastinum, but definitive diagnosis requires a CT angiogram or transoesophageal echocardiography. Control the heart rate <70 bpm (beta-blockers) and maintain the systolic BP 90–110 mmHg (GTN, SNP infusion). Seek urgent opinion from cardiothoracic surgeon.
- **Acute pericardial disease**—examine for friction rub and worsening chest pain on lying flat and improving when sitting forward. The characteristic ECG will show concave ST elevation across multiple chest and limb leads. A normal echocardiogram does not exclude pericarditis.

Investigations
- 12-lead ECG, CXR, FBC, U&Es, lactate, magnesium
- Consider:
  - ABGs (A–a gradient often raised in PE but otherwise non-specific baseline investigation)
  - troponin levels (may not rise for 6–10h after MI and can be elevated for reasons other than ACS in approximately one-third of patients, e.g. PE, AHF, or CVA)
  - serum D-dimer levels (only useful to help rule out PE if negative). Hospital inpatients may have positive D-dimers for other reasons
  - CT angiogram echocardiography, V/Q scan, abdominal ultrasound, Doppler ultrasound of legs (PE)

Risk factors
- Ischaemia/infarction—see pp26–7, 318–20
- Pneumothorax—undiagnosed rib fractures, chest wall or abdominal injury, CVC insertion
- DVT/PE risk—immobility, obesity, trauma, fractures, pregnancy, pelvic surgery
- Gallstones, biliary, or peptic ulcer disease
- Gastric distension—poor nasogastric tube placement

Exclusions
- Cardiac ischaemia/infarction, pulmonary embolus, pneumothorax, musculoskeletal.
- Referred pain from distended bladder, upper GI system (gastric distension or disease, laparoscopic banding problem, pancreatitis, biliary disease, ruptured viscus).

Paediatric implications
- Chest pain is not usually a feature of cardiac disease.
- Children have difficulty localizing pain. Discuss concerns with parents.
- Usually non-cardiac origin—common causes are musculoskeletal, pulmonary (infection, pneumothorax), or idiopathic (anxiety and hyperventilation in adolescents).

Special considerations
- Thrombolysis is usually contraindicated following surgery because of the bleeding risk.
- If MI is suspected, emergency cardiac catheterization ± coronary angioplasty should be considered prior to ICU/HDU admission.
- Pulmonary embolism can be extremely difficult to diagnose. Have a low threshold for further investigation to exclude PE.

Further reading
Erhardt, L., Herlitz, J., Bossaert, L. et al. (2002). Task force on the management of chest pain. *European Heart Journal*, **23**, 1153–76.

✪ Acute coronary syndromes (ACS)

(See also pp30–2)

Definition
Acute ischaemic myocardial injury.

Presentation
• Typical MI pain is a central crushing, pressing, or constricting pain or tightness, lasting longer than 20 min, and may radiate to the throat, jaw, arms, or epigastrium.
• Can be 'silent' or atypical (diabetics, elderly, epidural *in situ*, smokers, those who take NSAIDs).
• May present with new arrhythmias, heart failure, or cardiogenic shock.

Immediate management
• Initiate immediate resuscitation with attention to ABCs … Call for senior assistance early. MONA therapy (**M**orphine IV, **O**xygen, **N**itrates SL, **A**spirin (150–300 mg)).
• Establish continuous ECG, NIBP, SpO₂.
• Check temperature, maintain normothermia.
• Monitor 3-lead ECG and obtain 12-lead ECG—compare with previous records and stratify subsequent management. Patients with STEMI comprise 30% of patients with an ACS and require urgent reperfusion strategies. Thrombolysis is usually contraindicated following surgery, leaving urgent angioplasty as the option in tertiary centres. Patients with non-ST-segment-acute-coronary-syndromes (NSTEACS) should receive adjunctive therapy in accordance with their risk stratification.
• Maintain SaO₂ >94%.
• Give beta-blockers to keep heart rate 60–80 bpm (e.g. metoprolol 1–5 mg IV over 10 min Discuss with surgical and cardiological teams about further antiplatelet therapy (clopidogrel—300 mg PO) and heparinization (avoid LMWH in unstable patients at risk of bleeding), weighing up the individualized risks of postoperative bleeding with each patient.
• Maintain adequate systolic BP (100–130 mmHg) using GTN infusion (50 mg in 50 mL saline starting at 3 mL/h) if hypertensive. In hypotensive patients with an inferior STEMI, consider RV or posterior infarction. These patients may respond to cautious fluid boluses providing there are no signs of pulmonary congestion. Otherwise consider cautious use of vasopressors (dopamine, noradrenaline, or adrenaline) remembering they will increase myocardial oxygen demand and are potentially arrhythmogenic.
• Treat arrhythmias (drug therapy, pacing). Be aware of accelerated idioventricular rhythms that can be confused with VT or VF. It is relatively common (~10% STEMIs) within the first 24 hours of transmural myocardial infarction and is usually benign and self-limiting. It is characterized by bizarre widened QRS complexes at a rate of 60–110 bpm.
• Consider arterial line, CVP.

Subsequent management

- Correct electrolyte imbalances, especially potassium (aim >4 mmol/L) and magnesium (aim >1 mmol/L). Maintain good blood glucose control (5–9 mmol/L). Observe for complications (arrhythmias, heart block, heart failure, shock, acute mitral regurgitation).
- Arrange ICU admission (or CCU, according to hospital procedures).

Investigations

- 12-lead ECG for new ST-segment and T-wave changes or left bundle branch block (LBBB). The ECG is initially normal in 20% of patients with a MI.
- Troponin (may not rise for 6–10 h after MI).
- FBC, U&Es, magnesium, coagulation profile.

Risk factors

Known history of angina, unstable or poorly controlled hypertension, MI, any vascular disease, chronic renal insufficiency, lipid disorders, diabetes, obesity, hyperhomocysteinaemia, advanced age, family history of heart disease, abnormal ECG.

Exclusions

- ST-segment elevation can be seen when early repolarization occurs in normal patients, and is referred to as 'high take off'. It most commonly appears in leads V_2 and V_3 and has a concave upwards appearance.
- Non-ACS causes for ST elevation include pulmonary embolism, acute pericardial disease, left bundle branch block, hyperkalaemia, ventricular aneurysm, LVH, Brugada syndrome (an inherited arrhythmia presenting with ST segment elevation in leads V_{1-3} and RBBB).

Paediatric implications

- Causes include illicit drug use, coronary artery anomalies, perinatal asphyxia, myocarditis, Kawasaki syndrome, and obstruction of the coronary arteries following cardiac surgery.
- Infants present with non-specific symptoms, older children complain of prolonged, non-pleuritic chest or abdominal pain.

Special considerations

- Incidence is approximately 3% in patients undergoing non-cardiac surgery, but varies with the patient risk profile—the incidence doubles if the patient has known IHD.
- Mortality is higher than for patients presenting to emergency departments (15–20% vs. 12%).
- Troponin level will often be normal immediately following a period of ischaemic chest pain, therefore subsequent cardiac monitoring and repeat troponin levels may be required. Troponin-T usually peaks at 12 h and persists 4–7 days (normal <0.1 μg/L; 0.1–0.39 μg/L warrants further investigation; ≥0.4 μg/L suggests significant myocardial injury. Some centres now consider any rise to be significant).

Further reading

Acute Coronary Syndrome Guidelines Working Group. (2006). Guidelines for the management of acute coronary syndromes. *Medical Journal of Australia*, 184(8, Suppl), S1–S32. http://www.mja.com.au/public/issues/184_08_170406/suppl_170406_fm.html

Ryan, T.J., Antman, E.M., Brooks, N.H. *et al.* (1999). Update: ACC/AHA guidelines for the management of patients with acute myocardial infarction. A report of the American College of Cardiology/American Heart Association Task Force on Practice Guidelines (Committee on Management of Acute Myocardial Infarction). *Journal of American College of Cardiology*, **34**, 890–911.

☼ Acute heart failure (AHF)

Definition
AHF is a clinical syndrome representing inadequate systolic or diastolic heart function. If associated with anaerobic cellular metabolism, the terms 'circulatory failure' or 'shock' are often used.

Classification (European Society of Cardiology)
Hypertensive AHF—pulmonary oedema in the setting of relatively preserved systolic left ventricular function and often involving diastolic dysfunction.
Cardiogenic shock—evidence of tissue hypoperfusion, hypotension, oliguria ± pulmonary oedema
Decompensated AHF—mild to moderate signs and symptoms of heart failure that do not meet the definitions for either hypertensive or cardiogenic shock categories
High output failure—tachycardia, warm peripheries, pulmonary congestion with low to normal BP
Acute right heart failure—a low output syndrome with raised JVP, increased liver size, and peripheral oedema without pulmonary congestion.

Immediate management

- Initiate immediate resuscitation with attention to ABC.
- Call for senior assistance early. Many patients will respond quickly to therapy with well-directed management.
- Commence CPR if patient becomes unresponsive/pulseless. Establish patient monitoring with continuous 3-lead ECG, NIBP, and SaO_2 (and urinary catheter). Give early consideration to central venous access and arterial line.
- Maintain adequate oxygenation (SaO_2 >94%) with high flow oxygen, non-rebreathing mask, CPAP, or intubation. If the BP allows, position the patient as upright as possible.
- Attempt to normalize the heart rhythm and rate. Acutely decompensated patients with tachyarrhythmias will often need to be electrically cardioverted because most pharmacological agents are negatively inotropic and risk worsening the patient's condition. Amiodarone is probably the safest alternative (300 mg IV loading over 1 h). Digoxin (500 μg IV load) is positively inotropic but results in poor heart rate control in AHF. Bradycardic patients need to be pharmacologically (isoprenaline/dopamine/adrenaline) or electrically paced (external or transvenous).
- Aim for systolic BP 100–120 mmHg.
- If hypertensive (systolic BP >130 mmHg) reduce preload with GTN (50 mg in 50 mL saline, commence at 3 mL/h or topically 5 or 10 mg patches), plus furosemide 20–80 mg IV, CPAP (commence at 10 cmH$_2$O with 100% O_2) is an effective means of reducing the preload in hypoxic patients.

- If hypotensive (systolic BP <100 mmHg) increase afterload cautiously using vasopressors (dopamine/noradrenaline) ± very cautious fluid boluses. Adrenaline (1:10 000, 0–10 mL/h) or metaraminol are alternatives in the emergency setting until central access can be established. Optimize cardiac output. Consider inotropic drugs where end-organ perfusion is not adequate—dobutamine (250 mg in 50 mL beginning at 4 mL/h). Alternative infusions include dopamine, milrinone, and adrenaline. Be aware that all these drugs increase myocardial oxygen demand and are potentially arrhythmogenic.
- The use of morphine (1 mg IV) should be reserved for those patients with ongoing pain or undue anxiety. It conveys little additional advantage in reducing the preload.

Subsequent management

- Search for the underlying cause. Decompensation of pre-existing chronic heart failure, fluid overload, acute coronary syndromes, and acute arrhythmias are the most common causes. Undiagnosed or new valvular lesions (especially aortic stenosis), cardiomyopathies, or tamponade can be easily missed.
- Echocardiography (transthoracic, transoesophageal if intubated) is useful to establish segmental or global ventricular dysfunction or valvular pathology and monitor response to treatment.
- Correct electrolyte imbalances, especially potassium (aim >4 mmol/L) and magnesium (aim >1 mmol/L). Maintain good blood glucose control (5–9 mmol/L).
- Failure to respond to the above therapies warrants subsequent consultation and disposition with cardiology and intensive care. Further monitoring may be warranted with a Swan–Ganz catheter, pulse contour cardiac output (PiCCO), etc. Additional therapies may include an intra-aortic balloon pump or levosimendan. Cardiac catheterization may be indicated for acute MI. A bridging mechanical heart device (extracorporeal membrane oxygenation (ECMO) or left ventricular assist device (LVAD)) to recovery or cardiac transplant is rarely required.
- Specific management following resolution of acute heart failure will be tailored according to suspected cause, and may include:
  - afterload reduction—ACE inhibitors, angiotensin receptor blockers (ARB)
  - preload reduction—isosorbide mononitrate, and diuretics
  - aldosterone reduction—spironolactone
  - antiarrhythmic and heart rate control therapy—digoxin, amiodarone, permanent pacemaker (PPM), and implantable defibrillators, beta-blockers
  - anticoagulation—warfarinization for dilated cardiomyopathy or chronic AF

Investigations

FBC, U&Es, ABGs, Mg, blood sugar, lactate, troponin, CXR, 12-lead ECG, echocardiography

Risk factors

- Ischaemic heart disease; hypertension (systemic, pulmonary); myocardial, valvular, or pericardial disease or inflammation
- Obesity, sleep apnoea
- Drugs (e.g. beta-blockers) or excessive administration of fluids (IV, or during TURP), sepsis
- Acute neurological injuries (head or spinal cord injury, intracranial haemorrhage)
- Thyroid disease

Exclusions

- Non-cardiogenic pulmonary oedema—sepsis syndrome, allergic reactions, aspiration pneumonitis, multiple trauma, pancreatitis, etc.
- Hypervolaemia
- Pulmonary embolus, venous air embolism
- Tension pneumothorax, cardiac tamponade

Paediatric implications

Infants with heart failure may have tachypnoea, feeding difficulties, sweating, irritability, and laboured respirations. Hepatomegaly is common. Older children often have similar signs and symptoms to adults, although abdominal symptoms may predominate.

Special considerations

- Levosimendan (Simdax®) is a calcium-sensitizing agent with inotropic vasodilator properties used for the treatment of heart failure. It has an active metabolite with similar positive inotropic effects to the parent compound exerting pharmacological benefits for approximately 1 week. After initial small trials reported favourable results, larger trials (REVIVE II and SURVIVE) have been unable to produce a consistent benefit. Initiation of levosimendan should only be undertaken after discussion with a cardiologist or intensivist.
- B-natriuretic peptide (BNP) is a peptide hormone released in response to the mechanical stress of heart failure. It plays a homeostatic role as a systemic vasodilator and diuretic. While remaining relatively sensitive and specific for AHF, the diagnosis is normally established by clinical assessment. It may play a clinical role in COPD patients where differentiation between an exacerbation in emphysema and AHF can be difficult. False-positives occur in PE, pulmonary hypertension, liver and renal failure.

Further reading

The European Society of Cardiology. (2005). *Guidelines to the diagnosis and treatment of acute heart failure.* http://www.escardio.org/guidelines-surveys/esc-guidelines/Pages/acute-heart-failure.aspx

① Postoperative hypertension

Definition
BP more than 20% above baseline, systolic BP ≥140 mmHg or diastolic BP ≥90 mmHg.

Presentation
- Primary hypertension is usually asymptomatic.
- Patients with severe acute (systolic BP >160 mmHg or diastolic BP >115 mmHg) hypertension may have headache. Hypertension may precipitate myocardial ischaemia, resulting in chest pain.
- Immediate postoperative hypertension is common. Pain, arousal, and confusion are causative. Moderate hypertension is not usually life-threatening, but when combined with tachycardia is a cardiac stressor. Analgesia and beta-blockers are useful.

Immediate management

- Confirm pressure manually with appropriate-sized cuff, on more than one limb or, if using arterial line, check calibration, tubing, and height of transducer.
- Check oxygenation (SpO_2) and ventilation to exclude hypoxia, hypercapnia (use PACU capnography machine to sample $ETCO_2$, and consider ABGs measurement, especially if MH is suspected).
- Treat severe pain with IV opioids.
- Exclude bladder/bowel distension (especially if at risk for autonomic dysreflexia).
- Drug therapy includes:
  - labetalol 20–80 mg IV then infusion 0.5–4 mg/min
  - esmolol 0.5 mg/kg IV then infusion 50–200 µg/kg/min
  - hydralazine 5 mg IV to maximum 20 mg over 20 min
  - GTN infusion (50 mg/50 mL), start 3 mL/h IV and titrate to BP
  - sodium nitroprusside (25 mg in 50 mLs 5% glucose; 2–10 mLs/hr)
  - magnesium sulphate 2–4 g IV over 10 min, then infusion 1–2 g/h (maintain serum Mg >1.5 mmol/L)
  - phentolamine 1–2 mg IV prn, then infusion 5–30 mg/h
  - clonidine 25–150 µg slow IV

Subsequent management
Referral to physician for investigation and management of persistent hypertension, or to endocrinologist if thyroid disease, primary hyperaldosteronism (Conn's syndrome), or phaeochromocytoma is suspected.

Investigations
Check baseline levels Na^+/K^+/urea/creatinine/Hb, 12-lead ECG, urine for protein/blood.

Risk factors
- Untreated hypertension, hyperthyroidism
- Renal disease

- Preoperative omission of antihypertensive medications (especially clonidine, methyldopa, beta-blockers, and diuretics)
- Autonomic dysreflexia
- Pregnancy-induced hypertension
- Intraoperative drug use—MAOIs and intraoperative use of indirect sympathomimetics or opioids, or use of vasoconstrictors (cocaine, adrenaline, ephedrine).

Exclusions

- *Thyroid storm*—fever, tachycardia, atrial fibrillation, delirium, agitation or coma, vomiting, diarrhoea, muscle weakness (see pp270–1).
- *Phaeochromocytoma*—catecholamine-secreting tumours of the adrenal medulla may present after incomplete surgical removal or *de novo* with severe, paroxysmal, or sustained hypertension (see pp272–3).
- *Malignant hyperthermia*—see pp264–4.
- *Pre-eclampsia and eclampsia*—see pp156–8, 159.
- *Autonomic dysreflexia*—massive sympathetic response to a stimulus below the level of a chronic spinal cord injury (especially above T8). Triggers include bladder or hollow viscus distension or manipulation, temperature changes, surgery without adequate anaesthesia. Phenoxybenzamine is used preoperatively and phentolamine, nifedipine, and clonidine may be used in a hypertensive crisis. Beta-blocker only if tachycardia. (See pp204–5.)
- *Iatrogenic*—liberal use of adrenaline or other vasopressors during surgery; check intraoperative drug use. Phenylephrine eyedrops may cause hypertension during or before cataract surgery.
- Pain, agitation, anxiety.
- Full bladder, particularly elderly, confused/agitated males.

Paediatric implications

- Most hypertension in the recovery room is due to pain and is usually associated with tachycardia and agitation.
- Correct cuff size is important—cuff should completely encircle arm to ensure uniform compression. The inflatable bladder should cover at least two-thirds of the upper arm length and three-quarters of its circumference.
- Chronic hypertension in children is usually secondary to renal disease or vascular abnormalities, such as coarctation of the aorta. Adolescents may develop essential hypertension.
- If required, suitable agents for urgent control of BP include labetalol (1–3 mg/kg/h), SNP (0.5–0.6 µg/kg/min).

Special considerations

Sublingual nifedipine is no longer recommended, as sudden hypotension and cardiac ischaemia may result.

Further reading

Vaughan, C.J., Delanty, N. (2000). Hypertensive emergencies. *Lancet*, **356**, 411–17.

☼ Postoperative hypotension

Definition
BP more than 20% below baseline, systolic BP <90 mmHg or mean BP <60 mmHg.

Presentation
- Typically tachycardia, but dependent upon age and sympathetic/parasympathetic stimulation.
- Signs of reduced cerebral perfusion—altered mental state, nausea, vomiting.
- Weak or absent pulses (brachial, femoral, carotid), reduced urine output.

Immediate management
- ABC ... 100% O_2. If pre-arrest, intubate.
- Commence CPR if patient becomes unresponsive/pulseless
- ECG monitoring for heart rate, rhythm, ischaemia.
- Elevate patient's legs. IV access.
- Consider causes of pulseless electrical activity (PEA) since these can all cause severe hypotension (4Hs & 4Ts):
  - hypoxia, hypovolaemia, hypothermia, hyper/hypokalaemia
  - tension pneumothorax, toxins, thromboembolism, tamponade
- Correct fluid deficit with rapid IV fluid administration—colloid, Hartmann's, or saline. Consider vasopressors until suitable volume can be administered.
- Vasopressors:
  - ephedrine 6 mg IV boluses prn
  - metaraminol 0.5–1 mg IV prn
  - phenylephrine 25–100 µg IV prn
  - pre-arrest or unresponsive—adrenaline 50–100 µg IV prn
- Consider additional IV/CVC access. Massive blood loss warrants large-bore IV access (PAFC introducer sheath, rapid infusion line) and rapid infusion device ('Level 1'). Inform blood bank of urgent need for blood.
- **Anaphylactic/anaphylactoid reaction**—adrenaline IV in increments (50–100 µg) and infusion (5 mg in 50 mL saline) to maintain BP.
- **Severe blood loss**—see pp392–3.
- **Tamponade**—history of chest trauma or cardiothoracic surgery, distended neck veins, 'muffled' heart sounds (unreliable sign). Return to theatre for thoracotomy, pericardiotomy, or, if *in extremis*, pericardiocentesis.
- **Pneumothorax**—deviated trachea, hyperresonance, and reduced breath sounds (on one or both sides), needle thoracocentesis (2nd intercostal space, mid-clavicular line), then follow with chest tube/s (see pp48–9, 50–1, 448–50).

Subsequent management

- Persistent hypotension requires ICU/HDU admission and consideration of invasive haemodynamic monitoring (CVP ± PAFC), inotropic therapy.
- Specific therapy according to likely cause.
- Coronary angiography for new infarction/ischaemia.

Risk factors

- Most common postoperative cause is a combination of myocardial depression, vasodilatation, and relative volume deficit.
- *Hypovolaemia*—long fasting period, inadequate fluid administration, unrecognized fluid or blood loss, re-warming patient.
- *Inadequate cardiac output*—heart failure, tamponade, arrhythmias, myocardial ischaemia/infarction, pulmonary embolism (venous, air, or amniotic fluid), pneumothorax (chronic lung disease, recent CVC insertion or attempt), fluid overload (TURP syndrome, excessive fluid administration), aortocaval compression (pregnancy, abdominal tumour).
- *Reduced vascular resistance*—anaesthetic drugs, regional blockade (epidural, subdural, high or total spinal), sepsis (known or suspected infection), toxins, anaphylactoid reactions, drug overdose (mechanical pump problem or incorrect programming).
- Antihypertensive drugs—particularly ACE inhibitors.

Exclusions

- Do not delay treatment if there are other signs of low BP. Confirm hypotension by manually checking BP with appropriate-sized cuff, on more than one limb or, if using arterial line, checking calibration, tubing, and height of transducer.
- Check patient's preoperative BP.

Paediatric implications

- Hypotension is a late sign of circulatory failure in children. Earlier signs include tachycardia (up to 220 bpm in infants) and peripheral shutdown. Normal systolic BP can be calculated using the formula: BP = 80 + (age in years × 2). Correct cuff size is important.
- Give 10–20 mL/kg bolus of salt-rich fluid (lactated Ringers or normal saline) and assess response.
- The intraosseous route should be used early if IV access is difficult, and particularly if aged <6 years. Adrenaline dose for children in severe shock is 10 μg/kg (see pp 136–8, 470–2).

:✪: **Respiratory depression/failure**

Definition
Inadequate ventilation in a patient breathing spontaneously.

Presentation
- Variable, depending on underlying cause. May be:
  - reduced respiratory rate/volume if reduced ventilatory drive or neuromuscular function
  - tachypnoea and respiratory distress if reduced respiratory function
- Decreasing SpO_2, elevated $PaCO_2$, reduced frequency or abnormal pattern in CO_2 waveform, decreasing level of consciousness.

Immediate management
- Assess ventilation—quickly observe breathing pattern and frequency.
- Inspect airway and relieve obstruction with suction/Magill forceps—check for dentures, retained pharyngeal ('throat') pack, large clots (nasal, dental surgery).
- Stabilize airway with oral/nasal airway and jaw manoeuvres.
- Commence bag–valve–mask ventilation with O_2 if spontaneous ventilation inadequate.
- Monitor SpO_2. If bag–mask or spontaneous ventilation inadequate, consider tracheal intubation (or LMA insertion if appropriate).
- Check intraoperative drug administration (muscle relaxant, opioid, sedative, volatile use). Check for pupil constriction—if opioid overdose, consider ventilation ± naloxone (400 µg in 10 mL saline, administer 100 µg increments). If benzodiazepine overdose, consider flumazenil 0.2–1 mg in IV increments.
- Assess neuromuscular function clinically (grip strength, head lift >5 s) and electrically (nerve stimulator: normal train-of-four, sustained tetanus, equal double-burst stimulation). If inadequate neuromuscular function, consider neostigmine (maximum dose 70 µg/kg with glycopyrronium or atropine.

Subsequent management
- If unable to improve neuromuscular function, admit to ICU for ventilation.
- If chronic lung disease with CO_2 retention suspected, admit to ICU for ventilation or, if making borderline respiratory effort, admit to HDU for close monitoring of ventilatory function.
- Severe bronchospasm—see pp54–6.
- If history of head injury, neurosurgery or VP shunt *in situ*, perform rapid neurological examination (GCS, pupil inspection), obtain neurosurgical opinion, consider need for CT scan or re-operation.
- Upper airway problem—see pp80–4.

Investigations
ABGs, peripheral nerve stimulator, CXR

Risk factors

- Long duration or extensive surgery (e.g. thoracoabdominal incision)
- Underlying severe respiratory disease, especially with abdominal surgery
- Elderly or cachectic patient
- Large doses of muscle relaxants (especially in presence of renal or hepatic failure), sedatives, or opioids (remifentanil or other opioids in IV tubing at end of operation)
- Head injury, neurosurgery, VP shunt
- Obesity (especially morbid obesity: body mass index >35 kg/m^2)
- Hypothermia (temperature <35°C)
- Severe pain

Exclusions

- Residual anaesthetic effects (opioids, neuromuscular, sedatives)
- Heart failure
- Severe asthma/chronic lung disease
- Pneumothorax
- CNS disorder
- Phrenic nerve palsy with interscalene block

Paediatric implications

- Respiratory depression or failure can lead to early cardiorespiratory arrest in infants and children, and needs to be managed aggressively and rapidly.
- Infants under 3 months of age are very sensitive to opioids.
- Ex preterm babies can have episodes of apnoea/bradypnoea after anaesthesia.
- Monitor all babies <54 weeks' postconceptual age for at least 12h with apnoea monitor and pulse oximetry.
- Consider the use of caffeine (10 mg/kg IV) if <44 weeks' postconceptual age.
- Upper abdominal and chest wall surgery will limit respiratory effort.

:O: Hypoxia

Definition
SpO_2 <90% or PaO_2 <8 kPa (60 mmHg).

Presentation
- Low or falling pulse oximetry values, or difficulty in obtaining an SpO_2 reading.
- Cyanosis (may be seen if SpO_2 ≤85%, need ≥5 g/dL reduced Hb to detect cyanosis).
- Late signs include bradycardia or tachycardia, cardiac arrhythmias or ischaemia, decreased level of consciousness.

Immediate management
- Check ABC.
- Assess ventilation.
- Relieve obstruction, consider oral/nasal airways.
- Commence bag–valve–mask ventilation with oxygen. Observe bilateral chest movement.
- Monitor SpO_2, $ETCO_2$. Auscultate lungs (wheeze, absent breath sounds) and heart sounds.
- Consider tracheal intubation or LMA insertion if not responding.
- Use long suction catheter via tracheal tube to remove secretions.
- Most patients will respond to IPPV. Those who remain hypoxic, but in whom there are no signs of aspiration or pulmonary oedema, often have lung atelectasis/collapse. Diagnose on CXR. Re-expand by recruitment manoeuvres, suction, and PEEP.

Subsequent management
- Persistent or severe hypoxaemia will require admission to ICU/HDU.
- Therapy will include high-flow O_2 via face-mask/CPAP mask or IPPV, and other therapies according to diagnosis.

Investigations
- ABGs.
- Consider CXR after airway has been cleared, secured, and any tension pneumothorax treated.

Risk factors
- Long duration or extensive surgery (e.g. thoracoabdominal incision), resulting in atelectasis and lung collapse
- Large doses of muscle relaxants (especially in presence of renal or hepatic failure), volatile agents, IV sedatives or opioids
- Recent use of nitrous oxide
- Obesity (especially morbid obesity: body mass index >35 kg/m^2)
- Aspiration risk (non-fasted, late pregnancy, obesity, hiatus hernia, bowel obstruction or impaired gastric emptying, prior gastric surgery)
- Elderly or cachectic patient
- Hypothermia (temperature <35°C)
- Laryngeal disorder or disease; tracheal stenosis or injury

- Severe anaemia or methaemoglobinaemia
- Shock
- Burns victims (COHb)

Exclusions

- Problems with pulse oximeter—electrical interference, motion, ambient light, metHb, COHb, nail polish, skin pigmentation, methylene blue, indocyanine green, isosulfan blue/Patent blue (may also cause artefactual increase in metHb).
- Poor peripheral circulation.
- Hypoventilation due to any cause—airway obstruction, severe pain, drugs (opioids, sedatives, neuromuscular blockers), chest wall injury, fatigue.
- V/Q mismatch—pulmonary embolism, collapse.
- Hypotension.
- Heart failure.
- Congenital heart disease.

Paediatric implications

- Mild hypoxia in the recovery room is seen in children with a history of recent URTI, who develop V/Q mismatch intraoperatively. Generally resolves within 2 h after child awakens and begins coughing.
- Exclude congenital heart disease and right-to-left shunt.
- Untreated hypoxia can rapidly lead to bradycardia and cardiorespiratory arrest (see pp112–20).
- Respiratory reserve limited in neonates and infants due to:
  - reduced FRC
  - increased oxygen consumption

! Confusion

Definition
A state of inattentiveness and reduced capacity to think, with disorientation to time, place, person.

Presentation
- Disorientation, agitation, abnormal behaviour/movements, fighting with recovery room staff.
- Appear frightened or anxious.
- Picking at bed clothes, dressings, drains, or catheters.

Immediate management
- Treat hypoxia and hypotension (see pp332–3, 328–9).
- Reassure and 'orientate' patient to environment.
- Treat pain (see pp348–9).
- Clinical examination/bladder scan for distension and use catheter as needed; check balloon not inflated in urethra.
- Measure temperature—actively re-warm as necessary.
- Prevent patient from harming themselves or disrupting wounds, removing drains, dressings, catheters. Orderlies or other support staff may be required. Physical restraints remain a last resort.
- Rapid neurological examination seeking localizing signs. Perform GCS if regression of conscious state. If stroke or other neurological injury suspected, consult neurologist/neurosurgeon.
- Sedation if treatable cause(s) have been corrected and patient at risk of harming himself or others—incremental midazolam 1 mg IV, haloperidol 0.5 mg IV, or droperidol 1 mg IV can be used. If very restless in recovery, a low-dose propofol infusion may allow the patient to wake more slowly and improve. Physostigmine for anticholinergic syndrome, atropine for cholinergic syndrome (see below)
- Where appropriate, use familiar toys, family members, or known carers as support.

Subsequent management
- *Anticholinergic syndrome*—consider when confusion is associated with mydriasis, tachycardia, peripheral vasodilatation, dry skin, and facial plethora. Treatment with physostigmine 0.5–2 mg IV is diagnostic and therapeutic; repeat every 20–60 min (children 0.02 mg/kg IV or IM).
- *Cholinergic syndrome*—consider when confusion is associated with muscarinic effects such as bradycardia, miosis, sweating, blurred vision, excessive lacrimation and/or bronchial secretions, wheezing; or nicotinic effects such as tachycardia, hypertension, muscle weakness. Treat with atropine 1–2 mg (0.05 mg/kg in children).
- *Serotonin syndrome*—consider when confusion is associated with restlessness, myoclonus, hyperreflexia, tremor, shivering, sweating, fever, and other autonomic nervous system symptoms; following use of serotonin-enhancing drugs (SSRIs, MAOIs, tramadol, pethidine). Treatment is supportive—benzodiazepines may reduce patient

discomfort. Propranolol, cyproheptadine (4–8 mg PO 1–4-hourly) and ketanserin (10 mg IV) have also been used (see Further reading).

- **TURP syndrome**—see p290.
- **Hyponatraemia**—see p302.
- If longer term sedation is needed, consider haloperidol 2–10 mg IV/IM or lorazepam 1–2 mg IV/IM 4–6-hourly or droperidol 5–25 mg IM.
- Exclude hypothyroid coma (unlikely if normal preoperatively).

Investigations

- ABGs—hypoxia, CO_2 narcosis
- Glucose, U&Es—hyponatraemia, TURP syndrome, Ca^{2+} disorder
- Osmolality—TURP syndrome, SIADH, diabetes, or alcohol-related complications
- FBC—severe anaemia

Risk factors

- Dementia—note that early dementia may not have been detected preoperatively
- Common in elderly or intellectually impaired patient
- Alcohol withdrawal or drug abuse
- Diabetes, hepatic failure, encephalopathy, epilepsy
- Hypothyroidism, hyperparathyroidism
- Use of opioid/ketamine analgesia increases risk of hallucinations
- Benzodiazepines, anticholinergics, or acetylcholine esterase inhibitors
- Electroconvulsive therapy (especially bilateral)

Exclusions

- Dementia or preoperative confusion from any cause
- Deafness—locate hearing aid, or person trained in 'signing', or interpreter
- Full bladder
- Iatrogenic (ECT, neurosurgery, doxapram, anticholinergic, or acetylcholine esterase inhibitor drugs)

Paediatric implications

- Confusion/dysphoria following anaesthesia is common in the paediatric population and generally settles with time.
- Presentation—crying, screaming, agitation, doesn't recognize parents, doesn't make eye contact, won't settle with cuddling, possible evidence of hallucinations in older children. Causes include sevoflurane, ketamine, anxious child preoperatively, pain, hunger, midazolam premedication.
- Consider clonidine 0.5–1 µg/kg IV. If suspect midazolam as cause, consider flumazenil 5–10 µg/kg IV or clonidine.

Further reading

Jones, D. (2005). Serotonin syndrome and the anaesthetist. *Anaesthesia and Intensive Care*, **33**, 181–7.

Parikh, S.S., Chung, F. (1995). Postoperative delirium in the elderly. *Anesthesia and Analgesia*, **80**, 1223–32.

⊙ The unrousable patient

Definition
Failure to recover consciousness.

Presentation
- Patient does not recover consciousness after a reasonable period of recovery following general anaesthesia.
- Patient becomes unresponsive following admission to PACU.

Immediate management
- Check ABC ... 100% O_2.
- Treat hypoxia and hypotension (see pp332–3, 328–9).
- Measure temperature—actively re-warm as necessary.
- Anaesthetic history; check use of opioids (miosis, bradypnoea, apnoea), benzodiazepines (breathing but not awakening), other CNS depressants. Neuromuscular assessment with peripheral nerve stimulator.
- Reverse suspected drugs (naloxone, flumazenil, physostigmine).
- Give glucose 50% if hypoglycaemia is suspected.
- Rapid neurological examination seeking localizing signs. If stroke or other neurological injury suspected, arrange CT/MRI scan and consult neurologist/neurosurgeon.

Subsequent management
- Careful check of anaesthetic record; check used ampoules for drug error.
- According to diagnosis.
- Admit to HDU or ICU pending investigations.

Investigations
- Glucose, Na^+/K^+/ABGs
- CT or MRI scan to exclude stroke or other structural lesion, (later, EEG to exclude non-convulsive status epilepticus or metabolic/toxic encephalopathy).
- Osmolality (TURP syndrome, SIADH, diabetes, or alcohol-related complication)

Risk factors
- See 'Confusion'.
- Neurosurgery
- Carotid artery surgery or stenting
- Long, deep anaesthetics with excess volatile anaesthetics or TIVA
- Diabetes mellitus (hyperosmolar, hyperglycaemic coma; hypoglycaemia)

Exclusions
- Hypothermia:
  - *iatrogenic hypothermia*—long-duration surgery, use of cool irrigating fluids (TURP, abdominal washouts). Re-warm patient with hot-air warming blanket, warmed IV fluids

- *hypothyroid coma*—typically elderly women, with longstanding hypothyroidism, and may be precipitated by infection (pneumonia, UTI), trauma, heart failure, CVA, or drugs (amiodarone). Temperature usually <35.5°C, and there may be hypotension, hypoventilation, hypoglycaemia, hyponatraemia. Admit to ICU for ventilatory and cardiovascular support, temperature and glucose control, slow replacement of thyroid hormones
- Metabolic/toxic encephalopathy—hypoglycaemia, hyponatraemia, drug toxicity (e.g. benzodiazepines, illicit drugs), sepsis.
- Non-convulsive status epilepticus.
- Structural intracranial lesion compressing, or involving, brainstem.
- Stroke (ischaemic or haemorrhagic), subdural haematoma, tumour.
- *Pseudocoma*—usually a young patient with otherwise normal neuro-logical examination, resists eye-opening and does not allow arm to fall on face or genitalia.
- Muscle weakness or residual curarization (see pp340–1). Check neuromuscular function with peripheral nerve stimulator.

Paediatric implications

Consider—suxamethonium apnoea, opioid overdose, hyponatraemia, raised ICP, neurological condition (e.g. cerebral palsy).

Further reading

Mecca, R.S. (1991) Complications during recovery. *International Anaesthesiology Clinics*, **29**, 37–54.

ⓘ **Stroke**

Definition
Cerebral haemorrhage/infarction resulting in focal cerebral damage.

Presentation
New onset of focal neurological deficit or alteration in mental state.

Immediate management
- Maintain oxygenation—SpO_2.
- BP control—arterial line for uncontrolled hypertension or labile BP.
- Control ventricular rate in atrial fibrillation.
- Check glucose, U&Es, ECG.
- Neurological examination.
- CT or MRI scan to differentiate type of stroke.
- Carotid ultrasound (if carotid territory ischaemic event).

Subsequent management
- If acute thrombotic stroke <3 h old, consider thrombolysis with t-PA or aspirin in consultation with surgeon and neurologist.
- Admit to Stroke Unit for supportive treatment.
- Treat atrial fibrillation and other risk factors according to local protocols, and consider anticoagulation in consultation with surgeon and cardiologist.

Investigations
- Check glucose, U&Es, ECG.
- Neurological examination—CT or MRI scan to identify stroke lesion, distinguish infarction from haemorrhage, and help differentiate the aetiological subtype of ischaemic and haemorrhagic stroke (e.g. cardiac embolism, large artery disease, small artery disease). Carotid ultrasound (if carotid territory ischaemic event).
- ECG/echocardiography.

Risk factors
- Cerebrovascular disease (TIAs, migraine)
- Hypertension, smoking, hypercholesterolaemia, diabetes
- Atrial fibrillation, previous anterior myocardial infarction
- Carotid artery surgery or stenting, interventional neuroradiological procedures
- Cardiopulmonary bypass, induced hypotension

Exclusions

- Migraine—paroxysmal syndrome characterized by throbbing, pulsatile headache, photophobia, nausea (90%), vomiting (60%), aura (15–25%), and focal neurological signs (<5%). Administer anti-emetics and analgesics—aspirin (antiplatelet), NSAIDs, sumatriptan (or analogue), lidocaine infusion—and refer to neurologist.
- Partial epileptic seizures.
- Hypoglycaemia.
- Subdural haematoma.

Paediatric implications

Predisposing factors include blood dyscrasias, sickle cell disease, migraine, and neoplasia.

Further reading

Kam, P.C.A., Calcroft, R.M. (1997). Perioperative stroke in general surgical patients. *Anaesthesia*, **52**, 879–83.

The European Stroke Initiative Executive Committee and the EUSI Writing Committee (2003). European stroke initiative recommendations for stroke management—Update. *Cerebrovascular Diseases*, **16**, 311–37.

① Residual neuromuscular blockade

Definition
Unexpectedly prolonged neuromuscular blockade following anaesthesia.

Presentation
- Poorly supported or obstructed airway with inadequate breathing/cough, poor hand-grip, head-lift <5 s.
- 'Floppy', struggling, jerky, or agitated patient, pseudo-sedation (eyes closed).
- Low SpO_2.

Immediate management
- Assess ventilation; if inadequate, commence BLS with bag–mask ventilation and oxygen; apply pulse oximeter.
- If ventilation adequate, consider jaw support, oral/nasal airway insertion, and assist ventilation as needed with patient on side. Reassure patient, encourage slow inspiratory breaths, and stay with patient until return of full neuromuscular function.
- Apply nerve stimulator and check train-of-four (TOF) or double-burst stimulation (DBS). Absence of fade indicates adequate neuromuscular function. A post-tetanic count can be used when the TOF shows no twitches (reversal is likely when the post-tetanic count is ≥10).
- Administer further or first dose of reversal agent (max. dose neostigmine 70 µg/kg with glycopyrronium 10 µg/kg) if indicated.
- If neuromuscular function does not return after reversal, or there are features of Phase II (mixed) blockade, consider IV anaesthesia and tracheal intubation. Transfer to ICU for ventilation.
- If the patient is conscious but partly paralysed, reassure and consider sedation with small doses of midazolam or propofol.
- Establish/maintain normothermia and normocarbia.

Subsequent management
- Pseudocholinesterase genotyping 3 days after suxamethonium, mivacurium, or neostigmine exposure (8 weeks after blood administration) with follow-up by anaesthetist, counselling, and biochemical testing of family members. Organize 'Medic Alert' bracelet or other disease identification system.
- Referral to neurologist for patients with suspected neuromuscular disease.
- Explain episode to patient later if they have any recall. Some are terrified and assume this will occur again.

Investigations
- Apply peripheral nerve stimulator and test for residual paralysis.
- Baseline U&Es, Ca^{2+}, Mg^{2+}, ABGs, core temp. (tympanic).

Risk factors
- Hypothermia/acidosis.
- Known neuromuscular disease (e.g. myasthenia gravis) or symptoms (unexplained weakness) in patient or family.
- Excessive use of neuromuscular blockers or repeated use of suxamethonium (>10 mg/kg).
- Use of aminoglycoside antibiotics (gentamicin, amikacin, tobramycin, neomycin), anticholinesterases (echothiophate eye drops with suxamethonium), or magnesium infusion.
- Renal or hepatic impairment (with reduced metabolism/clearance of certain neuromuscular blockers).
- Cholinesterase deficiency (hepatic disease, malnutrition, carcinomatosis, pregnancy, cardiopulmonary bypass) or reduced activity (abnormal genotypes).
- Lithium therapy.
- Verapamil.

Exclusions
- Psychiatric disturbance
- Respiratory depression (see pp330–1)
- Neurological problems, e.g. myasthenia gravis or myasthenic syndromes (Eaton–Lambert syndrome), stroke, laryngeal nerve palsy
- Hypothyroidism, myxoedema coma
- Hyper-, hypokalaemia (e.g. hypokalaemic paralysis—rare clinical syndrome of systemic weakness with low K^+)
- Hyperparathyroidism with hypercalcaemia, hypocalcaemia

Special considerations
- Attempted reversal of mivacurium before neuromuscular function starts to return may result in prolonged duration of action and neuromuscular blockade.
- Do not try to reverse neuromuscular drugs when there are no signs of recovery on the TOF.
- Successful reversal of neuromuscular blockade appears to be dependent upon intracellular pH, therefore correct respiratory acidosis.
- Consider use of sugammadex for reversal of non-depolarizing neuromuscular blockade, especially rocuronium.

Further reading
Lenz, A., Hill, G., White, P.F. (2007). Emergency use of sugammadex after failure of standard reversal drugs. *Anesthesia and Analgesia*, **104**(3), 585–6.

① Oliguria/acute renal failure (ARF)

Definition (also see Further reading)

- **Oliguria**—reduced urine production:
  - *significant:* when urine is reduced to <0.5 mL/kg for 6 h
  - *severe:* when less than 0.3 mL/kg for 24 h
- **ARF**—deterioration of renal function over hours/days that results in failure to excrete waste products of metabolism.

Presentation

May present as polyuria, oliguria, or anuria. Often classified according to site of lesion: prerenal, renal, or postrenal.

Immediate management

- Hourly urine output measurement via urinary catheter (exclude blocked catheter by flushing with 50 mL saline via a bladder syringe).
- Maintain normovolaemia.
- Estimate fluid loss and calculate fluid balance:
  - fluid challenge (250–500 mL over 15 min)—repeat according to response; avoid >1 L positive fluid balance
  - CVC insertion and maintain CVP at 10–12 cmH$_2$O
- Maintain BP at normal levels (MAP >70 mmHg) or higher if patient usually hypertensive. Vasopressors may be necessary.
- Optimize cardiac output, consider dobutamine.
- Treat life-threatening electrolyte disturbances.

Subsequent management

- Acute hyperkalaemia (K$^+$ >6.5 mmol/L)—see pp296–7.
- TURP syndrome—see pp290–1.
- Stop or avoid nephrotoxic drugs.
- Consider mannitol/furosemide to promote some diuresis and make fluid management easier.
- Refer to nephrologist or intensivist for further management of prerenal or intrinsic ARF.
- Refer to urologist for postrenal obstruction. Suprapubic catheter or percutaneous nephrostomy may be necessary.

Investigations

- U&Es, FBC, coagulation screen, and consider creatine kinase (rhabdomyolysis).
- ABGs.
- Urinary Na+ and osmolality. In prerenal ARF the kidney will attempt to retain Na+ (urinary sodium <20 mmol/L) and concentrate urine (SG >1.015). These patients may benefit from more fluid boluses. In acute tubular necrosis (ATN) the kidney will begin to lose this ability (urinary sodium >20 mmol/L and SG <1.015). Newer renal biomarkers such as cystatin C and NGAL have failed to make a significant impact on clinical management of ARF at present.

Risk factors

- The 'vulnerable' kidney—patients with diabetes, hypertension, vasculopathy, and increasing age with a normal creatinine often have a reduced nephron capacity and impaired renovascular response to even modest changes in BP. 75% of the kidneys' nephrons need to be impaired before a patient's GFR begins to decline.
- Pre-existing chronic kidney disease—glomerulonephritis and/or nephrosclerosis.
- Prerenal—hypotension, hypovolaemia/dehydration, cardiac or liver failure.
- Renal—nephrotoxins (antibiotics, contrast agents, NSAIDs, ACE inhibitors, ciclosporin, myoglobin), sepsis, obstructive jaundice, ABO blood transfusion reactions.
- Postrenal—renal tumours, stones, prostate tumours.
- Surgery—aortic, renovascular, prolonged procedures, cardiopulmonary bypass.
- Consider preloading with saline for patients at risk of renal failure (chronic kidney disease, prolonged fasting, NSAID use) and acetylcysteine for prevention of contrast-induced nephropathy.

Exclusions

- Catheter problems (poorly positioned, obstructed, or kinked urinary catheter). Irrigate catheter to relieve obstruction, dislodge clots or debris.
- If a urinary catheter is not present, or cannot be easily inserted, the presence of a distended bladder should be sought by palpation and/or abdominal ultrasound. Cystoscopy with ureteric stent insertion, suprapubic catheter insertion, or percutaneous nephrostomy may be indicated, according to level and type of obstruction.

Special considerations

- **Contrast nephropathy** is a leading cause of in-hospital acute renal failure. Patients with known renal impairment and diabetes are at greatest risk. At present, the most robust evidence suggests a modest fluid load with isotonic sodium bicarbonate (3 mL/kg for at least 1 hour before contrast followed by 1 mL/kg until 6 h post-procedure) may be beneficial. The role of N-acetylcysteine remains uncertain but can be given in conjunction with sodium bicarbonate (1200 mg bd for 24 h before and 48 h after contrast).
- **Drugs**. Diuretics can be used following appropriate volume replacement. Osmotic (mannitol), loop (furosemide), and thiazide diuretics (and renal dose dopamine) confer no benefit in reducing the incidence of acute renal failure, dialysis, or mortality in oliguric patients. Their role lies in attempting to optimize fluid balance and stratifying patients who respond to diuretics into a more favourable outcome group. Mannitol is most useful in rhabdomyolysis or intracerebral oedema.
- **Abdominal compartment syndrome** occurs in the setting of a raised intra-abdominal pressure (IAP) and end-organ dysfunction. A raised IAP may lead to renal and splanchnic hypoperfusion, respiratory embarrassment by inhibiting downward/caudal diaphragmatic movement, reduced venous return to the heart, raised intracranial pressure, and

bacterial translocation. This occurs with acute pancreatitis, large retroperitoneal bleeds, emergency AAA surgery, and abdominal trauma
surgery. Urinary manometry is the more reliable method of monitoring
IAP. Specific IAP urinary manometry kits exist. Alternatively, connect
a manometer to an 18G needle and insert it into a urinary catheter
(which has been clamped distally) with 50 mL of sterile saline in the
bladder, to achieve an accurate reading. Zero reference point is pubic
symphysis. IAP scale is:

- normal   <10 mmHg
- mild elevation   10–20 mmHg
- moderate elevation   20–30 mmHg
- severe elevation   30 mmHg.

Measure the IAP every 2–4h. Consider surgical decompression if IAP
>25 mmHg and evidence of end-organ dysfunction.

Further reading

Recent attempts to achieve a consensus definition for ARF have resulted in the RIFLE criteria; this
defines acute kidney injury (AKI) into three grades of severity based on serum creatinine and/or
urine output and two outcomes based on the duration of renal impairment. See: Acute renal
failure—definition, outcome measures, animal models, fluid therapy and information technology
needs: the Second International Consensus Conference of the Acute Dialysis Quality Initiative
(ADQI) Group. Bellomo, R., Ronco, C., Kellum, J.A. et al. (2004). *Critical Care*, **8**, R204–R212.

http://ccforum.com/content/8/4/R204

① Severe postoperative nausea and vomiting (PONV)

Definition
Persistent nausea ± vomiting despite first-line drug therapy.

Presentation
- Patient reports feeling of nausea.
- Attempted ('dry-retching') or actual vomiting of gastric contents.

Immediate management
- Check heart rate and blood pressure (nausea often precedes detection of hypotension).
- Fluid therapy, correct electrolyte disturbance.
- Treat pain and severe anxiety.
- Drug therapy (treatment cascade will differ according to local protocols):
  - $5HT_3$ antagonists (ondansetron 4 mg IV, tropisetron 2 mg IV, dolasetron 12.5 mg IV, granisetron 1 mg IV)
  - phenothiazine (prochlorperazine 10–12.5 mg IM)
  - metoclopramide 10 mg IV (not with gastric/bowel obstruction)
  - butyrophenone (droperidol 0.5–1 mg IV—not available in UK, haloperidol 0.5–2 mg IV)
  - steroids (dexamethasone 4–8 mg IV)
  - antihistamines (cyclizine 25–50 mg slow IV, promethazine 12.5–50 mg IM/slow IV)
  - anticholinergics (hyoscine hydrobromide 0.3–0.6 mg IM/SC/IV)
  - benzodiazepines have been used preoperatively or (rarely) as a low-dose postoperative infusion (midazolam 0.5–1 mg/h) for intractable PONV
  - small dose of propofol (10–20 mg IV)
- Consider NG tube if there is gastric outlet obstruction, bowel obstruction, severe retching/vomiting

Subsequent management
- Withhold oral fluids and continue IV therapy.
- Administer anti-emetics regularly or add to IV fluids.
- Monitor electrolytes, renal and hepatic function.
- Consider drug side-effects.
- Try alternative opioids for analgesia. Consider regional analgesia/ketamine infusion and NSAIDs if patient intolerant of all opioids used.
- Consider acupuncture (P6 point on wrist).
- Document severe PONV for future anaesthesia.

Risk factors
- *Patient factors*—baseline risk is 10%. Female sex, history of PONV or motion sickness, non-smoker, post-op. opioids. Each additional risk factor increases baseline risk to 20%, 40%, 60%, 80%.

- *Anaesthetic factors*—use of certain drugs: opioids, tramadol, N_2O, etomidate, ketamine, neostigmine. Duration of anaesthesia, with each 30 min increasing risk by 60%.
- *Surgical factors*—laparoscopic surgery, laparotomy, breast/plastic/strabismus surgery, gastric dilatation (gastric outlet obstruction, poor bag–mask ventilation).

Exclusions

- Hypotension—see pp328–9.
- Gastric dilatation—difficult bag–mask ventilation, NG tube incorrectly positioned, unrelieved bowel obstruction.
- CNS problem—raised or low ICP, migraine, head injury, neurosurgery, CSF leak. Consider neurosurgical opinion if changed level of consciousness or new CNS signs.
- Consider myocardial ischaemia/infarction. Perform 12-lead ECG.

Paediatric implications—drug therapy

- Ondansetron 0.1 mg/kg IV to maximum of 4 mg
- Dexamethasone 0.2 mg/kg IV
- Metoclopramide 0.1 mg/kg IV

Special considerations

PONV (the 'big little problem') is associated with adverse effects (raised intracranial and intraocular pressure), but aggressive perioperative management can reduce morbidity (wound dehiscence, pain), recovery room, and hospital stay.

Further reading

Gan, T.J., Meyer, T.A., Apfel, C.C. et al. for the Society for Ambulatory Anesthesia Guidelines for the Management of Postoperative Nausea and Vomiting (2007). *Anesthesia and Analgesia*, **105**(6), 1615–28.

① Severe postoperative pain

Definition
Severe pain on emergence from anaesthesia or on regression of regional blockade. Pain score ≥7 and consistent behavioural score (grimacing).

Presentation
- Patient distress, anger, crying, or reluctance to move
- Tachycardia, hypertension, sweating, or other sympathetic responses. Agitation, especially in elderly or intellectually impaired
- Inadequate respiratory effort with arterial desaturation (abdominal/chest wounds)

Immediate management
- Titrate opioid to analgesia with repeated boluses of: fentanyl 10–30 µg IV, morphine 1–3 mg IV, or tramadol 50 mg slow IV (if severe try morphine/alfentanil mix (10 mg morphine/1 mg alfentanil in saline to 10 mL) 1–3 mL IV).
- Consider clonidine (1–2 ug/kg IV) if associated agitation
- Consider paracetamol 1 g PO/PR/IV.
- Unless contraindicated, give NSAID—diclofenac 100 mg PR (or Dyloject®—injectable diclofenac, bolus IV) or parecoxib 40 mg IV.
- Consider ketamine 10–15 mg IV single bolus for intractable pain, or if patient has implanted opioid antagonist.
- Consider pethidine (25–50 mg IV) or hyoscine butylbromide (Buscopan®) if visceral pain (urologic, intestinal, or biliary surgery).
- Consider pregabalin (75–100 mg PO) if significant preoperative pain (neuropathic pain component)
- Consider temporary use of Entonox® until effect of other analgesics is felt.
- Consider regional analgesia (intercostal or nerve block, epidural, paravertebral).
- Exclude new or untreated pathology (surgical review if original diagnosis in doubt or possible new pathology, such as compartment syndrome or iatrogenic nerve damage).

Subsequent management
- If there is still significant pain after high-dose morphine, a small dose of midazolam (1 mg) may improve matters—watch respiration and conscious level.
- Consider clonidine 1 µg/kg up to 50 µg as an adjuvant, observe BP and for sedation.
- Acute Pain Service to manage postoperative opioid/ketamine infusions or regional block, neuraxial or interpleural infusions, treat complications, and maximize use of multi-modal analgesic therapy.

Investigations
Exclude new or untreated pathology. Check history of opioid use/abuse.

Risk factors
- Preoperative opioid use
- Poor control of pain prior to surgery
- Inadequate intraoperative analgesics or exclusive use of remifentanil
- Implanted opioid antagonist (e.g. naltrexone) or mixed opioid agonist/antagonist (e.g. buprenorphine, which has a ceiling effect)
- Visceral pain, including bladder spasm (neostigmine) and biliary spasm (morphine)

Exclusions
- Severe anxiety or psychiatric disturbance.
- Acute confusional state.
- Consider full bladder, glucose, or metabolic problem if agitated.
- Opioid-seeking behaviour (advisable to give patient the benefit of doubt, give analgesics, and seek specialist help later).
- Exclude new or untreated pathology, such as compartment syndrome, nerve damage, or ischaemia from any cause—consider surgical review if original diagnosis in doubt or possible new pathology.

Special considerations
- Always exclude hypoxia following opioid administration.
- *Chronic preoperative opioid use or abuse*—patients may require high opioid dosages that exceed standard protocols. A dedicated pain service can assist with perioperative analgesic therapy.
- *Elderly or intellectually impaired patient*—pain assessment may be difficult and agitation or confusion can be the only indication of pain.
- *Cultural differences*—some cultures show little behavioural evidence of pain. Assessment should include ability to move, breathe deeply, or cough.
- *Severe anxiety*—titrate clonidine 25–50 µg IV every 5 min prn to achieve sedation (maximum 2 µg/kg) or midazolam 1 mg IV every 5 min prn to achieve sedation.

Paediatric implications
Pain scores in preverbal children are difficult. Use observational pain scoring tools (e.g. CHIPPS scale for 0–23 months, FLACC scale for 2–7 years), then self-reporting tools appropriate for age (e.g. Faces pain scale for 4–12 years), and standard VAS scales for older children and adolescents.

Further reading
Büttner W, Finke W. (2000). Analysis of behavioural and physiological parameters for the assessment of postoperative analgesic demand in newborns, infants and young children: a comprehensive report on seven consecutive studies. *Paediatric Anaesthesia*, **10**, 303–18. [CHIPPS scale]

Hicks CL, von Baeyer CL, Spafford PA, van Korlaar I, Goodenough B. (2001). The Faces Pain Scale-Revised: toward a common metric in pediatric pain measurement. *Pain*, **93**, 173–183.

Joshi, G.P., White, P.F. (2001). Management of acute and postoperative pain. *Current Opinion in Anaesthesiology*, **14**(4), 417–21.

Merkel SI, Voepel-Lewis T, Shayevitz JR, Malviya S. (1997). The FLACC: a behavioral scale for scoring postoperative pain in young children. *Pediatric Nursing*, **23**, 293–7.

Rowlingson, J.C. (2001). Acute postoperative pain management. *Anesthesia and Analgesia*, **92**(Suppl.), 78–85.

① Epidural problems

Definition

Any problem related to the epidural technique, catheter, or drugs.

Presentation

Pain, hypotension/bradycardia, headache, nausea/vomiting, itch, shivering, postdural puncture headache, urinary retention.

Immediate management

Hypotension/bradycardia
- Associated with total spinal, dural puncture, subarachnoid, or subdural catheter position, high block.
- Nausea/vomiting often precedes hypotension (especially parturients).
- Stop infusion.
- Lay patient flat, elevate legs.
- Give ephedrine 3–6 mg IV (alternatives include metaraminol 0.5–2 mg IV, phenylephrine 100 µg IV (or 5 mg in 50 mL saline at 0–30 mL/h IV), adrenaline 20–100 µg IV).
- Give atropine 0.6–1.2 mg IV (glycopyrronium 0.2–0.4 mg IV) if bradycardia.
- Rapid IV fluid administration (crystalloid 1000 mL or colloid 500 mL).

'Total' spinal—see pp246–7.

Local anaesthetic toxicity—see pp236–8.

Wound pain
- Perform 'ice mapping' to determine extent and quality of block—is the block 'patchy' with missed dermatomes?
- Perform catheter aspiration test (absence of CSF or blood, but may be false-negative in 50% of cases).
- Consider adjusting catheter position if block too high, too low, or unilateral—withdraw catheter using aseptic technique but leave at least 3 cm in the epidural space.
- Administer test dose of local anaesthetic if BP normal, and repeat to achieve analgesia. Consider higher concentration LA ± opioids—if hypotension/bradycardia develop, give opioids only (fentanyl 50–100 µg, or pethidine 50–100 mg, or diamorphine 2.5 mg).
- Consider adding clonidine 1 µg/mL to LA solution to treat patchy block.
- Supplement regional analgesia with systemic adjuvant (paracetamol, NSAIDs) or opioid analgesics and remove opioid from epidural solution.

Nausea/vomiting
- Treat hypotension.
- If epidural infusion includes an opioid, give anti-emetics IV according to protocol. Consider naloxone 0.1 mg IV ± naloxone infusion (naloxone 400 µg added to maintenance IV fluids).
- If symptoms persist, remove opioid from epidural infusion, maintain epidural with local anaesthetic.

Shivering
- Treat hypothermia with hot-air warming blanket.
- Warm IV fluids.
- Pethidine 25 mg IV or tramadol 25 mg IV or clonidine may be useful.

Postdural puncture headache(PDPH)
- Postural headache relieved by lying and exacerbated by sitting or standing.
- Risk can be reduced if intrathecal catheter introduced for 24h at the time of dural puncture. This should be meticulously labelled as 'intrathecal'.
- Give simple analgesics.
- Caffeine may be effective.
- 85% of PDPH resolve by 6 weeks.
- Definitive treatment is epidural blood patch performed by experienced personnel; success rate is 70–98%.

Subsequent management
- *Urinary retention*—according to local protocol, the bladder may be catheterized as a single-shot, or an indwelling catheter may be left *in situ* until the epidural catheter technique is discontinued.
- *Tachyphylaxis*—if sensory block recedes more quickly than expected in patients with an epidural infusion, try an alternative local anaesthetic. Regular testing of sensory level and appropriate increases in infusion rates of the epidural infusion can maintain an effective block. In general, if there are no problems of hypotension or excessive block, an infusion rate of 10 mL/h (lumbar) or 7 mL/h (thoracic) will help to prevent a sudden contraction in block.
- *Itching*—consider use of naloxone (100 µg IV prn), promethazine (25–50 mg IM), or removing opioid from epidural mixture. Low-dose propofol and ondansetron have been reported to be beneficial.

Investigations
MRI if epidural haematoma suspected.

Risk factors
- Previous back surgery, obesity, kyphoscoliosis
- Inexperienced anaesthetist, multiple attempts at insertion, poor technique

Exclusions
- *Subarachnoid (spinal) catheter/inadvertent dural puncture*—should be suspected with high block, hypotension, and bradycardia. Treat symptomatically, prepare for airway management if large dose of local anaesthetic has been given or block is ascending. Remove catheter.
- *Subdural catheter*—should be suspected when a higher than expected block occurs 15–30 min after injection of local anaesthetic. Remove catheter.

- *Epidural haematoma*—should be suspected if sensorimotor block persists 6 h after surgery—urgent investigation with MRI indicated and proceed with surgical drainage as necessary (see pp242–3).

Further reading

Wheatley, R.G., Schug, S.A., Watson, D. (2001). Safety and efficacy of postoperative epidural analgesia. *British Journal of Anaesthesia*, **87**, 47–61.

Emergency department problems

Neil Rasburn

☼ Major trauma

Definition

Major injury to head/chest/abdomen/pelvis/spine/limbs

Presentation

- Depends on severity of injury.
- Patient may be awake or unconscious.
- A confused patient may worsen injuries by moving.
- The same clinical picture can arise from different injuries, e.g. loss of consciousness (LOC) can result from significant head injury, CVE or medical coma, major blood loss or primary cardiac arrest.

Immediate management

- ABC … At the scene, healthcare staff may have followed the MARCH protocol (Massive haemorrhage control, Airway, Respiratory, Cardiovascular, Haemorrhage).
- 100% oxygen via a non-rebreathing mask..
- IV access with two large-bore (14–16G) cannulae.

Airway

- Cervical spine immobilization with either a hard collar or manual in-line stabilization.
- Establish an airway with simple manoeuvres and then consider definitive airway if:
  - correction of hypoxaemia required
  - severe head injury
  - confusion/fluctuating LOC requiring head CT—'GCS of 8, time to intubate'
  - major traumatic injury, GA required on humane grounds ± major surgery imminent
- Rapid sequence induction with cricoid pressure—protect cervical spine as above.
- Awake fibreoptic intubation not recommended if patient non-compliant or there is trauma to the airway, consider surgical tracheostomy.

Breathing

- Identify major thoracic injuries. Tension pneumothorax should be diagnosed clinically (see pp50–1).
- If pneumothorax, haemopneumothorax, flail segment, or fractured ribs present consider tracheobronchial injury, pulmonary contusion, diaphragmatic injury, cardiac contusion/tamponade, and mediastinal disruption. Injury to the 1st rib is an indication of major forces involved in the trauma.

Circulation

- Major external haemorrhage should have been stemmed with direct pressure.
- Adequate IV access should be secured with at least two short, large-bore cannulae (14G).
- Check pulse rate and depth. Assess peripheral perfusion.

- Blood pressure should be low enough not to exacerbate bleeding but high enough to maintain major organ perfusion (MAP 50–60 mmHg).
- Hypotension may be a late sign of hypovolaemia, particularly in young and fit patients.
- Deteriorating conscious level in the absence of primary head injury is suggestive of a blood loss of >30% total blood volume.
- Arterial cannulation will allow monitoring of acid–base status and give an indication of how effective the resuscitation has been. Central venous saturations of <70% may suggest inadequate circulating volume but requires central venous access. This may be a short, large-bore cannula if it is also to be used for rapid fluid resuscitation.

Disability

- Assess with the GCS and observe the pupils. Any change in the GCS requires reassessment of Airway, Breathing, and Circulation.
- The patient's neurology should always be assessed and documented prior to intubation. The motor component of the score gives the best indication of outcome.

Exposure

- Examine patient completely and then cover up to reduce heat loss.

Fluids

- Initial fluid resuscitation with crystalloid or colloid is appropriate; adequacy of replacement is judged by cardiovascular parameters, urine output, and cognitive function.
- Rapid response suggests losses are <20 % blood volume and there is no further ongoing bleeding.
- A transient response suggests losses are 20–50% of normal blood volume.
- Minimal or no response to volume resuscitation suggests concealed bleeding, tamponade, tension pneumothorax, embolism, spinal cord injury, cardiogenic cause, or sepsis.
- Consider in the context of age, drug therapy and other comorbidities.
- Fluid should be replaced carefully. Overly aggressive infusion may exacerbate further bleeding and inadequate resuscitation may compromise vital organ perfusion.
- A rapid infusor should be available and all products should be warmed.

Subsequent management

Secondary survey follows the primary survey and resuscitation, and involves head-to-toe systematic assessment. It may include reassessment of the primary survey and additional imaging/blood tests:

- The need for laparotomy should be assessed rather than concentrating on an absolute diagnosis. Examination, including PR, should be followed by FAST (see below) if available.
- Consider chest injuries including pulmonary/cardiac contusion, major vessel transection/rupture, and diaphragmatic/oesophageal rupture.
- Pelvic injuries can bleed profusely: stabilization is critical and may need to precede laparotomy. Consider urethral injury.

- Cervical spine injuries—monitor for loss of motor function, loss of sensation, altered pattern of ventilation, hypotension with bradycardia, loss of signs of peritoneal irritation.
- Limb injuries should be assessed for vascular and neurological deficit, compartment syndrome—pale/pallor/paraesthesia/pressure from swelling/pulseless (late sign). Urgent surgical decompression may be required.
- Potential further management issues include massive blood loss, long surgical procedures with other serious injuries (e.g. head injury—see below).
- Surgical procedures need to be performed in order of importance.

Investigations

Essential initial investigations in the multi-trauma patient:
- Crossmatch/FBC/U&Es/clotting/LFT
- CXR (supine):
  - lungs—look for evidence of aspiration or contusion
  - pleura—look for haemopneumothorax
  - heart shadow—if enlarged suspect pericardial tamponade
  - pneumomediastinum/pneumopericardium/SC emphysema—suspect major airway injury
  - ribs—if upper ribs fractured then patient at high risk of major intra-thoracic trauma
  - correct placement of lines and tubes
- Lateral cervical spine X-ray indicated for:
  - head injury
  - severe maxillofacial injury
  - mechanism of injury, e.g. sudden deceleration
  - spine pain/tenderness
  - cervical spine X-ray checklist—need to see from C1 to C7/T1 interspace, look for alignment of the anterior and posterior vertebral lines, the spinolaminar line and the tips of the spinous processes, compression of any bones including C1 peg, equal disc spaces, and normal appearance of soft tissue in the prevertebral space
- CT scan of head/chest/abdomen/pelvis as indicated, the films can be used to look at thoracolumbar spine for possible injury
- Focused Assessment with Sonography for Trauma (FAST)—looking at abdominal injuries
- ECG

Special considerations
- Severe head injury—see pp182–5

Risk factors
Motorcyclists, cyclists, pedestrians, alcohol or drug usage

Further reading
Advanced Trauma Life Support® guidelines: available at http://www.facs.org/trauma/atls/index.html

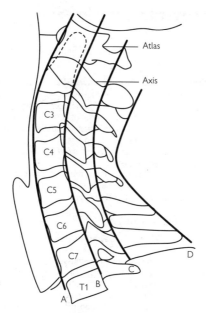

Lateral cervical spine X-Ray

A = Anterior vertebral line
B = Posterior vertebral line
C = Spinolaminar line
D = Tips of spinous processes

☠ Drug overdose

Definition
Intentional or non-intentional consumption of drugs/medication in excess of their therapeutic index.

Presentation
- It may not be obvious what has been taken.
- Presentation can vary from no signs or symptoms to significant cardio-vascular disturbance and decreased level of consciousness.
- Polypharmacy is common, the medication consumed may also have been combined with alcohol and illicit drugs.
- In the UK drug overdose is responsible for 6,300 suicides per annum, and 20% of deaths in young people.
- 140,000 para-suicides occur per annum, these are most common in young females 14–19 years old. The most common method is poisoning and paracetamol accounts for 50% of cases.

Immediate management
- Always follow an ABC protocol, assess neurology, and conduct a full examination.
- Obtain history from the patient and witnesses—'**when?**', '**what?**', '**quantity?**'—past medical history, drug history, psychiatric history.
- Initial management is supportive: correct hypoxia, hypotension, dehydration, hypo/hyperthermia, acidosis, and control seizures.
- Monitor temperature, pulse, respiration, BP, ECG, oxygenation, and GCS.
- The aims of management are to decrease absorption, increase excretion ± administer specific antidotes.
- Methods of decreasing absorption include:
  - gastric lavage—only if within 1 h of overdose; **never** with corrosives; intubate if decreased consciousness level.
  - Activated charcoal—50 g single or repeated dose (also increases elimination). Activated charcoal **does not** bind heavy metals, ethanol, or acids.
- Methods of increasing elimination include:
  - multiple doses of activated charcoal (quinine and phenobarbital)
  - charcoal haemoperfusion (barbiturates and theophylline)
  - diuresis
  - urinary alkalinization (tricyclics)
  - dialysis

Investigations
- Always check blood glucose, paracetamol, and salicylate levels.
- FBC, U&Es, LFT, clotting, bicarbonate, ABGs, ECG, CXR.
- Blood and urine for toxicology screening, specific blood levels.

Paediatric implications
Accidental overdose may have occurred.

Specific management of toxins
Paracetamol
- Most common drug in overdose, few signs or symptoms early on.
- Hepatic and renal toxin (centrilobular necrosis), higher risk if liver enzymes are induced (phenobarbital, phenytoin, carbamazepine, barbiturates, rifampicin, alcohol) or if glutathione-depleted (HIV, starvation, cachexia, cystic fibrosis).
- Just 150 mg/kg or 12 g in an adult can be fatal.
- Treatment is with N-acetylcysteine (NAC), i.e. a glutathione precursor and a source of sulphydryl groups allowing conjugation to non-toxic metabolites.
- NAC dose regime is 150 mg/kg in 200 mL of 5% glucose over 15 min, then 50 mg/kg over 4 h, then 100 mg/kg in 1 L of 5% glucose over 16 h. Side-effects include flushing, wheeze, hypotension, and anaphylactoid reaction. Alternative to NAC is methionine PO (<12 h).
- Use nomogram for calculating paracetamol toxic dose (Fig. 11.1).
- *Presentation less than 4 h since ingestion:*
  - give activated charcoal
  - wait 4 h before checking plasma drug levels unless there is another clinical reason for checking earlier
- *Presentation 4–8 h since ingestion:*
  - check paracetamol and salicylate levels, assess risk using paracetamol nomogram (Fig. 11.1)—if additional risk factors are present (see above) NAC treatment will be triggered by lower plasma paracetamol concentration
  - start treatment <8 h post ingestion. Do not delay treatment if 150 mg/kg or 12 g consumed by an adult or if plasma concentration not available in <12 h
  - measure INR, ALT, U&Es, bicarbonate after NAC. If results are normal, patients usually fit for discharge with advice to return if they have symptoms of nausea or abdominal pain
- *Presentation 8–15 h since ingestion:*
  - start NAC.
  - bloods—for paracetamol and salicylate levels, INR, ALT, creatinine, bicarbonate.
  - if level above treatment line, continue NAC and admit for observations and serial blood tests.
  - if level low stop NAC unless other bloods are abnormal
- *Presentation 15–24 h since ingestion:*
  - much more likely to develop severe liver damage. Prognostic accuracy of paracetamol level is debatable, but if above treatment level then risk of serious liver damage is high. There is still benefit in starting NAC even after 24 h

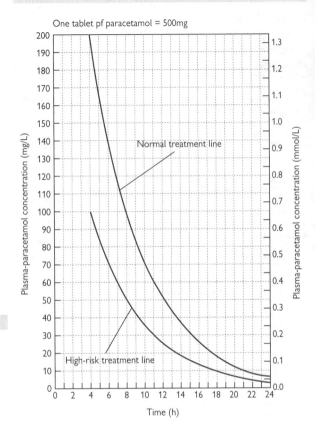

Fig. 11.1 Paracetamol poisoning nomogram.

Aspirin

- Treatment is likely to be necessary if single dose ingestion exceeds 100 mg/kg and/or if patients are young or elderly (<10 yr or >70 yr).
- Early features—hyperventilation, sweating, tinnitus, tremor, nausea/vomiting, and hyperpyrexia.
- Metabolic features—hypo/hyperglycaemia, hypokalaemia, respiratory alkalosis, metabolic acidosis.
- Other—renal failure, pulmonary oedema, seizures, coma and death
- Specific management:
  - bloods—salicylate level after 2 h >700 mg/L (5.1 mmol/L) is potentially lethal; 500 mg/L considered moderate to severe poisoning
  - U&ES, glucose, bicarbonate, ABGs
  - activated charcoal
  - rehydrate, monitor glucose, correct metabolic acidosis (with 8.4% sodium bicarbonate), and monitor K^+
  - monitor urinary pH and alkalinize urine to a pH >7.5 with bicarbonate if plasma salicylate level >500 mg/L
  - consider haemodialysis if plasma salicylate level >700 mg/L before rehydration, or if renal failure or pulmonary oedema are present

Tricyclic antidepressants (TCAs)

- Absorbed in GIT, reach peak levels between 2 and 4 h after ingestion.
- 10 mg/kg can be fatal.
- Pharmacodynamic effects include:
  - Na^+ channel blockade—QRS complex >100 ms
  - alpha-1 adrenoreceptor blockade—vasodilatation, widened pulse pressure, decreased pupillary size
  - myocardial action potential repolarization is prolonged due to potassium efflux blockade—QT interval increased
  - anticholinergic, antihistamine effects (see below).
- Clinical effects:
  - initial symptoms can be trivial but may deteriorate rapidly, most major problems occur within the first 6 h
  - sinus tachycardia, hot dry skin, dry mouth, urinary retention, hypotension, and hypothermia
  - dilated pupils, nystagmus, squint, ataxia, decreased level of consciousness, coma, seizures, increased tone, variable reflexes
  - prolonged PR, QRS, and QT, and ventricular dysrhythmias
- Management:
  - supportive—check airway, maintain ventilation, correct hypoxia and hypercarbia. IV crystalloids for hypotension
  - activated charcoal
  - if QRS >100 ms or dysrhythmias are present—use IV boluses of sodium bicarbonate aiming for a pH of 7.45–7.5 (no higher), avoid antidysrhythmic drugs
  - beware of fluid overload and excess sodium bicarbonate, consider inotropic support for refractory hypotension
  - **do not** use flumazenil if benzodiazepine also taken—can be fatal
  - need to continue monitoring ECG, BP, SpO2, respiratory rate, GCS

Selective serotonin-reuptake inhibitors (SSRIs)
- Absorbed in GIT with a peak plasma concentration occurring 3–8 h after ingestion.
- Lipophilic and have long half-lives (4–9 days).
- Clinically:
  - decreased GCS, ataxia, hyperreflexia, hyperthermia
  - hypertension, ventricular tachycardia and bradycardia
- Management:
  - activated charcoal and IV fluids for hypotension
  - ALS protocols for ventricular dysrhythmias
  - haemodialysis is not indicated
  - benzodiazepines for CNS manifestations

Benzodiazepines
- Often taken in combination with other medications.
- Management:
  - supportive, maintain adequate ventilation and cardiovascular support
  - flumazenil is a specific antidote but is not licensed for overdose treatment in the UK. May require an infusion as half-life is shorter than benzodiazepines. May induce seizures.

Other specific toxins

Table 11.1 Specific antagonists

Overdose drug	Specific antagonist
Benzodiazepines	Flumazenil
Opioids	Naloxone
Iron	Desferrioxamine
Lead	Sodium EDTA
Digoxin	FAB (digoxin-specific antibody fragments)
Calcium channel blockers	Calcium
Ethylene glycol	Ethanol
Lithium	Dialysis

☠ Massive gastrointestinal bleed

Definition

Bleeding from any point in the GI tract. Upper GI causes (in order of frequency) are peptic ulcer disease, gastric erosions, oesophageal varices, Mallory–Weiss tears, and oesophagitis. Lower GI causes include diverticulosis, angiodysplasia, cancer/polyps, rectal disease, and irritable bowel disease

Presentation

- Haematemesis is present in 50% of upper GI bleeds, haematochezia (bright red blood per rectum) is present in 80% of all GI bleeds, and melaena occurs in 70% of upper GI bleeds and 30% of lower.
- Class 1   10–15% blood loss—physiological compensation
- Class 2   15–30%—postural hypotension, reduced urine output
- Class 3   30–40%—tachycardia, tachypnoea, confusion
- Class 4   >40%—as above + no urine output and coma

Immediate management

- ABC ... 100% oxygen and IV access (two 14–16G cannulae).
- Intubate if there is an aspiration risk such as altered mental state or massive upper GI bleed.
- Correct haemodynamics with crystalloid/colloid initially—10 mL/kg bolus. Give blood after 30–40 mL/kg if still unstable.
- Appropriate resuscitation and management can positively affect outcome as 20–40% of the circulating volume is normally present in the splanchnic circulation.
- Mortality is usually from comorbid conditions (MI, organ failure, aspiration, and sepsis).
- Rapid correction of haemodynamics results in fewer MIs and fewer deaths.
- Bleeding stops spontaneously in 80% of cases.
- Correct platelets if <50 × 10^9/L and clotting if INR >1.5.
- Start a proton pump inhibitor (PPI) IV if necessary (e.g. omeprazole 40 mg slow IV).
- If varices are likely, consider terlipressin 1 mg 6-hourly IV to decrease portal blood flow. Antibiotics (e.g. ceftriaxone 2 g IV od) should also be considered as sepsis increases portal pressure and antibiotic prophylaxis in variceal bleeding does reduce risk of re-bleeding and mortality. Give before endoscopy as the procedure causes a bacteraemia in up to 50% of patients.

Subsequent management

- Endoscopy should be considered if the patient remains unstable and there is risk of ongoing bleeding (80% of ulcers and 60% of varices stop bleeding spontaneously).
- May require GA, in an already unstable patient, if agitated, or there is increased risk of aspiration. Consider invasive monitoring.
- Ensure adequate blood products available.

- Beware of re-bleeding post endoscopy, consider repeating procedure, or a Sengstaken–Blakemore tube can be used if varices are present.
- Sengstaken–Blakemore tubes should only be used in intubated patients and should be placed by experienced staff (risk of oesophageal rupture).
- Consider high-dose PPI infusion post endoscopy (e.g. omeprazole 80 mg slow IV, followed by 8 mg/h for 72 h).
- Intra-abdominal surgery is required for 10% of bleeding peptic ulcers.

Investigations
FBC/U&Es/LFT/clotting (including fibrinogen), ABGs, ECG, CXR

Risk factors
- Liver disease, alcohol
- Clotting abnormalities
- Use of anticoagulation medications/NSAIDs
- Comorbidities—liver/heart/renal disease

Exclusions
Massive haemoptysis, upper airway bleeding

Special considerations
Complications of massive blood transfusion

Further reading
Ramrakha, P., Moore, K. (2006). *Oxford Handbook of Acute Medicine*. Oxford University Press, Oxford.

:⚙: Chemical, biological, and radiation injuries

Definition
Biological, nuclear, radiological, incendiary, chemical, or explosive injury.

Presentation
Depends on type of exposure—explosive and chemical injuries tend to be immediate, whereas biological and radiation exposure can take some time to reveal any symptoms. In a major incident, patients will be triaged at the scene and decontamination should commence prior to moving patients away from the scene (Hot Zone) and to hospital.

Chemical injuries

Immediate management
- ABC management should be adhered to, but personal safety is important. Personal Protection Equipment (PPE) should be worn and information on initial decontamination should be sought.
- All attempts should be made to determine the identity of the hazardous material. Responders should obtain assistance in identifying the chemical(s) from container shapes, placards, etc.
- Potential for secondary contamination—Victims who were exposed only to gas or vapour and have no gross deposition of the material on their clothing or skin are unlikely to carry significant amounts of chemical beyond the 'Hot Zone' and are unlikely to pose risks of secondary contamination to hospital personnel. However, victims whose skin or clothing are covered with liquid or solid chemical or those who have chemical vapour condensate on their clothes or skin may contaminate hospital personnel and the emergency department by direct contact or by vapour.
- If the victim has ingested a chemical, toxic vomitus may also pose a danger through direct contact or off-gassing vapour.
- Patients who are able and cooperative may assist with their own decontamination. Remove and double-bag contaminated clothing and personal belonging.
- Flush exposed or irritated skin and hair with plain water for 3–5 min. For oily or otherwise adherent chemicals, use mild soap on the skin and hair. Rinse thoroughly with water.
- Flush exposed or irritated eyes with plain water or saline for at least 5 min. Remove contact lenses if present and easily removable without causing additional trauma to the eye. If a corrosive material is suspected or if pain or injury is evident, continue irrigation while transferring the patient to the Critical Care Area.
- In cases of ingestion, **do not** induce emesis. Administer 125–250 mL of water to dilute stomach contents if the patient is conscious and able to swallow. Immediately transfer the patient to the Critical Care Area.

Subsequent management
Can be split into different agents.

Nerve agents (e.g. Sarin)
- Structurally related to organophosphates and inhibit anticholinesterases (AChE).
- Predominantly, they are liquids at room temperature with high lipid solubility.
- Classical presentation of nerve agent poisoning is cholinergic toxic syndrome, and muscarinic features predominate—salivation, bronchoconstriction, bronchorrhoea, bradycardia, diarrhoea, urination, lacrimation, and dilated pupils.
- Treatment follows ABC principles—death occurring from bronchoconstriction, vocal cord paralysis, bradycardia, or convulsions. Airway management is vital and then early administration of antidotes.
- Non-depolarizing agents cause prolonged paralysis and once AChE is irreversibly inactivated, reversal with neostigmine is ineffective. Suxamethonium causes prolonged paralysis and ketamine increases secretions and should be used with caution.
- Pyridostigmine is a reversible antagonist of AChE. Pretreatment improves survival after nerve agent exposure.
- Atropine antagonizes the muscarinic effects, but nicotinic receptors are unaffected and muscle weakness or paralysis does not improve.
- Pralidoxime reverses nicotinic receptor dysfunction and reduces paralysis if given as an infusion.
- Diazepam is indicated to prevent seizures and minimize secondary brain injury.

Blistering agents (vesicants, e.g. mustard gas)
- May be a latent period of between 2 and 12 h following exposure before symptoms appear, vapour exposure causes most casualties.
- Respiratory symptoms include tracheobronchitis with bronchospasm, epithelial necrosis, pulmonary oedema, and haemorrhage. Intubation may be required as an emergency intervention. Pseudomembrane formation can cause obstruction.
- Ocular symptoms including pain, lacrimation, and oedema require saline irrigation and petroleum jelly to limit closure.
- Skin becomes oedematous and painful. Fluid loss can be considerable from blisters and full thickness burns. Surgical debridement may be required.
- High-dose exposure can suppress the bone marrow and death can result from secondary infection.
- No specific antidote exists to mustard agents.

Blood agents (e.g. hydrogen cyanide)
- Metabolic poisons usually result in rapid death.
- Tachypnoea, confusion, and dizziness are rapidly followed by convulsions, coma, and cardiac arrest.
- Arterial blood gas analysis shows a metabolic acidosis with a raised lactate level. Mixed venous oxygen saturations are raised due to decreased oxygen uptake.

- Treatment is organ-supportive.
- Sodium nitrite (300 mg) converts haemoglobin to methaemoglobin and binds cyanide. Sodium thiosulphate (12.5 g) given simultaneously provides sulphur groups and increases the detoxification of cyanide.
- Dicobalt edetate (300 mg followed immediately after with 50 mL glucose 50% infusion, may be repeated) combines with cyanide forming inert compounds.

Choking agents (e.g. industrial gases)

- Low doses cause eye pain, lacrimation, cough, and bronchospasm.
- High doses induce laryngospasm, extensive tissue necrosis, and alveolar leakage (up to 1 L/h) resulting in pulmonary oedema and respiratory failure.
- Clinical picture of ARDS results.
- Treatment involves bronchodilators, steroids, and prophylactic antibiotics.
- There is no antidote.

Toxins (e.g. ricin and botulinum)

- Ricin inhibits protein synthesis, resulting in death.
- Botulinum toxin permanently inhibits the presynaptic release of ACh at peripheral cholinergic synapses. Recovery occurs after the formation of new terminal boutons which can take months. Treatment is supportive, but an antitoxin is under development.

Incapacitating agents (e.g. Kolokol-I)

- Opioid-based agent causing airway obstruction, apnoea, and decreased level of consciousness in seconds and lasting for hours.
- Reversed by naloxone.

Biological injuries

Immediate management

- Biological agent exposure results in unusual casualties, sometimes with minimal trauma. A history of unusual spray, liquid, or vapour should be sought.
- Effects may be immediate, or more likely delayed ranging from several hours to weeks, the time delay being due to an incubation period. May lie dormant in the environment for weeks/years.
- The agents do not penetrate unbroken skin, in contrast to chemical agents.
- Usually the agents need to be inhaled or ingested to cause disease, do not evaporate, are more toxic than chemical agents by weight, and are undetectable by senses.
- The initial determination of a biological attack must focus on whether the agent is infectious or not. An infectious agent can cross the entire microbiological spectrum (bacteria, virus, rickettsia, yeasts, fungi, prions, etc.) especially when used as a weapon.
- Indications of exposure to an infectious agent may include disease in close family relations, friends, work, and common associations, pets, or surrounding animal contacts. Also consider any other respiratory or bodily fluid contacts with people or animals that have same signs and symptoms at any stage of the suspected disease.

- Non-infectious agents can be viewed as hazardous (chemical) materials to the extent that the release, unless supplemented with other releases, can be dealt with through decontamination and medical treatment. However, it is important to note that biological agents, just like chemical agents, may be extremely persistent depending on the conditions and the mechanism of dispersal. Anthrax has been known to persist for 50 years. It is important to remember when responding to these incidents that bio-agents may be 1000 times more potent.

Subsequent management

- Supportive management initially. Treatment depends on causative agent, which may be: bacterial, e.g. anthrax (antibiotics); viral, e.g. Ebola (vaccine and antivirals); or biotoxins, e.g. ricin (antidotes).
- Significant illness and multi-organ failure can result, but usually not in the emergency setting.
- Investigations include FBC, U&Es, LFT, blood/sputum cultures, CXR.

Radiation injuries

Immediate management

- Cannot be detected without a radiological survey requiring specialist equipment.
- It is highly unlikely that a contaminated patient would pose a risk to healthcare providers but masks should be worn, outer garments removed when leaving contaminated area, and regular body surveys undertaken.
- Remove contaminated clothing, double-bag, and store in lead containers, handle clothing with forceps.
- Wash wound with water and then soap and water starting from edge and working inwards.
- Gastric lavage may be considered.
- Radiation experts may recommend administration of radionucleotide-specific decorporation agents such as Prussian blue, DTPA, or bicarbonate.

Subsequent management

- Symptoms may be immediate or delayed.
- Vomiting—time after exposure:
  - <10 min: possible lethal dose
  - 10–30 min: very severe
  - <1 h: severe
  - 1–2 h: moderate
  - >2 h: mild
- Higher doses are associated with bone marrow suppression, gastrointestinal destruction, cardiovascular and neurological effects requiring organ support.
- Cutaneous lesions can be immediate or delayed and can themselves be lethal.
- Fluid and electrolyte balance is vital.

- Investigations include FBC, U&Es, LFTs.
- The rate of decline of the absolute lymphocyte count is a marker of severity of exposure.

Investigations

- Routine laboratory studies for all exposed patients in a chemical, biological, or radiological incident include FBC, glucose, U&Es, LFTs, ECG monitoring, CXR, and pulse oximetry (or ABG measurement).

Special considerations

- Explosions may result in blast injury or smaller devices may release shrapnel which cause multiple puncture sites, internal bleeding, and risk of infection from unusual causative organisms.
- Patients may suffer multiple injuries and appear to require urgent life-saving intervention, but personal safety must be remembered if bioterrorism is suspected.
- May be multiple admissions requiring a hospital major incident plan.

Paediatric implications

- Because of their larger surface area:body weight ratio children are more vulnerable to toxicants absorbed through the skin.

Further reading

Advanced Life Support Group, (2005). Major Incident Medical Management and Support: The Practical Approach in the Hospital. WileyBlackwell, Oxford.

Baker, D.J. (2002). Management of casualties from terrorist chemical and biological attack: a key role for the anaesthetist. British Journal of Anaesthesia, **89**, 211–14.

✪ Management following cardiac arrest

Definition
Management of patients with return of spontaneous cardiac output (RSCO) following cardiac arrest.

Presentation
- Resuscitated patients with RSCO.
- Bradycardia with pulse <60/min.
- Evidence of circulatory shock, which is frequently seen post cardiac arrest.
- GCS <9 with no other reason for coma.
- If available history of resuscitation—early intervention is associated with improved prognosis.

Immediate management
- ABC ... 100% O_2. Intubate if GCS <9.
- Cardiology review with echocardiography if possible, consider CT head.
- Insert arterial line and preferably obtain central venous access.
- Target MAP 80–100 mmHg, with a lower goal if acute coronary syndrome (ACS) present, chronic heart failure (CHF), or shock.
- If MAP <80 mmHg and CVP <8 mmHg, give a fluid challenge of 250–500 mL crystalloid. If there is no change, further fluid boluses can be administered if the CVP <18 mmHg. If the target MAP is not reached, dobutamine should be considered if the ejection fraction is low, and noradrenaline if the ejection fraction is normal. An intra-aortic balloon pump should be considered if hypotension persists.
- MAP >80 mmHg—consider GTN or furosemide if evidence of CHF. Esmolol should be commenced if there is a persistent tachycardia or ACS with normal ejection fraction and central venous saturation ($ScvO_2$) is >65%.
- Once target MAP has been achieved the venous saturation should be measured ($ScvO_2$). A value of <65% suggests shock or inadequate organ perfusion. CVP should be optimized up to 18 mmHg, transfuse packed cells if Hb <10 g/dL, commence dobutamine if not already initiated, consider cardiac output monitoring if CVP >15 mmHg or vasopressors escalating.
- Once MAP, CVP, and $ScvO_2$ goals achieved, monitor serial lactate as a marker of tissue perfusion.
- Serial ECG—if ischaemic changes present, discuss with cardiology regarding intervention.

Subsequent management
- Stabilization needed for transfer to intensive care or catheter lab, if primary intervention is indicated.
- Consider therapeutic cooling. This should be instituted as soon as possible following RSCO, goal temperature is 32–34°C for 24 h. Evidence suggests it is most effective for patients with VF as an initial rhythm.

Non-VF patients should also be treated if the duration of cardiac arrest was short. Circulatory shock is no longer considered a contra-indication.
- Patients should be sedated and paralysed to prevent shivering.
- Allow passive re-warming after 24h period.

Investigations
- FBC, clotting, U&Es, LFTs, TFTs, G&S, troponin
- CXR
- Serial ECG
- CT head
- Core temperature

Risk factors
- Ischaemic heart disease
- Recent myocardial infarction
- Electrolyte disturbance
- Hypoxia
- Thromboembolic disease
- Cardiac tamponade
- Hypothermia
- Hypovolaemia
- Tension pneumothorax

Exclusions
- Patients with DNAR orders or very significant comorbidities.
- Prolonged resuscitation with very poor response despite maximal intervention.

Special considerations
Therapeutic hypothermia:
- Insufficient evidence exists to support cooling paediatric patients, pregnant patients, or patients with a primary coagulopathy.
- Plasma glucose increases.
- Plasma potassium, magnesium, and phosphate all decrease.
- Risk of infection increases.
- Hypotension and hyperkalaemia on re-warming.

Further reading
Bernard, S.A., Gray, T.W., Buist, M.D., Jones, B.M., Silvester, W., Gutteridge, G., Smith, K. (2002). Treatment of comatose survivors of out-of-hospital cardiac arrest with induced hypothermia. *New England Journal of Medicine*, **346**(8), 557–63.

Hypothermia after Cardiac Arrest Study Group. (2002). Mild therapeutic hypothermia to improve the neurologic outcome after cardiac arrest. *New England Journal of Medicine*, **346**(8), 549–56.

Nolan, J.P. et al. (2003). Therapeutic hypothermia after cardiac arrest: An Advisory Statement by the Advanced Life Support Task Force of the International Liaison Committee on Resuscitation. *Circulation*, **108**, 118–21.

☼ Decreased level of consciousness— requiring anaesthetic input

Definition
Altered mental state, combative, confused, not protecting own airway, Glasgow coma score of <9.

Presentation
Usually these will be patients who have presented to A+E or have acutely deteriorated on the ward. GCS <9. One of the most common referrals for the on-call anaesthetist is to intubate patients for transfer to the CT scanner.

Initial management
- History is paramount.
- Common causes of decreased GCS and request for CT scan include: cerebrovascular event (ischaemia, intracerebral bleed, subarachnoid/extradural bleed); metabolic disorders; postictal state (new onset seizures); systemic infections; meningitis; brain tumours; encephalopathy; trauma; following cardiac arrest.
- ABC ... 100% O_2.
- Airway manoeuvres. A definitive airway may be required—RSI.
- Exclude hypoxia as a cause for low GCS, ventilate to normal/low $PaCO_2$.
- Circulation—may be hypotensive or hypertensive depending on cause. Hypotension should be corrected and a cardiac cause excluded. Maintain adequate cerebral perfusion pressure (70–100 mmHg). If the patient is unstable consider arterial cannulation prior to transport.
- Neurological assessment is vital. Evaluate GCS (with particular attention to motor score as a prognostic factor). Pupil responses should be noted and any focal signs.
- Serum electrolytes and glucose should be corrected.
- If the patient is to be intubated and ventilated, initiate contact with the ward/unit where they are to be managed following the CT scan.
- Intra-hospital transfer to CT scanner.

Subsequent management
- If there is evidence of intracerebral or extradural bleed/SAH/tumour, the patient needs urgent referral to neurosurgery and may require further intra-hospital or inter-hospital transfer.
- 85% of strokes are ischaemic, currently less than 10% are thrombolysed but this management is evolving. Time from initial event to thrombolysis is paramount, so prompt referral and action is required.
- HDU/ITU for other appropriate medical causes.
- If there has been a catastrophic event, extubation in A+E and palliative care must be considered after consultation with family and appropriate teams.

- CT normal and/or postictal, consider meningitis and encephalitis. Appropriate antibiotic cover with CNS penetration and aciclovir if the latter suspected. Consider lumbar punctures (LP) if no evidence of raised intracranial pressure.
- If patient paralysed, ongoing seizures may be masked.

Investigations
- BP (possibly invasive), HR, ECG, FBC/U&Es/LFTs/clotting, SpO_2, $ETCO_2$, ABGs, LP.

Risk factors
- Hypertension, ischaemic heart disease, and peripheral vascular disease are risk factors for stroke.
- Decreased conscious level following thrombolysis or antiplatelet treatment may signify the onset of an intracranial bleed.
- Beware of requests for sedation for CT. These patients may require emergency airway control and intubation at any point. Access to the patient's airway will be much more difficult in transit or in the CT scanner.
- Normal CT head does not exclude raised intracranial pressure—important when considering LP.

Paediatric implications
- Children presenting to hospital with decreased level of consciousness without a history of trauma can pose a diagnostic challenge given the wide variety of causes and the frequent lack of clues as to diagnosis.
- Children can make significant demands on intensive and high dependency resources.
- A recent UK population-based study found a 40% mortality associated with non-traumatic coma as defined by a GCS of 12 or less for at least 6 h, with an estimated annual incidence of 30/100 000 children and 160/100 000 in the first year of life.

Special considerations
- Malignant cerebral oedema following major infarcts (particularly middle cerebral artery) may now be considered for decompression by hemi-craniectomy, particularly if the patient is <65 years of age.
- These patients may have a reduced GCS 48 h post-event and need urgent referral to neurosurgery.

:⚙: Sepsis

Definition

There is a defined pathway:

Organism→Systemic inflammatory response syndrome (SIRS)→Diffuse endothelial disruption and microcirculation defects→Global hypoxia and organ dysfunction→Severe sepsis→Multi-organ dysfunction and refractory hypotension→Septic shock.

Presentation

- SIRS—core temperature <36°C or >38°C; HR >90 bpm; RR >20/min or $PaCO_2$ <4.0 kPa (30 mmHg); WBC <4 × 10^9 or >12 × 10^9.
- Severe sepsis—elevated creatinine; elevated INR (DIC); GCS <12; lactate >4 mmol/L; hypotension that responds to fluid.
- Septic shock—as above **plus** hypotension that does not respond to fluid (500 mL bolus).
- Common causes of sepsis in the medical patient include pneumonia, meningitis, septic arthritis/cellulitis, meningitis, UTI, cholangitis, and infective endocarditis. Surgical sepsis includes intra-abdominal sepsis of any cause, ischaemic limbs, and invasive procedures/burns/trauma or any mechanism of bypassing the body's defence system.

Initial management

- Six initial steps:
  - administer high-flow oxygen
  - take blood culture specimens—at least two sets, one should be percutaneous and the other via any vascular device that has been in place for <48 h. Urine, sputum, and pus, etc. should also be cultured
  - commence antibiotics—broad spectrum to cover most likely pathogens, preferably two agents initially and administered within 1 h of diagnosis of sepsis. In the case of life-threatening sepsis of unknown origin consider tazocin 4.5 g IV tds, gentamicin 4 mg/kg IV od, and add metronidazole 500 mg IV tds if anaerobes implicated or intra-abdominal source suspected. Review with the results of any positive cultures. Consider antifungal agents
  - measure serum lactate and haemoglobin to maintain levels between 7 and 9 g/dL.
  - resuscitate with fluid, 20 mL/kg bolus volumes. There is no evidence of benefit of any particular colloid/crystalloid. Failure to respond indicates the need for invasive monitoring and early goal-directed therapy
  - measure and improve poor urine output. ARF in association with severe sepsis has a mortality of between 50 and 70%.
- Early goal-directed therapies to be achieved within 6 h:
  - insert CVP line and aim for CVP of 8–12 mmHg (12–15 mmHg if already mechanically ventilated)
  - urine output 0.5 mL/kg/h (catheterize)
  - central venous oxygen saturation of >70% or mixed venous saturation of >65%

- If mixed venous saturation not achieved, consider:
  - further fluid challenge (1000 mL crystalloid or 500 mL colloid over 30 min). The rate of infusion may need to be increased if sepsis-induced tissue hypoperfusion is evident, but care must be taken if cardiac filling pressures increase with no haemodynamic improvement
  - transfusion of packed red blood cells if haematocrit <30%
  - dobutamine infusion to a max. of 20 µg/kg/min
- Target MAP of >65 mmHg:
  - noradrenaline or dopamine are the first-line agents of choice
  - vasopressin (0.03 units/min) may be subsequently added to nor-adrenaline in non-responders. Adrenaline can also be considered if blood pressure responds poorly to first-line agents
  - **do not** use dopamine for renal protection
  - insert an arterial line at the earliest opportunity
- Inotropes:
  - consider dobutamine if there is cardiac dysfunction
  - do not aim for supranormal cardiac index

Subsequent management
- Transfer to ITU should be arranged for patients who require this level of support. Further management and delivery of care bundles should be carried out in an ITU setting, but aspects can be started in the emergency department.
- Steroids—consider when hypotension responds poorly to fluid therapy and vasopressors (up to 300 mg/day IV hydrocortisone), ACTH stimulation test is not recommended.
- Blood product administration:
  - packed RBCs if Hb <7 g/dL, aiming for a level >9 g/dL if there is concurrent MI, severe hypoxaemia, worsening lactic acidosis or cyanotic heart disease
  - FFP should only be used to correct laboratory clotting abnormalities if there is bleeding or a planned invasive procedure with a risk of bleeding
- Platelets should be transfused if the count is below 5×10^9/L, if the count is between $50-30 \times 10^9$/L and there is significant risk of bleeding, or if the count is <50×10^9 and an invasive procedure is planned.
- Ventilatory strategies—aim for a peak airway pressure of <30 cm/H_2O with a target tidal volume of 6 mL/kg or less. Permissive hypercapnia can be tolerated to facilitate lower tidal volumes and peak pressures. Manage patient in a semi-recumbent position
- Glucose—monitor blood glucose, but tight control (<8.3 mmol/L) should be instituted on ITU.
- Deep vein thrombosis prophylaxis—use either low-dose unfractionated heparin or low molecular weight heparin unless contraindicated (the latter in high-risk patients). A compression device should be used if heparin is contraindicated, and a combination of both compression device and heparin in high-risk patients.
- Stress ulcer prophylaxis with H_2-blocker or a proton pump inhibitor depending on local guidelines.

Investigations
- FBC, U&Es, LFTs, clotting
- ECG, CXR
- Blood cultures, MSU
- CVP monitoring
- Serial ABGs, venous saturations
- Urine output

Risk factors
Extremes of age, neutropenic patients, intra-abdominal cause of sepsis, pneumonia as a common cause, indwelling devices as a focus.

Paediatric implications
(See also pp136–9)

- Fluid resuscitation with 20 mL/kg over 5 min. Repeat up to 40–60 mL/kg.
- Blood pressure is an unreliable marker of adequacy of resuscitation.
- Use dopamine if fluid resuscitation not effective. Noradrenaline and adrenaline should be used for shock refractory to dopamine. Dobutamine should be used for low cardiac output states.
- Inhaled nitric oxide (NO) is useful for neonates with postpartum pulmonary hypertension and sepsis.
- Therapeutic endpoints:
  - CRT<2 s
  - warm peripheries
  - urine output >1 mL/kg/h
  - normal mental status
  - decreasing lactate level
  - central venous oxygen saturation >70%

Special considerations
Early consultation with ITU is important.

Further reading
Surviving sepsis guidelines www.survivingsepsis.org

Equipment problems

Jules Cranshaw and Kim J. Gupta

:✪: **Breathing system disconnection**

Definition
Failure of gas delivery from the anaesthetic machine to the patient due to unintentional disconnection in the breathing system.

Presentation
- *If the patient is breathing spontaneously*—the reservoir bag empties; CO_2 waveform changes; there is a fall in FiO_2 which may cause a fall in SaO_2; there is a fall in FiAA (if volatile used) which may cause the patient to wake up.
- *If the patient is on IPPV*—the ventilator bellows empties; no chest movements or breath sounds detectable; alarm sounds for low airway pressure, $ETCO_2$ apnoea, low expired tidal volume/minute volume; change heard in ventilator sounds; smell of inhaled anaesthetic agent (if in use); may be an audible gas leak.

Immediate management
- If a disconnection is not found immediately:
  - switch to manual ventilation with 100% oxygen
  - close APL valve
  - depress oxygen flush (it may then be possible to hear and identify a leak at the point of disconnection)
- If reservoir bag fills:
  - squeeze bag and check adequate chest expansion
  - observe capnograph
  - check that arterial oxygen saturation improves
- If ventilation adequate:
  - check for leaks in the breathing system and airway device/ETT seal
- If ventilation unsuccessful:
  - abandon breathing system and ventilate with a self-inflating reservoir bag (attached to cylinder oxygen when able)
- If ventilation still unsuccessful:
  - check the airway device/endotracheal tube for displacement
- If necessary:
  - remove the airway device/endotracheal tube and ventilate with a face mask
  - maintain anaesthesia intravenously

Subsequent management
A methodical check includes connections between the airway device/endotracheal tube and breathing system; side-stream sampling ports; connections between filters; condensers; humidifiers; pressure sensor; flowmeter; oxygen analyser; PEEP valve; CO_2 absorber; reservoir bag; and inspiratory/expiratory limb connections.

Risk factors
- Inadequate check of breathing system prior to use
- Moving the patient's head or the operating table
- Sharing the airway with a surgeon/endoscopist

- Changing components of the breathing system, e.g. CO_2 absorbers, sampling lines
- Re-filling vaporizers
- Using the fresh gas outlet as an oxygen source without reconnecting the breathing system
- A machine/workstation returning from a service/repair

Exclusions

- Loss of patent airway with supraglottic airway device
- Endotracheal tube/supraglottic airway cuff leak, tear, or surgical puncture
- Placement of nasogastric tube in trachea
- Tracheobronchial leak
- APL valve unintentionally open/stuck open when ventilating with a Bain system
- Leaking or incorrectly seated CO_2 absorber housing
- Active gas scavenging system ports occluded, causing negative pressure in breathing system
- Ventilator/breathing system pressure relief valve set too low or stuck open
- Fresh gas flow too low, not switched on, or supply failure
- Ventilator failure or not switched on

Paediatric implications

Uncuffed endotracheal tube diameter too small.

Special considerations

- If the patient is breathing spontaneously:
  - the alteration in capnograph trace depends on the site of disconnection. If the sampling port is in a section of circuit disconnected from exhaled gas, there will be complete loss of the waveform. Otherwise, it will detect a variable amount of rebreathing of carbon dioxide
  - if air is entrained, there may be a fall in inspired/expired oxygen, inhalational agent or a rise in inspired/expired nitrogen
- If patient is positive-pressure ventilated:
  - bag-in-bottle ventilators—ascending bellows collapses (bag generates 2–4 cmH$_2$O PEEP); descending bellows fall to a fully expanded position and may not reveal disconnection
  - minute volume dividers—continue to function if disconnection is distal
  - many ventilators do not have a visible reservoir, e.g. Penlon Nuffield 200
- Low pressure/volume alarms:
  - breathing system low pressure alarms are mandatory during IPPV. The alarm trigger limit should be set just below the maximum inspiratory pressure. This alarm is not infallible since resistance distal to the sensor (e.g. partial obstruction at the point of disconnection) may mean that the alarm limit is not reached. Therefore the optimum location of the alarm sensor is the Y-piece
  - volumetric devices should usually be located in the expiratory limb

Further reading

Raphael, D.T., Weller, R.S., Doran, D.J. (1988). A response algorithm for the low-pressure alarm condition. *Anesthesia and Analgesia*, **67**(9), 876–83.

① Pipeline oxygen supply failure

Definition
Insufficient pipeline oxygen delivery to the anaesthetic machine.

Presentation
- Oxygen failure alarm sounds and pressure gauge falls.
- Oxygen and linked flowmeters fall, emergency oxygen flush fails, pipeline oxygen-driven ventilators stop.
- Audible escape of gas if pipeline connection leaking.

Immediate management
- Turn on the reserve oxygen cylinder *fully*, since the flow from partially opened valves may decrease with cooling as oxygen flows out.
- Check that the pressure gauge indicates a full or adequately filled cylinder. Verify pressure failure on the pipeline pressure gauge.
- Switch to manual ventilation to preserve cylinder oxygen, if ventilator uses oxygen as a driving gas.
- Use low oxygen flows to preserve available oxygen. If using a circle system close the APL valve to preserve potentially useful oxygen reserves.
- Check for disconnection between the pipeline and wall and re-attach it if possible.
- Check oxygen analyser confirms return of oxygen flow.

Subsequent management
- Disconnect the pipeline supply. If the pipeline supply has failed, re-establishment may result in a temporary flow of gas that is contaminated, or the wrong gas may be reconnected at source. As the regulated pipeline pressure is greater than the regulated cylinder pressure, the restored flow will take priority.
- Inform the surgeon what has happened and make a plan to expedite surgery.
- Inform other hospital areas where pipeline oxygen is used and the department responsible for the central oxygen supply.
- Arrange for an appropriate number of oxygen cylinders to allow completion of surgery. Find out when the oxygen supply is likely to be reliably restored.
- If the cylinder oxygen supply runs out, allow the patient to breathe room air or ventilate using a self-inflating reservoir bag—administer intravenous anaesthesia. Using air alone may render the patient hypoxaemic and should not be used until necessary.

Risk factors
- No machine check performed
- Failure to reconnect pipeline after machine check
- Unfamiliar pipeline connections
- Loss of power to an anaesthetic workstation
- Recent machine or pipeline maintenance, repair, or replacement
- Exhausted hospital central oxygen source

- Fault during refilling of central oxygen source
- Construction work in hospital

Exclusions

- Obstruction or large gas leak within the anaesthetic machine, e.g. around vaporizers or within the ventilator
- Kink or obstruction in supply hose
- Anaesthetic workstation power failure

Paediatric implications

IPPV cannot be delivered via an Ayre's T-piece in the event of a gas failure.

Special considerations

- If the fresh gas flow to a Mapleson breathing system is interrupted, rebreathing occurs quickly. By contrast, a closed circle system acts as a temporary oxygen reservoir and the absorber prevents CO_2 accumulation. However, be aware that a continuing fresh gas flow containing air from some anaesthetic workstations will pressurize the system and wash out oxygen already present.
- Oxygen supply failure in older anaesthetic machines is heralded by a 'Bosun's' or 'Ritchie' whistle-type alarm. These activate if the supply pressure falls by 50%, sound for at least 7 s, and are silenced by restoring the oxygen supply. Additional fail-safe mechanisms simultaneously stop or adjust the flow of nitrous oxide preventing the delivery of hypoxic mixtures.
- Modern anaesthetic workstations employ electronic oxygen supply pressure alarms and complex carrier gas management systems in the event of oxygen failure. Some continue to deliver pipeline air even after oxygen pipeline failure.
- Some ventilators are driven by oxygen pipeline supply and stop if it fails. However, some anaesthetic workstations will reroute other available pipeline gases at sufficient pressure to continue driving the mechanical ventilator in this event.

Further reading

Anderson, W.R., Brock-Utne, J.G. (1991). Oxygen pipeline supply failure. A coping strategy. *Journal of Clinical Monitoring*, **7**(1), 39–41.

⊙ Ventilator failure

Definition
Unplanned cessation of automatic positive pressure ventilation.

Presentation
- Bellows stop moving (but may not empty); ventilator cycling stops (may be audible); chest movements stop; absent breath sounds on auscultation.
- Loss of normal breathing system pressure trace; loss of normal capnograph waveform; apnoea, low tidal and minute volume alarms sound.
- Switching to manual ventilation restores the *status quo*.

Immediate management
- Check ventilator is switched on.
- Check manual/ventilator selector switch is set correctly.
- Switch to manual ventilation with a simple breathing system.
- Maintain adequate minute ventilation and anaesthesia until another suitable checked ventilator is available. Consider allowing return of spontaneous ventilation if appropriate, or call for another ventilator.
- If the reservoir bag will not fill or empties quickly consider:
  - inadequate fresh gas flow settings?
  - oxygen pipeline failure (and thus ventilator driving gas failure)
  - disconnection or large leak in breathing system
  - unintentional extubation, displacement of airway device, and endotracheal tube cuff leak
- If the reservoir bag fills, but there is resistance on squeezing:
  - consider the causes and management of high airway pressure

Subsequent management
- Clearly label and remove a faulty ventilator from use until inspected and repaired.
- If the ventilator is an integral component of an anaesthetic workstation, the whole workstation should be taken out of service.
- The anaesthetist with responsibility for equipment should be informed and the critical incident logged.
- A qualified/certified person should examine the equipment with the authority of the manufacturer.
- Events related to design faults, system faults, and persistently recurring problems should be reported to manufacturers and the National Patient Safety Agency (NPSA) and Medical Devices Agency division of the Medical and Healthcare Products Regulatory Agency (MHRA).
- If there is a potential manufacturing problem (a batch of components might be faulty), other anaesthetists should be informed.

Risk factors
- Unfamiliarity with ventilator
- Inadequate machine check
- Interruption of power supply

- Power surge and disruption of ventilator programming
- Recent anaesthetic machine service
- Brand new equipment

Exclusions

- Ventilator not switched on.
- Manual/ventilator switch incorrectly set or faulty.
- Improper assembly or failure of ventilator, breathing system, pressure sensors, or pressure relief valves.
- Ventilator, anaesthetic workstation, or general power failure.
- Ventilator performance or settings insufficient for patient characteristics.
- Inappropriate ventilator settings causing pressure relief valve to open:
  - excessive tidal volume for inspiratory time
  - excessive inspiratory flow
  - pressure relief threshold too low
- Bellows or ventilator mechanism stuck.
- Failure of secondary driving gas to some anaesthetic workstation ventilators.
- High airway pressures—see pp388–9.
- Large leaks or inadequate fresh gas flow.

Special considerations

- Oxygen pipeline supply-driven ventilators may stop if the pressure falls. Some will automatically switch to other piped gases, remaining at sufficient pressure.
- Low-pressure, apnoea, low tidal/minute volume alarms may sound if the ventilator stops at end expiration.
- Continuous positive airway pressure alarm may sound if it fails in inspiration.
- Ventilators were involved in 27% of perioperative equipment failures in one French survey. Even though ventilator failure might seem a problem intrinsic to a complex piece of equipment, data from the ASA Closed Claims Project database suggests that ventilator *misuse* might contribute to an approximately equal number of deaths. Focusing on fixing a problem with a ventilator can detract from the simple necessity of providing adequate ventilation by hand.

Further reading

Bourgain, J.L., Baguenard, P., Puizillout, J.M., Ankri, J.C., Damia, E., Billard, V. (1999). The breakdown of anesthesia equipment survey. *Annales Françaises d'Anesthesie et de Reanimation*, **18**(3), 303–8.

⚠ Power failure

Definition
Loss of electrical supply to the operating theatre.

Presentation
- AC power failure alarms sound on devices with charged back-up batteries.
- Devices without charged back-up batteries stop working: anaesthetic workstations (potentially stopping fresh gas flow); monitors; electronically managed ventilators; infusion devices; warming devices; essential surgical instruments (e.g. diathermy); cardiopulmonary bypass machines (may need to be hand-cranked); electrically powered operating tables and beds.
- Lights may go out (in theatres without windows, or at night, darkness may be absolute).
- Theatre air-conditioning, heating, laminar flow systems fail.

Immediate management
- Call for help and light if necessary (daylight, torches, pen-torches, laryngoscopes, mobile phones). Do not use naked flames.
- Check mechanical flowmeters (fluorescent or back-lit) or electronic flowmeters (if display remains), listen and feel for fresh gas flow at the common gas outlet.
- If fresh gas flow has stopped, temporarily continue low-flow spontaneously breathing anaesthesia with a closed circle system if equilibrated.
- Alternatively, use a self-inflating reservoir bag with cylinder O_2 and maintain anaesthesia intravenously.
- Check ventilator is still functioning (if in use).
- Begin manual ventilation if necessary.
- Maintain clinical monitoring as far as possible:
  - visual—chest rise/fall, cyanosis, pupil size, movement, sweating
  - tactile—pulses (peripheral or at surgical site), capillary refill time
  - auditory—stethoscope, sphygmomanometer
- Easily available battery-powered monitors include: oxygen analysers; pulse oximeters; defibrillator ECG; transport monitors

Subsequent management
- Obtain information about duration of theatre power failure.
- In a hospital-wide power failure, information may be best disseminated by a designated crisis manager rather than potentially bombarding a busy engineering department with calls.
- If necessary, continue with a pneumatic anaesthetic machine and ventilator if pipeline gas supplies or cylinders allow.
- Under difficult circumstances it may be safer to establish spontaneous ventilation.
- Be aware of battery life—especially infusion pumps.
- If infusions need to be titrated and electric pumps fail use volumetric burettes and measure drop rates.
- Ask surgical team to finish as quickly as possible or abandon operation.

- Reallocate personnel and resources to areas where they are needed.
- Elective work should be cancelled until a reliable power supply has been restored.
- A hospital disaster plan may have to be initiated.

Risk factors

- Lack of back-up batteries or inadequate battery maintenance
- Injudicious unplugging of theatre equipment—lack of charge
- Emergency generator tests
- Hospital construction work
- Natural disaster

Exclusions

- Workstation unintentionally unplugged or switched off.
- Workstation electronic failure; failure of electrical leads and fuses.
- Isolated socket power failure.
- Isolated theatre power failure (get help from other theatres).
- Circuit breaker (if fitted) has opened (consider why it has tripped— there may be a potentially dangerous electrical problem).

Special considerations

- Power failure ranges from a problem with the anaesthetic workstation to hospital-wide—including back-up generators. Modern machines have integrated battery back-up, but the effects of mains power failure depend on the type. Fresh gas flow and volatile delivery may continue but other functions (e.g. monitoring) may cease immediately. Emergency oxygen flush should still work.
- Power fluctuations (lights may flicker) are also capable of causing electronic equipment to switch off or 'hang' in an inoperable state.
- If a workstation needs to be restarted, it will be inoperable until its auto-testing process is complete. The start-up may include leak and compliance tests of the breathing system. These should be cancelled. They are time-consuming and require the breathing system to be disconnected from the patient and occluded. If the circuit is connected to a patient during these tests, there is a risk of barotrauma.
- Pneumatically driven anaesthetic machines and ventilators may continue to function if pipeline supplies are intact or on cylinder oxygen (see 'Pipeline supply failure', pp382–3).
- Operating lights (some have back-up batteries), diathermy, laparoscopic camera and gas delivery equipment, microscopes, lasers and some drills may stop, as well as theatre air conditioning and heating. Only some hospital areas and power sockets may be supplied with power from an emergency generator.

Further reading

Mitchell, J. (2001). Complete power failure 1. *Anaesthesia*, **56**(3), 274.

Tye, J.C., Chamley, D. (2000). Complete power failure. *Anaesthesia*, **55**, 1133–4.

Welch, R.H., Feldman, J.M. (1989). Anesthesia during total electrical failure, or what would you do if the lights went out? *Journal of Clinical Anesthesia*, **1**(5), 358–62.

✪ High airway pressure

Definition

An abnormally high positive pressure in the breathing system. A peak inspiratory pressure of >30 cmH$_2$O may be considered high.

Presentation

- High measured airway pressure, high airway pressure alarm, audible leaks, abnormal cycling sounds from ventilator, sound of ventilator pressure relief valve.
- Low tidal volume and minute volume alarm, poor chest expansion.
- Diminished cardiac output secondary to raised intrathoracic pressure.

Immediate management

- Switch to manual ventilation with 100% oxygen.
- Squeeze the reservoir bag and verify difficult ventilation.
- Scan the breathing system and the airway device/endotracheal tube for obvious obstructions (e.g. Boyle–Davis gag or foreign body).
- Check the filter/HME (heat-moisture exchanger) for any soiling/obstruction—if in doubt remove/replace.
- If there are signs of light anaesthesia (laryngospasm/coughing/straining/biting with occlusion of the airway device/endotracheal tube) deepen anaesthesia intravenously.
- If ventilation is inadequate, exclude breathing system obstruction by assessing ventilation with an alternative system (e.g. self-inflating reservoir bag) connected directly to the airway device/endotracheal tube.
- If ventilation is still difficult, the problem lies in the airway device/endotracheal tube or the patient:
  - check the airway device/ETT is in the right position and patent
  - manipulate and replace if necessary
  - an appropriately sized suction catheter or a gum-elastic bougie should pass easily through the whole length of the airway device
  - proceed to check for specific patient causes of high airway pressure

Subsequent management

- Auscultate for bronchospasm, examine chest movement, neck veins, tracheal position, and for flushing, urticaria, subcutaneous emphysema. Check for cardiovascular changes while squeezing the reservoir bag.
- Consider:
  - endobronchial intubation
  - bronchospasm—pp54–6
  - tension pneumothorax—pp50–1
  - lung/lobar collapse
  - subtotal obstruction of the airway device/ETT
  - anatomical/pathological obstruction of the airway
  - opioid-induced chest wall rigidity
  - acute pulmonary oedema—pp52–3

Investigations

- CXR, ABGs, fibreoptic bronchoscopy

Risk factors

- Cleaning or re-assembly of the circle system
- Contamination of breathing system (particularly filter/HME) with condensate, secretions, blood
- Inadequate breathing system check
- Re-use of single-use equipment
- Loose debris on anaesthetic workstation (e.g. cannula caps, needle covers)
- Is airway pressure appropriate for clinical situation:
  - obesity, severe restrictive lung or chest wall disease?
  - patient position, e.g. steep Trendelenburg (beware endobronchial migration of endotracheal tube)?
  - endotracheal tube resistance, e.g. microlaryngoscopy tube?
  - raised intra-abdominal pressure, e.g. pneumoperitoneum, ileus?

Exclusions

- Surgical team applying retractors or leaning on the patient
- Airway pressure alarm malfunction or inappropriate setting
- Ventilator settings inappropriate (excessive tidal volume or inspiratory flow, excessively short I:E ratio or long I:E ratio with gas trapping)
- Mechanical ventilator/manual ventilation selector in the wrong position
- Ventilator malfunction—expiratory/PEEP valve, pressure-limiting valve
- Clogged filter/HME—condensate, blood, gastric contents, oedema
- Occult obstruction—kink, foreign body, sputum, clot, secretions
- APL valve stuck or unintentionally closed (especially after switching from mechanical ventilation)
- Circle expiratory/inspiratory valve stuck closed
- Malfunction of scavenging system
- Oxygen flush depressed inadvertently or stuck open
- Failure of flow restrictors or machine regulators allowing gas under high pressure to enter breathing system

Special considerations

- Diagnosing the equipment problem can wait if it can be eliminated.
- Capnography and clinical examination may be the only early indicators of inadequate ventilation during pressure-limited ventilation. Expired CO_2 may rise or fall, depending on the cause of the high airway pressure.
- During IPPV, expiratory resistance (e.g. an obstructed APL valve, circle expiratory valve, ventilator expiratory valve, or scavenging system) may be diagnosed by raised peak inspiratory pressure, abnormal end-expiratory pressure, or abnormal distension of the reservoir bag during manual (or spontaneous) ventilation.
- Intrathoracic pressure is released by disconnecting the breathing system, unless generated by sub-total obstruction or a 'one-way valve' effect in an airway device.

Further reading

Carter, J.A. (2004). Checking anaesthetic equipment and the Expert Group on Blocked Anaesthetic Tubing (EGBAT). *Anaesthesia*, **59**(2), 105–7.

Keith, R.L., Pierson, D.J. (1996). Complications of mechanical ventilation. A bedside approach. *Clinical Chest Medicine*, **17**(3), 439–51.

Miscellaneous problems

John Isaac

Mark Stoneham

Colin Berry

✚ Massive haemorrhage

Definition
Replacement of total blood volume in less than 24h or replacement of blood faster than 1 mL/kg/min.

Presentation
- Hypovolaemic shock.
- Blood loss usually obvious, but can be hidden.

Immediate management
- *ABC … 100% O₂.*

- *Stop bleeding*—apply direct pressure, clamp arterial supply, aortic clamp.
- *Call for help*—a team approach is needed.
- *IV access*—14G × 2, consider using PA catheter sheath (8.5 Fr) in a central vein.
- *IV fluids*—increasing circulating volume is the first priority. Use colloid in preference to crystalloid, warmed as soon as practicable.
- *Re-assess vital signs*—pulse, BP, colour, peripheral perfusion.
- *Order blood products*—designate a named individual to take and label blood sample. Consider likely need for red blood cells, platelets, FFP, cryoprecipitate. Contact the blood bank and warn them, it will speed things up.
- *Warn theatres* if surgery is likely—prepare fluid warmers, inotropic infusions, transducers.
- *Anaesthesia*—if required, use rapid sequence induction. Consider etomidate (0.1–0.3 mg/kg) or ketamine (1–2 mg/kg). Have intravenous infusions running maximally. Be prepared for hypotension on induction.

Subsequent management
- Arterial line, central line, and urinary catheter after definitive treatment started.
- Continue to monitor haematocrit, arterial pH, clotting (Table 13.1).
- Administer FFP once the INR >1.5 and platelets once the platelet count <75 × 10⁹/L if actively bleeding.
- Remember, platelets can be given via any *fresh* giving set, but a platelet-giving set has reduced dead space, allowing minimal wastage.
- Use near-patient testing whenever available (blood gases, haematocrit, Ca²⁺, Hemocue®, Coagucheck®, thromboelastography).
- Inform ICU early.

Investigations
ABGs, haematocrit, clotting screen, crossmatch, U&E

Risk factors
- Surgery (vascular/obstetrics/major cardiothoracic/major GI/major orthopaedic)
- Trauma (especially blunt body-cavity trauma)
- Oesophageal varices in patients with liver disease
- Ruptured aortic aneurysm

- Coagulopathy—congenital (e.g. haemophilia), acquired (e.g. patient taking clopidogrel)
- Blind traumatic procedures (e.g. liver biopsy)

Exclusions
- Dehydration
- Sepsis
- Anaphylaxis
- Heart failure

Paediatric implications
- Get help from experienced colleague. Paediatricians can come to theatre!
- Intraosseous infusion (<6 years), external jugular or femoral vein may help with access.
- Work out blood volume (80 mL/kg)—see also pp130–1.
- Give fluid boluses in aliquots of 10 mL/kg.
- Titrate according to vital signs.
- Keep warm.

Special considerations
- Hypothermia impairs coagulation, so *keep warm*.
- Hypocalcaemia may occur during very rapid transfusion, causing hypotension. Treat with IV calcium gluconate 10 mL 10%, or calcium chloride 3.5 mL 10% (adult doses).
- During emergency laparotomy, packing abdomen and closing can help control bleeding.
- Haematologist may help—particularly if underlying coagulation problem.
- There is no place for a 'formula' approach in the use of blood products in the management of massive haemorrhage. Use 'near patient' or laboratory testing to guide transfusion.
- Some cases of massive haemorrhage may benefit from specific drug therapy.
- Recombinant factor 7 (NovoSeven®) 2.4 mg has been reported to be effective in severe haemorrhage unresponsive to standard treatments. It is unproven and expensive. Consult a haematologist.
- A 'Cell Saver' should be used whenever possible—avoid in contaminated cases. Needs to be set-up ready and with someone to operate the machine.

Table 13.1 Target values

Hb	7–8 g/dL unless good reason to be higher (severe CVS/respiratory disease)
Platelet count	>75 × 10^9/L if actively bleeding (or >100 × 10^9/L if multiple trauma/CNS injury)
Prothrombin time (PT)	<1.5 times control
Partial thromboplastin time (PTT)	<1.5 times control
Fibrinogen	>1.0 g/L

⑦ Using blood products

Red cell transfusion

- Blood loss of >30% can usually be treated with crystalloid or colloid solutions (depending on initial Hb concentration). Blood loss of >50% will require red cell transfusion.
- Target red cell transfusion to maintain Hb >7 g/dL (CVS disease >9 g/dL).
- Use available near-patient testing frequently (blood gases, haematocrit, Hemocue®).
- Use Group O-negative blood if anaemia is immediately life-threatening (i.e. Hb <5 g/dL with ongoing bleeding). An alternative is uncrossmatched group-compatible blood. This can be issued by the blood bank immediately.
- Transfusing SAG-M O-negative blood carries a minimal risk of ABO mismatch as there is so little residual plasma in the bag. Transfusing group-specific blood carries a small risk of the transfused cells being haemolysed due to recipient antibodies. The risk of serious morbidity or mortality from either strategy is very low, and should be weighed against the risk of delaying transfusion until crossmatched red cells become available.

Fresh frozen plasma, platelets, cryoprecipitate

- Coagulation deteriorates after 3–5 L of blood loss. Anticipate changes and measure coagulation regularly. Use near-patient testing if available (Coagucheck®, thromboelastography).
- Transfuse FFP and platelets as clinically indicated until coagulation screen available.
- Prolonged PT and PTT will correct with fresh frozen plasma (FFP) transfusion.
- Fibrinogen <1 g/L with continuing haemorrhage may require cryoprecipitate transfusion.
- There may be considerable delay in obtaining platelets, so you need to plan in advance for their use.
- Platelets are indicated when <75 ×10^9/L if patient is actively bleeding (100 ×10^9/L if multiple trauma, CNS disease, or when ineffective due to disease/drugs).
- Transfuse using a standard blood- or platelet-giving set, provided the line has not previously been used for blood transfusion.
- Thawed FFP can be stored safely for 24 hours in a blood fridge (4°C).

Other information (Tables 13.2, 13.3)

Table 13.2 Cost of various blood products

Product	Cost/unit (UK, 2008)
SAG-M blood	£140
Platelets (adult pack)	£230
Fresh frozen plasma	£36
Cryoprecipitate (10 pack)	£230

Table 13.3 Estimated risk of viral infection/unit transfused (UK)

	Allogeneic blood	Fresh frozen plasma
Hepatitis B	<1/200 000	<1/10 million
Hepatitis C	<1/200 000	<1/2 million
HIV	<1/3 million	<1/10 million

☼ Acute transfusion reactions

Definition
Acute reaction to blood product transfusion.

Presentation
- Fever, urticarial rash, dyspnoea, wheeze.
- Anaphylactic shock—see pp256–8.

Immediate management
- Stop the transfusion—keep the IV line open with saline.
- Check and record vital signs, including temperature.
- Check for respiratory signs—dyspnoea, tachypnoea, wheeze, cyanosis.
- If severe, institute ABC … 100% O_2.
- Provide further management according to the developing clinical features.
- Check the identity of patient and blood/product unit and documentation.
- Check blood gases or SpO_2.
- Be prepared to manage full-blown anaphylactic shock.
- Multi-organ failure may ensue—ICU if indicated.

Subsequent management
- Notify blood bank, they will want the unit returned along with a blood sample from the patient.
- Consult a haematologist.
- Inform the Hospital Transfusion Committee.
- The blood bank will report the case to SABRE and SHOT if appropriate.

Investigations
- SpO_2
- Clotted sample for transfusion lab.

Risk factors
- Inability to label patient accurately at time of admission (e.g. patient unconscious).
- Failure to complete request form—name, address, ID number, date of birth missing.
- Labelling mistakes in the laboratory.
- Use of single wrist label (often removed during surgery) rather than multiple limb labels. If you remove a wrist label to insert catheters, secure it around the patient's ET tube and replace it on a limb prior to discharging the patient from your care.
- Correct matching of blood units with the issue form, but failure to match the issue form with the patient.
- Hurried or incomplete checking of blood products with patient. More likely in emergency situations or at night.

Table 13.4 Acute transfusion reactions

Acute reaction	Cause	Timing/incidence	Outcome/management
Acute intravascular haemolysis	ABO-incompatible blood	First few mL transfused Occurs 1/600 000 units	10% mortality, from DIC, renal failure. Maintain BP and urine output
Febrile non-haemolytic reactions	Patient anti-leucocyte antibodies react with leucocytes in transfusion. Incidence reduced by leucodepletion	Within hours 1–2% of RBC transfusions	0% mortality Paracetamol
Urticaria	Patient IgE to allergens in transfusion	During transfusion 1% of transfusions	0% mortality Chlorphenamine 10 mg IV
Anaphylaxis	Patient IgE or IgG response. IgA-deficient patient may have anti-IgA antibodies vs. transfused blood	Immediate Very rare	Life-threatening. As for anaphylaxis
Infective shock	Bacterial contamination of product with: Pseudomonas, Yersinia, Staphylococcus spp.	During first 100 mL 1/500 000 units	High mortality. As for septic shock
TRALI (transfusion-related acute lung injury)	Donor plasma antibodies to patient leucocytes	<4 h Rare	Some mortality. As for acute lung injury

Exclusions
- Sepsis
- Drug reaction
- Shock from other cause

Special considerations
- If the only feature is a rise in temperature of less than 1.5°C from baseline or an urticarial rash:
  - recheck that the correct blood is being transfused
  - give paracetamol for fever
  - give antihistamine for urticaria
  - recommence the transfusion at a slower rate
  - observe the patient more frequently than routine practice
- *TRALI* (transfusion-related acute lung injury)—cannot be distinguished clinically from other forms of acute lung injury, and usually presents within 4h of transfusion with pulmonary oedema, hypoxaemia, and bilateral infiltrates on chest X-ray. It can occur in response to red cell transfusion but is more common following FFP or platelet administration. It is due to donor plasma antibodies to patient leucocytes. Treatment is supportive, and the outcome can be fatal. The recent practice of limiting the use of plasma for resuspending concentrated blood products (e.g. platelets) from only male donors should reduce the incidence of TRALI.
- *Infection*—bacterial infection of blood products occurs very rarely, but carries a high mortality. Platelets carry the highest risk, since they are stored in a semi-permeable bag at 22°C. The risk of bacterial infection from platelet transfusion is estimated at 1/12 000 units transfused. Overall, the risk from all components is estimated at 1/500 000 units transfused.

✪ Burns

(See also 'Paediatric Burns', pp132–4)

Definition

Tissue damage as result of exposure to heat, electrical energy, or caustic agent.

Presentation

- Inhalational burns cause tachypnoea, airway obstruction, and pulmonary oedema.
- Surface burns cause hypovolaemia, pain, and may produce constrictive bands.
- COHb poisoning causes nausea and vomiting, tachycardia, angina, chorea, and convulsions.

Immediate management

Primary care ABC

- **A**pproach with care as a first responder (fire, smoke, electrical shock risk); stop the
- **B**urning process by removing objects that retain heat (e.g. plastic, metal jewellery).
- **C**ontamination—not all burns are due to heat. Protect against chemical contamination of the unit and staff.

Secondary care ABC

- **A**irway injury—signs suggestive of inhalational burns include: hoarseness; cough; sooty sputum; singed nasal hair; facial burns; mucosal injury. If in doubt, intubate early since airway oedema may make this impossible. Anticipate a difficult intubation (see pp68–74) but *do not delay*. Suxamethonium is safe initially. Leave the ETT long and uncut because oedema may displace it later.
- **B**reathing—is the patient breathing spontaneously? Burns caused by electric shock are associated with transient respiratory muscle paralysis. Give high-flow 100% oxygen as tissue oxygenation may be compromised by carbon monoxide poisoning despite normal SaO_2 and PaO_2. High respiratory rate may indicate lower airway damage predisposing to later pulmonary oedema, or it may indicate smoke inhalation with metabolic poisoning.
- **C**irculation—check output and rhythm. Electrical burns may cause dysrhythmias by inducing VF or damage to the conducting system. BLS/ALS if necessary. Establish IV access in an unburnt area if possible. The femoral triangle is often spared. Fluid resuscitate to normovolaemia.
- Check for severe occult injuries sustained during escape from the fire (e.g. by jumping), especially if adequate fluid resuscitation is difficult to achieve.

Subsequent management

- Cover exposed burns with 'cling-film'. This limits evaporative loss, conserves heat, and reduces infection risk. Gram-negative sepsis is a major complication.
- Burn area: There are three simple methods of rapidly estimating burn area:
  - Wallace's 'rule of nines'—quick and useful for medium-sized burns, but a tendency to overestimate burn extent by counting erythema (Fig. 13.1)
  - Lund and Browder charts (see p133)—most accurate method if used carefully. Takes into account relative changes in surface area with age
  - palmar surface = 0.8% of BSA. Useful for very small areas of burn (<15%). This relates to the *patient's* hand, including fingers. Also useful for widespread burns >85% (counting unburnt area)
- Parkland formula for fluid management: assuming normovolaemia initially:
  - 24h fluid requirement (mL) = 4 × BSA of burn (%) × body weight (kg)
  - 50% should be given in the first 8 h. Type (crystalloid/colloid) is not critical.
- Insert a urinary catheter to assess adequacy of fluid replacement (urine output >1 mL/kg/h).
- Circumferential chest wall burns—restrictive picture may require escharotomies.

Investigations

- Carbon monoxide poisoning (COHb >20%)—ABGs will appear normal. SaO_2 will appear normal because both COHb and oxyhaemoglobin absorb at 940 nm. Bench co-oximetry utilizes an additional wavelength of red light, allowing differentiation.
- Cyanide poisoning (>50 ppm)—causes unexplained metabolic acidosis and high venous oxygen saturation. Common with combustion of plastics. Treat with O_2.
- ECG—for evidence of ischaemia/dysrhythmia/conduction abnormality.
- U&Es—patients may develop hyperkalaemia from release of intracellular K^+.
- Inhalation burns are best documented by later fibreoptic bronchoscopy. CXR is of little help initially as positive findings appear late.

Risk factors

Inhalational injury should be suspected if there is a history of exposure to smoke, particularly if fire occurred in a confined space, or there is a reduced conscious level.

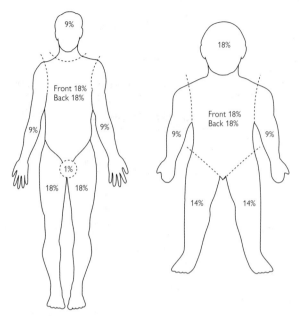

Fig. 13.1 Rule of nines burns assessment (see also p132).

Exclusions

Airway injury—careful observation is required following an inhalational injury as severe airway obstruction can develop after a 'free period' of 3–8h.

Special considerations

- It is easy to confuse full-thickness burns with unburnt skin. Full-thickness burns look dry, waxy/leathery, and are insensitive, but do not bleed on pinprick.
- Following a burn injury, suxamethonium causes acute hyperkalaemia, due to the extra-junctional migration of acetylcholine receptors. It is safe within the first few hours, but subsequently should not be used for the following 12 months.
- Resistance develops to non-depolarizing relaxants, persisting up to 10 weeks.
- Renal failure may occur secondary to initial hypovolaemia and myoglobinuria.
- While there is no benefit in prophylactic antibiotic or steroid therapy, steroids may be required along with aminophylline if severe bronchospasm develops.

- Enteral feeding has been shown to protect against gut translocation of toxins and micro-organisms, and to reduce the incidence of sepsis.
- Some advocate avoidance of central lines (another portal for infection).

Further reading

Hettiaratchy, S., Papini, R. (2004). ABC of Burns—Initial management of a major burn (assessment and resuscitation). *British Medical Journal*, **329**, 101–3.

⊙ Inoculation injury

Definition
Object or substance contaminated by blood or other body fluids breaches the integrity of the skin or mucosa (needlestick or subcutaneous exposure), or comes into contact with the eyes, mouth, broken skin (mucocutaneous exposure).

Presentation
- Usually 'needlestick' injury in the anaesthetic setting.
- Hollow, blood-containing needles present the highest risk to anaesthetists.

Immediate management
- Wash the wound liberally with soap and water but without scrubbing.
- Exposed mucous membranes, including conjunctivae, should be irrigated copiously with water or saline (remove contact lenses).
- If puncture wound, free bleeding should be encouraged gently, but wound should not be sucked.
- Hospitals should have an 'inoculation injury' protocol and pack.
- Report the exposure *immediately* to Occupational Health and seek urgent advice on further management and treatment. Local protocols will indicate from whom advice should be sought if the exposure occurs outside normal working hours.
- If postexposure prophylaxis (PEP) is recommended, it should ideally start within 1 h of the exposure.

Subsequent management
- Further management will involve assessing the potential risk from the patient, seeking consent from the patient to testing for bloodborne viruses (this should **not** be undertaken by the exposed healthcare worker), and testing the healthcare worker in a similar fashion.
- In most circumstances of hepatitis B and HIV exposure, postexposure prophylaxis (PEP) will be offered.
- Expert advice should be sought from Occupational Health.

Investigations
Occupational Health

Risk factors
- The major hazard associated with inoculation injuries is the transmission of bloodborne viruses: hepatitis B, hepatitis C, and HIV.
- In the healthcare setting, transmission most commonly occurs after percutaneous exposure to a patient's blood. The risk of transmission to a healthcare worker from an infected patient following such an injury is:
  - 1 in 3 when a source patient is infected with hepatitis B and is 'e' antigen-positive
  - 1 in 30 when the patient is infected with hepatitis C virus
  - 1 in 300 when the patient is infected with HIV

- The transmission risk after a mucocutaneous exposure is lower than that of percutaneous exposure. The risk of acquiring HIV after a single mucocutaneous exposure from an infected patient is less than 1 in 2000.

Paediatric implications

Parents need to give consent for their child to undergo blood testing.

Special considerations

- Always employ 'Universal Precautions':
  - wear gloves
  - handle sharps carefully—do not re-sheath needles
  - dispose of sharps in sharps bin immediately after use. Do not over-fill sharps bin
  - discard disposable syringes and needles wherever possible as a single unit
- Hepatitis B immunization—all healthcare workers who perform exposure-prone procedures should be immunized against hepatitis B and have their response to the vaccine checked. Advice should be obtained from the Occupational Health Service.
- Postexposure prophylaxis (PEP) with hepatitis B immunoglobulin and/or antiretroviral drugs should be recommended to healthcare workers if they have had a significant occupational exposure to blood or another high-risk body fluid from a patient, or other source either known to be Hep B/HIV infected, or considered to be at high risk of Hep B/HIV infection, but where the result of testing has not or cannot be obtained. PEP should ideally commence within 1 h of the exposure.

Further reading

UK Health Departments (1998). *Guidance for Clinical Health Care Workers: Protection against infection with blood-borne viruses; Recommendations of the Expert Advisory Group on AIDS and the Advisory Group on Hepatitis.* http://www.dh.gov.uk/assetRoot/04/07/68/16/04076816.pdf

UK Health Departments (2004). HIV *post-exposure prophylaxis—Guidance from the UK Chief Medical Officers' Expert Advisory Group on AIDS.* http://www.advisorybodies.doh.gov.uk/eaga/prophylaxis-guidancefeb04.pdf

☼ Bone cement implantation syndrome (BCIS)

Definition
CVS collapse in response to the insertion of methyl methacrylate cement during hip arthroplasty procedures.

Presentation
Hypotension, hypoxaemia, cardiac arrhythmias, and cardiac arrest.

Immediate management
- ABC ... 100% O_2
- IV fluids
- IV ephedrine (6 mg boluses), α-agonists (e.g. metaraminol 0.5 mg boluses) and/or adrenaline (10–50 µg boluses)

Subsequent management
Usually transient reaction which stabilizes. In unfit patients sudden deterioration may progress rapidly if not managed aggressively.

Investigations
- 12-lead ECG to exclude cardiac event.

Risk factors
- Clinical experience suggests that the syndrome is rare in healthy patients.
- It is more common in:
  - elderly patients
  - those with reduced myocardial reserve
  - dehydrated patients
  - poor surgical technique
- Commonest scenario is relative hypovolaemia in a patient having regional block technique—keep ahead with fluids in patients likely to be at risk.

Exclusions
- Massive pulmonary embolus—prolonged hypoxaemia
- Myocardial infarction or cardiac failure—more prolonged hypotension, pulmonary oedema, little response to fluids and vasopressors, known risk factors
- Anaphylaxis

Special considerations
- Bone cement implantation syndrome (BCIS) has been attributed to many things:
  - one component of the cement is a liquid monomer which causes vasodilatation and tachycardia when it reaches the circulation

- mixing of the cement produces an exothermic reaction, and heat may cause bone marrow and blood cells to release thrombotic and vasoactive substances
- embolization of air, fat, bone marrow, and bone debris can occur when the prosthesis is impacted
- Intravasation of air, fat, bone marrow, and bone debris occurs during the implantation of the femoral prosthesis, and the embolization of these elements into the right heart can be demonstrated clinically using transoesophageal echocardiography (TOE). It is suggested that these microemboli may lead to acute pulmonary hypertension and right ventricular failure. As with most embolic phenomena, TOE reveals many patients with microemboli, some of whom develop transient hypoxaemia, but very few of whom develop full-blown BCIS.

① Extravasation of anaesthetic agents

Definition
Leakage of fluid from a vein into the surrounding tissue.

Presentation
Effects range from mild discomfort and discoloration, through to tissue necrosis with damage to tendons and nerves, compartment syndrome requiring fasciotomy, reconstructive surgery, and even amputation.

Immediate management
- There is no proven definitive treatment for extravasation injury. There is some evidence that early treatment may improve outcome.
- Stop injecting.
- Leave the cannula *in situ*.
- Assess risk of solution injected.
- Hyaluronidase breaks down hyaluronic acid in connective tissue and is used to increase the permeability of tissues to injected fluids (e.g. hypodermoclysis). Subcutaneous infiltration of hyaluronidase (15 units/mL saline) at 5–10 sites along the leading edges of the extravasation has been used successfully. Another approach is to deliver the hyaluronidase into the cannula. Total dose should not exceed 1500 units.
- Topical cooling and topical warming have both been advocated, although there is little evidence that either is beneficial.

Subsequent management
- The extravasation injury should be clearly documented in the patient's notes.
- The patient should be given a full explanation of events and an apology.
- The site should be observed closely for the first few days.
- Local blistering suggests partial-thickness injury.
- Firm induration suggests eventual ulceration.
- A plastic/reconstructive surgeon should be consulted early.
- Surgery is usually indicated if full-thickness skin necrosis occurs.
- The injury should be reported on a 'Green Card' to the National Extravasation Information Service (www.extravasation.org.uk).

Investigations
Clinical diagnosis

Risk factors
- Site of cannulation—antecubital fossae and dorsi of the hand or foot are the most common sites of extravasation injury. Joints and creases should be avoided as these represent a 'small tissue space', often containing nerves and tendons.
- Patient factors include diabetes, rheumatoid, Raynaud's disease, peripheral vascular disease, lymphoedema, recent surgery to limb, recent radiotherapy to limb.
- Type of drug—the following are all high risk in extravasation injury:

- high pH (e.g. thiopental, etomidate, phenytoin)
- vasopressors (e.g. adrenaline, noradrenaline)
- high osmolality (e.g. mannitol, calcium chloride, potassium chloride, sodium bicarbonate, parenteral nutrition, some antibiotics)
- cellular toxicity (e.g. chemotherapy)

Exclusions

Intra-arterial injection leads to severe burning pain in the conscious patient. Blanching, hyperaemia, and cyanosis *of the distal limb* can occur depending upon the drug injected.

Special considerations

- Beware IV cannulae inserted prior to arrival in the anaesthetic room. Always test cannulae with a saline flush prior to use, or insert a new one.
- Always use a test dose of 1–2 mL of induction agent and assess the patient and the site of injection.
- Check the cannula if the patient complains of excessive pain at induction. The cannula may well be in an intact vein if using propofol or etomidate, as pain upon injection is common.
- If possible, position the limb so that the cannulation site can be directly inspected throughout the surgical procedure.
- Distrust a positional IV cannula. It may have tissued and fluid may be entering the perivenous space. If the drip does not run freely, assume it has tissued until you can confirm otherwise. Never give drugs via a positional cannula. Insert a new cannula at a different site.

Further reading

www.extravasation.org.uk

① Intra-arterial (IA) injection

Definition
Injection of an intravenous drug into an artery.

Presentation
- IA injection leads to severe burning pain in the conscious patient.
- Blanching, hyperaemia, and cyanosis of the distal limb can occur.

Immediate management
- Stop injecting immediately.
- Leave the cannula in place.
- Inject lidocaine 100 mg and papaverine 40 mg in 10–20 mL saline via the cannula.
- Regional blockade of the upper limb (brachial plexus block or stellate ganglion block) has been used in attempt to reduce arterial vasospasm.
- The patient will need systemic analgesia.
- Formal anticoagulation with IV heparin and subsequently with oral warfarin should be considered.
- Use of intravenous epoprostenol (prostacyclin) has been described.
- Seek early guidance from a vascular surgeon.

Subsequent management
- Many approaches have been described but none is proven.
- No specific treatment recommendations can be given on the available evidence. The few studies available are animal models with small sample sizes.
- Formal thrombolysis using urokinase has been described, although an animal model studying intra-arterial thiopental injection (using intra-arterial urokinase as a therapy) showed a detrimental effect.
- IA *thiopental*—causes severe pain and blanching of the distal limb. There is profound constriction of the artery caused by local noradrenaline release. Thiopental may crystallize in arterioles. Thromboses occur and these may embolize to distal parts of the limb, e.g. individual digits.
- IA *fentanyl*—has been injected into a conscious patient without causing any symptoms, signs, or sequelae.
- *Propofol*—leads to severe distal hyperaemia lasting between a few hours and 12 days. Full recovery is the norm.

Investigations
- Overall diagnosis is clinical, and requires a high index of suspicion.
- Transduce pressure from the cannula and take blood sample for ABGs. If cannula is kinked, or patient has AV fistula, these tests will not be diagnostic.

Risk factors
- Inadvertent IA injection is a rare complication of anaesthesia.
- It can occur due to mistaken injection into an arterial line port, especially if lines are not properly marked or labelled.

- It occurs with cannulae inserted into the antecubital fossa (brachial artery) or into an aberrant radial artery.
- The arterial vascular anatomy of the upper limb is extremely variable, and you cannot assume that arteries occur only as they do in an anatomy text.
- IA injection has been described into cannulae placed in the dorsum of the hand.

Exclusions
- Pain on (IV) injection is common with many anaesthetic induction agents.
- Extravasation from a tissued cannula can cause pain, discoloration, and blanching (see pp408–9).

Special considerations
- Always check for a pulse in the vessel that you intend to cannulate. Ideally this should be performed prior to a tourniquet being applied.
- Ensure that any applied tourniquet is not so tight as to occlude arterial flow in the limb.
- Attaching a drip and allowing it to run prior to induction does not preclude intra-arterial placement of the cannula, but may demonstrate backflow of arterial blood.
- Take great care with all arterial line ports. Label them appropriately, or tape them closed while in theatre.
- Give a test dose of 1–2 mL of induction agent and assess the patient's response before proceeding.

Further reading
Ghouri, A.F., Mading, W., Prabaker, K. (2002). Accidental intra-arterial drug injections via intravascular catheters placed on the dorsum of the hand. *Anesthesia and Analgesia*, **95**, 487–91.

⑦ What to do in the event of fire

Definition
Fire occurring in the theatre suite or Critical Care Unit.

Presentation
- Most hospitals are now fitted with two-stage fire alarms. When a fire occurs, the alarm will sound continuously in the affected area, but will ring intermittently in adjoining areas.
- Persons in an area where the alarm is sounding intermittently need not evacuate, but should make provisional preparations. Staff should prepare patients and visitors for evacuation should the alarm change to a continuous sound.

Immediate management
- The person in charge of the department must first determine the exact location of the fire by instructing staff to carry out a rapid visual check of the area.
- If the fire incident is minor and can be tackled safely by staff, then total evacuation may be unnecessary and the procedures being carried out within the department may continue.
- If the fire incident is serious, and is within or threatens the department, and cannot be tackled by staff with fire extinguishers, then the safety of staff and patients is paramount. All work should stop and all non-essential persons must be evacuated to an adjoining safe area. While the speedy evacuation of patients is essential, staff must not compromise their own safety to do this.
- In the event that fire/suffocation is imminent, identify staff and resources that will be required to safely evacuate the patient (e.g. self-inflating bags, oxygen, etc., including an oxygen supply for the staff).
- Consider the most practical route of evacuation (lifts should not be used, stairs are impassable on ward or ITU beds, but mattresses can be used to move a patient down a stairwell).
- Establish a route of communication to the outside (telephone, mobile phone, radio, runner).
- Firemen are trained and equipped to rescue people from burning buildings ... doctors are not.
- It may be that a ventilated patient has a better chance of surviving suffocation if left in the unit than if moved through a smoke-filled exit route.
- Staff should not risk their lives by staying with a patient who cannot be evacuated.

Risk factors

- Of basic importance to the fire strategy in hospitals is the principle that, should a fire occur, it is rapidly detected, an alarm is given, and the fire brigade is called.
- The immediate and total evacuation of a hospital in the event of fire is usually neither desirable nor necessary.

Special considerations

- NHS Trusts have a responsibility for ensuring that all new staff (including agency staff) receive basic fire training immediately upon taking up their first appointment. The training should include instruction on the action to take in the event of a fire and the emergency evacuation procedures applicable to their actual places of work.
- Fire extinguishers used to come in standard colours according to the type of extinguishing agent. New European legislation decrees that all fire extinguishers must now be red. You should, however, find a colour-coded label fixed to the front of the extinguisher to denote the type of extinguishing agent contained within.
- All staff should seek training in the operation of fire extinguishers available in their workplace.

:☼: Bleeding following tonsillectomy

Procedure	Re-operation to treat bleeding from adenoid or tonsil
Time	0.5–1 h
Pain	*/**
Position	Supine
Blood loss	May be significant, but difficult to estimate. Crossmatch 2 units
Practical techniques	RSI, ETT, IPPV

Presentation

- Haemorrhage may be early (haemostasis failure) or late (infective).
- Patient may have lost significant amount of blood, but difficult to esti-mate due to swallowing/vomiting.
- Decision to take patient back to theatre should be made by a senior surgeon. Delay should be avoided, but IV resuscitation will be required.

Immediate management

- ABC … 100% O_2. Reassure the patient and relatives.
- Ensure senior anaesthetist available.
- Check Hemocue and start IV resuscitation with large-bore IV access.
- If hypotensive, use colloid (20 mL/kg).
- Ensure crossmatched blood available.
- May be residual narcosis due to opioids and previous GA. Exclude hypovolaemia as cause.
- RSI is usual. Cricoid pressure does not stop blood trickling down pharynx, but does limit the risks from a stomach full of blood.
- Alternatively, left side, head down, and gaseous induction—not recommended.
- Intubation will be difficult due to blood and oedema. Have suction and difficult intubation aids to hand.
- Following surgery, use large orogastric tube to empty stomach.
- Extubate awake, on left side, head down.
- In some patients with adenoidal bleeding a pack may be left *in situ* until the following morning.

Subsequent management

Keep in recovery/HDU for several hours to ensure bleeding has stopped and resuscitation is adequate.

Special considerations

Intubation will be more difficult than at first operation—do not underestimate risks.

⚙: Bleeding following thyroid surgery

Procedure	Return to theatre post thyroid surgery. Haemorrhage may cause airway obstruction
Time	1 h
Pain	*/**
Position	Supine, slight head-up tilt
Blood loss	500–1000 mL
Practical techniques	GA with ETT, may be difficult intubation

Presentation

- Thyroid surgery followed by bleeding into the tissues of the neck.
- More common following large tumour resection (bleeding risk and tracheomalacia).
- The whole neck may be distended and oedematous.

Immediate management

On ward

- If stridor and respiratory embarrassment present—remove skin stitch/clips and sutures holding strap muscles together. Manually remove haematoma.
- If respiration is not impaired, accompany the patient to theatre and allow surgeon to remove the haematoma under local anaesthesia.

Theatre

- After decompression, the patient will need anaesthesia for haemostasis. Intubation may be difficult due to oedema of the upper airway, caused by venous obstruction.
- Consider awake fibreoptic intubation or inhalational induction using oxygen and halothane/sevoflurane.
- *In extremis*—either trial of direct laryngoscopy or awake tracheostomy.
- If airway obstruction has been severe, keep intubated overnight and give dexamethasone 8 mg IV.

Subsequent management

Tracheostomy may be required in a few cases.

Special considerations

- Surgeon should palpate the trachea (partly withdraw the ET tube) to assess degree of tracheomalacia before extubation.
- When decompressing the neck as an emergency procedure, remember that the haematoma may be beneath the muscle layer and simply opening the skin wound may not be sufficient.

☠ Bleeding following carotid endarterectomy

Procedure	Opening of neck wound, evacuation of haematoma and haemostasis. Airway obstruction can be life-threatening
Time	1 h
Pain	*
Position	Supine, head up
Blood loss	<1000 mL, crossmatched 2 units from earlier operation
Practical techniques	If the CEA was performed under regional anaesthesia, the block may still be working sufficiently or can be topped up. Alternatively: ETT, IPPV intubation may be difficult

Presentation
Carotid endarterectomy (CEA) earlier in the day. Subsequent distension of the neck which will ultimately compromise the airway. The quoted incidence is 1–4% of CEA patients, most within 4h after surgery. It increases mortality significantly.

Immediate management
- ABC ... 100% oxygen.
- Reassure the patient, sit up.
- Neck wound—if stridor or complete airway obstruction is impending, get surgeon to open the neck wound immediately.
- Return to theatre.
- Call for help and difficult airway trolley.
- Intubation may be difficult, but with no time for awake fibreoptic intubation—emergency tracheostomy may be required.
- Consider adrenaline nebulizer (5 mg, 5 mL of 1:1000)—this may help to reduce airway oedema, provided it does not delay the patient getting to theatre.

Subsequent management
- Once airway secure, management is straightforward.
- Administer dexamethasone (8 mg).
- Patients intubated due to airway obstruction should be kept intubated overnight on ITU to allow the oedema to settle.
- Significant bleeding requiring transfusion is uncommon. However, check the Hb and coagulation.

Further reading
Self, D.D., Bryson, G.L., Sullivan, P.J. (1999). Risk factors for post-carotid endarterectomy hematoma formation. *Canadian Journal of Anesthesia*, **46**, 635–40.

:☠: **Emergency aortic aneurysm repair**

Procedure	Emergency repair of ruptured abdominal aortic aneurysm
Time	3–6 h
Pain	**** (ventilated post-op)
Position	Supine, arms out (crucifix)
Blood loss	1000–10 000 mL (crossmatch 8 units packed RBC, order platelets and FFP). Very suitable for autotransfusion
Practical technique	ETT, IPPV, arterial + CVP lines, Level-1® fluid warmer or equivalent

Presentation

- Two different clinical presentations:
  - rupture—exsanguinating patient
  - retroperitoneal leak—hypotensive but stable
- Ultrasound or CT scan if time available
- True ruptured AAA has an *in-hospital* mortality of at least 50%. Survival uncommon >80 years and if CPR has been necessary preoperatively.

Immediate management

- ABC ... 100% oxygen.
- Anaesthetic history—allergies, medications, cardiac history.
- IV access—two 14G or PAFC sheath.
- Crossmatch—8 units packed red cells and warn blood bank about platelets and FFP.
- Fluids—if hypotensive, warmed fluids and vasopressors to a systolic pressure of 90–100 mmHg.
- Ephedrine 3–6 mg boluses or metaraminol 0.5–1 mg boluses.
- Adrenaline 100 µg boluses—if resistant hypotension or imminent cardiac arrest.
- Avoid hypertension, coughing, or straining.
- Analgesia—IV morphine for pain.
- Inform theatre—phone ahead, fluid warmers (Level-1® if available), pressure transducers and drugs including vasopressors and inotropic infusion (adrenaline 2 mg in 40 mL = 50 µg/mL). Induction will be in theatre.
- Go directly to theatre.
- Relatives—speak to (or have someone else speak to) them.

Perioperative

- Induce in theatre.
- Assign one assistant to manage IV fluids, including organizing supply of fluid/blood.

- Arterial line pre-induction (upper limbs only). Central venous access only if time permits (more commonly after cross-clamp). Urinary catheter.
- Talk to the patient while he is being draped, and preoxygenate.
- IV infusions running maximally with pressure bags.
- When surgeon ready *and blood available* induce with a suitable hypnotic, e.g. propofol/remifentanil, etomidate/fentanyl, or ketamine with suxamethonium. As soon as intubation is confirmed, surgeons can start.
- Treat further hypotension with rapid infusion of IV fluid and vasopressors/inotropic agents.
- Clamping the aorta usually allows some measure of haemodynamic stability for the first time. However, collaterals will continue to bleed.
- IV fluids/blood to maintain Hb 8 g/dL. Platelets and FFP as indicated—if in doubt, give them. Use thromboelastography to guide blood replacement therapy.
- Unclamping the aorta is hazardous. Fill to CVP >10 mmHg and mildly hyperventilate to a $PaCO_2$ of 4.2 kPa—but combination of metabolic acidosis, relative hypovolaemia, vasodilatation, and myocardial stunning will usually necessitate inotropic support. Start adrenaline infusion (2 mg/40 mL at 1–10 mL/h). Consider giving calcium gluconate (10 mL 10%) and bicarbonate if pH <7.1 (but not simultaneously!).
- Adjunctive therapy for renal protection may include:
  - mannitol (25 g)
  - furosemide (20–80 mg)
  These drugs may increase urine output but there is no evidence that they reduce the incidence of renal failure.
- Hypothermia is a particular hazard, warm *all* fluids and use warm air blower on upper body (contraindicated on lower body during cross-clamp). Monitor temperature.
- NG tube (orogastric if severe coagulopathy present).

Subsequent management
- Overnight ventilation in ITU.
- Hypothermia, renal impairment, blood loss, and coagulopathy are common postoperative problems.

Special considerations
- Epidural analgesia rarely appropriate.
- Oesophageal Doppler can be misleading during cross-clamp period.
- Be prepared to use group-compatible, non-crossmatched blood if necessary.
- If the bleeding cannot be stopped, the surgeon may pack the abdomen and transfer the patient to ITU. Consider giving recombinant factor 7 (NovoSeven) 2.4 mg which has been shown to be effective in some cases of uncontrolled bleeding.

Further reading
Brimacombe, J., Berry, A. (1993). A review of anaesthesia for ruptured abdominal aortic aneurysm with special emphasis on pre-clamping fluid resuscitation. *Anaesthesia and Intensive Care*, **21**, 311–12.

☼ Sick laparotomy

Procedure	Emergency laparotomy in ASA 3 or greater
Time	1–4 h
Pain	****
Position	Supine
Blood loss	500 mL +
Practical techniques	GA, ETT, arterial, CVP lines Preoperative resuscitation± epidural

Presentation
- Usually perforated viscus or bowel ischaemia/obstruction
- Septic—tachycardia, hypotension, hypovolaemia

Immediate management
- Review patient on ward—ABC ... 100% O_2.
- Define current surgical problem and premorbid condition.
- Examine patient and check FBC, U&Es, coagulation, amylase, cross-match, ECG.
- ABGs if dyspnoeic—base deficit/raised lactate usually a sign of inadequate resuscitation.
- Make a judgement—delay for resuscitation vs. early surgery.
- Resuscitate according to determined goals (HR, BP, CVP, ABGs, BE, UOP).
- Use best place for optimization (ICU, HDU, Recovery).
- Discuss condition and timing of surgery with surgical team.
- Consider need for invasive monitoring (CVP, arterial line, oesophageal Doppler).

Preoperative optimization
- Review as early as possible.
- ABC—oxygenation. Intubate and IPPV if required. May need transfer to ICU if signs of organ dysfunction are present and surgery not urgent.
- Ensure adequate resuscitation, particularly oxygenation and circulating volume. Decide on appropriate resuscitation goals. Measures of tissue oxygenation and oxygen delivery are best indicators of resuscitation.
- Replace volume with Hartmann's solution, 0.9% saline, or colloid. Most patients are hypovolaemic and many will need CVP monitoring. Other monitors such as 'measurement of systolic pressure variation' or oesophageal Doppler may give more useful clinical information.
- Failure to reach resuscitation goals with fluids alone is an indication for inotropes or vasopressors (if septic, first-line agent is noradrenaline).
- Antibiotic therapy depending on the diagnosis.

- Timing of surgery is crucial. Daytime surgery by senior staff whenever possible. This also allows time for pre-optimization. However, delaying patients with ischaemic bowel or bleeding will cause substantial deterioration.
- Sodium bicarbonate is occasionally needed for acidotic patients in renal failure or with hyperkalaemia. Use for severe metabolic acidosis only (pH <7.15) is controversial. Normally acidosis improves with resuscitation.

Resuscitation goals

- HR <100 bpm
- MAP >65 mmHg
- CVP 8–12 cmH$_2$O
- Mixed venous SaO$_2$ >70%
- Hb 7–9 g/dL (possibly higher for ischaemic heart disease)
- Urine output >0.5 mL/kg/h
- pH normal
- Lactate normal or falling (<2 mmol/L)

Perioperative

- Large-bore venous access and intra-arterial monitoring prior to induction.
- Epidural according to diagnosis, experience, and patient's wishes (better for pain and weaning, no survival benefit, more postoperative hypotension). Top up cautiously in theatre.
- RSI—thiopental, propofol, etomidate according to condition. Give steroid cover if using etomidate (single dose of 50–100 mg hydrocortisone IV). Some induce with ketamine (1–2 mg/kg slowly IV) if marked hypotension or cardiovascular instability.
- Standard ETT anaesthesia—some anaesthetists use air/O$_2$, to avoid N$_2$O (gaseous distension, PONV).
- Vasopressors should be prepared in case severe hypotension follows induction. Metaraminol (0.5–1 mg) if HR >60 bpm, otherwise ephedrine. Raising the patient's legs may temporarily improve BP.
- If inotropes are required, start early—choice depends on cardiac output vs. vasodilatation. For vasodilatory shock use noradrenaline (4 mg/40 mL, 5–10 mL/h). For a mixed picture use adrenaline (2–4 mg/50 mL, 5–10 mL/h). Dobutamine (5–10 µg/kg/min) is occasionally used, but tachycardia and vasodilatation may be problematic. Vasopressin is a useful second-line vasoconstrictor (4 units/h), which may be given with noradrenaline in resistant cases.
- In patients unresponsive to vasopressors, give hydrocortisone 200 mg in case of adrenal failure.
- CVP monitoring is usually necessary, with particular attention to volume status. Oesophageal Doppler or PAFC can help guide therapy.
- Ventilation may prove difficult in theatre, with high inflation pressures due to abdominal distension and pulmonary oedema/ARDS. Aim for tidal volume 6 mL/kg, PEEP 5–12 cmH$_2$O, peak airway pressure <30 cmH$_2$O. Allow some CO$_2$ retention if necessary.

Subsequent management
- ICU/HDU for anyone who is physiologically compromised.
- Prolonged stay in recovery for all others.
- Analgesia.
- Oxygen for 3 days at 3–4 L/min nasal/facemask delivery.

Special considerations
- Mortality—up to 30%, highest in unfit patients, and those in whom surgery is delayed. Patients who are very unlikely to survive should be identified ahead of time and the desirability of surgery discussed with the consultant surgeon and consultant anaesthetist, who should take personal responsibility for the decision.
- Maximal effort in the perioperative period, produces benefits long into the postoperative period.

Further reading

Arenal, J., Bengoechea-Beeby, M. (2003). Mortality associated with emergency abdominal surgery in the elderly. *Canadian Journal of Surgery*, **46**, 111–16.

Dunser, M.W., Mayr, A.J., Ulmer, H. *et al.* (2003). Arginine vasopressin in advanced vasodilatory shock. *Circulation*, **107**, 2313–19.

Rigg, J.R.A., Jamrozik, K., Myles, P.S. *et al.* (2002). Epidural anaesthesia and analgesia and outcome of major surgery: a randomised trial. *Lancet*, **359**, 1276–82.

Wilson, R.J.T., Davies, S.J. (2004). Preoperative optimization of the high-risk surgical patient. *British Journal of Anaesthesia*, **93**, 121–8.

☼ Ludwig's angina (angina maligna)

Procedure	Incision and drainage of oropharyngeal abscess. Establishment of definitive airway.
Time	1 h
Pain	*/**
Position	Supine
Blood loss	
Practical techniques	Awake tracheostomy Awake fibreoptic intubation Gas induction

Ludwig's angina is characterized by a severe soft-tissue infection of the floor of the mouth and neck.

Presentation

- Progressive swelling of the neck, mouth, and face over a period of a few days. May follow dental treatment or result from dental caries in adults (50–90%).
- Elevation of tongue potentiates risk of airway obstruction.
- Without antibiotics and airway management, mortality in excess of 50%. 8–10% quoted mortality even in treated cases.
- Presentation may be accelerated by rapidly increasing pain, dysphagia, or respiratory distress.
- Infection characterized by brawny induration with multiple abscesses.
- Dysphagia may cause drooling of secretions and dehydration.
- Signs of systemic sepsis, including pyrexia, tachycardia, and hypotension.
- Spread of infection via cervical fascia and retropharyngeal space to mediastinum may result in mediastinitis and pulmonary abscess formation.

Exclusions

Other causes of stridor, including epiglottitis, inhaled foreign body, tumour.

Immediate management

- ABC ... 100% O_2.
- Assess airway for signs of obstruction. If stridor or other difficulties are present, call for trained, senior airway specialists (consultant anaesthetist and consultant ENT surgeon).
- Sit patient upright and give humidified 100% O_2. Reassure patient.
- Transfer patient to a critical care area near operating theatres.
- Consider anticholinergics (e.g. glycopyrronium 200 µg) to reduce secretions.
- Nebulized adrenaline (5 mg in saline) may reduce swelling and provide temporary improvement while theatre is planned.

- Intravenous antibiotics.
- Morbidity in the event of aspiration is reduced by giving ranitidine (50 mg IV) or omeprazole (40 mg slow IV)
- Plan immediate airway intervention if:
  - stridor
  - hypoxia—SaO_2 <95% on oxygen
  - progressive respiratory distress
  - tachypnoea
  - can't speak
- Airway obstruction may progress rapidly. *Intubate at an early stage before it becomes more difficult.*
- Intubation should only be attempted with surgeon scrubbed and ready for immediate tracheostomy. The following options are possible:
  - awake tracheostomy—technically difficult in swollen neck and perceived risk of spreading infection. Cricothyroidotomy is likely to be even harder as swelling spreads from above. Midline anatomy may be difficult to define
  - awake fibreoptic intubation—beware complete obstruction after spraying the airway with local anaesthetic. Presence of intubating scope and tube in already compromised airway may also convert partial into complete obstruction. Consider exploratory nasendoscopy to view cords prior to intubation
  - O_2 and sevoflurane/halothane gas induction—possibly easiest for maintaining oxygenation during airway manipulation

Subsequent management
- Intensive care management is likely to be needed.
- Appropriate antibiotics.
- Surgical management of abscesses—usually multiple incisions and drainage.
- Mediastinoscopy may be indicated if spread of infection to thoracic inlet is suspected.
- Treat cause—dental caries.

Paediatric considerations
- Fewer children require tracheostomy.
- Less likely to require surgical incision and drainage.
- Mortality similar to adults.

Special considerations
A potential problem is contamination of the airway with pus on intubation. Have suction immediately at hand and checked!

Practical procedures

Nicky Ross and Bruce McCormick

ⓘ Intubating laryngeal mask airway (ILMA)

Definition
Variant of LMA that is wide and short enough to allow passage of a specialized endotracheal tube (ETT) into the trachea. Success rate for intubation is 88% in routine cases.

Indications
Elective use
• Anticipated difficult intubation where ventilation is not a problem.

Emergency use
• Failed intubation—see pp68–79.

Contraindications
Absolute
• Limited mouth opening, severe trismus.

Relative
• Does not guarantee ventilation will be possible—does not replace fibreoptic intubation.
• Cervical spine injury.
• Prior radiotherapy or abnormal neck anatomy (use fibreoptic guidance).

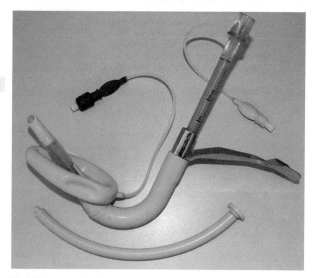

Fig. 14.1

Equipment checklist

For example, LMA-Fast Trach™ (Intavent):

- Comprises standard LMA cuff (sizes 3, 4, 5), mounted on rigid stainless-steel airway tube with 15 mm proximal connector. Shaped to optimize alignment of mask with glottis.
- Diameter of all sizes of ILMA allows passage of specialized size 7.0, 7.5, or 8.0 mm silicone, reinforced ETTs.
- ETT tip is rounded to ease blind passage between cords and minimize laryngeal trauma.
- Stabilizing rod aids removal of ILMA over ETT after placement.

Preparation

- Patient anaesthetized.
- Use size 4 (<70 kg) or 5 (70 kg or greater) ILMA for males, and size 4 for females.
- Check that stabilizer is present in pack (alternative is bougie with several layers of tape applied to one end).
- Apply lubricant to posterior surface of ILMA and completely deflate cuff.
- Check chosen lubricated ETT fits smoothly into ILMA, removing it before use.

Technique

- Head in neutral position.
- Holding device by handle, insert ILMA.
- Inflate ILMA cuff to recommended volume and elevate entire device without tilting, to achieve best seal. Ventilate patient via breathing circuit.
- Adjust position to achieve best capnography trace (a long horizontal plateau on expiration).
- Alternatively, confirm position using bronchoscope or transilluminate neck using lightwand.
- If correctly positioned, patient can be intubated blindly by passing lubricated ETT through ILMA. If necessary, rotate ETT 90° anticlockwise to negotiate right arytenoid cartilage. Attach 15 mm connector to ETT, confirm correct positioning in standard way and oxygenate patient. The LMA can either be left in position for the duration of the case or removed.
- Remove ILMA using tube stabilizer with 15 mm connector unattached.

Troubleshooting—failed intubation using ILMA

- If it is not possible to intubate the patient after two attempts, check ILMA position and glottic orientation with fibrescope, or try larger ILMA. Some anaesthetists prefer to mount the ETT on a fibrescope routinely.
- Avoid prolonged intubation attempts, which will cause bleeding and swelling. Emergency cricothyroidotomy should not be delayed if oxygenation is inadequate.

Complications

Sore throat, hoarse voice, epiglottic oedema, oesophageal intubation (5%, one death reported related to oesophageal rupture).

Paediatric implications
- The smallest available ILMA is a size 3, which may be used for children of about 25 kg upwards.
- Intubation of children smaller than this may be achieved through a standard LMA, although correct LMA positioning is more difficult with the smaller LMA sizes (Table 14.1):

Table 14.1 Paediatric LMA sizes

Size 2.5	20–30 kg
Size 2	10–20 kg
Size 1.5	5–10 kg
Size 1	<5 kg

Intubation through a classical LMA
- The fenestrations of the laryngeal aperture of the LMA may need to be cut away to allow passage of the ETT.
- Position laryngeal mask in the normal fashion and use as a guide for blind intubation by passing an appropriately sized endotracheal tube through laryngeal mask.
- Recommended maximum tube sizes are (Table 14.2):

Table 14.2 Maximum ETT size vs. LMA size

Laryngeal Mask size	ETT size (ID, mm)
1	3.5
1.5	4.0
2	4.5
2.5	4.5
3	5.0
4	6.0 cuffed
5	7.5 cuffed

- In about 70% of cases the ETT will be guided directly into the trachea (but only 50% with cricoid pressure applied).
- The ETT can be stabilized in position as the LMA is removed, using the plunger from a 5 mL syringe.
- Fibreoptic bronchoscopy may both enhance placement and confirm correct positioning. Mount the ETT on the fibrescope, which is then used as a bougie for insertion of the tube. The scope and then the laryngeal mask are removed.
- Another alternative is to insert an airway exchange catheter (Cook®) through the LMA. After removal of the LMA, oxygenation is possible while an ETT is railroaded over the catheter. A gum elastic bougie can be used, but without the facility for oxygenation during the exchange.

Further reading

Kihara, S., Watanabe, S. *et al.* (2000). Segmental cervical spine movement with the intubating laryngeal mask during manual in-line stabilization in patients with cervical pathology undergoing cervical spine surgery. *Anesthesia and Analagesia*, **91**, 195–200.

☠ Cricothyroidotomy

Definition
Insertion of a cannula or needle through the cricothyroid membrane.

Indications
• Last resort in failed intubation in order to achieve oxygenation.
• Bronchial toilet in patients with poor clearance of sputum (e.g. 'Mini-Trach®').
• Administration of supplemental oxygen.
• Administration of nebulized drugs.

Contraindications
Relative
• Unclear or distorted anatomy.
• Surgical cricothyroidotomy not recommended in children <12 years.

Anatomy
• Cricothyroid membrane lies between thyroid cartilage superiorly and cricoid cartilage inferiorly.
• Palpate anterior part of neck in the midline. Most prominent cartilaginous point is thyroid cartilage. With index finger, palpate downwards until you feel a hollow between the thyroid cartilage and cricoid cartilage—the cricothyroid membrane (Fig. 14.2).

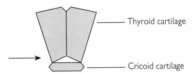

Thyroid cartilage

Cricoid cartilage

Fig. 14.2 Cricothyroid membrane (arrow).

Needle/cannula cricothyroidotomy
Description
• Technique of choice for inexperienced anaesthetists needing to oxygenate a patient in an emergency.
• Allows oxygenation via a 14G cannula for a max. of 30 min.
• Oxygenation achieved via Sanders injector or, where not available, using the system below.
• Ventilation is not achievable and hypercapnia will occur.
• ENT surgeon should be called urgently to carry out emergency tracheostomy.
• Cannula can be upgraded to a wider bore airway using formal cricothyroidotomy kit (see below).

Equipment checklist

- Antiseptic solution.
- Scalpel blade (not essential).
- 14G cannula attached to 10 mL syringe containing 3–4 mL sterile saline.
- Simple system for connecting cannula to oxygen delivery device. This should usually be a Sanders injector or Manujet® (a Sanders injector with a pressure gauge and adjustable driving pressure) attached to cannula by Luer lock (Fig. 14.3).
- Where an injector is not available, the following alternative should be immediately available, fully assembled:
  - cut the drip chamber off an IV giving set and attach the open end to the common gas outlet of the anaesthetic machine using the connector from a size 3.0 mm endotracheal tube. Attach the other end of the IV tubing via its Luer lock to a 3-way tap and then the cricothyroidotomy cannula (Fig. 14.4).

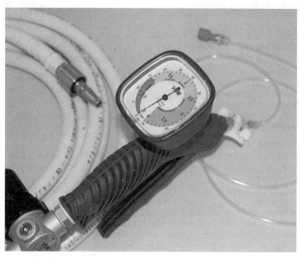

Fig 14.3 Manujet (VBM, Germany).

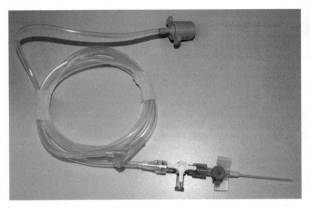

Fig. 14.4 Alternative oxygen delivery system.

Preparation

Only preparation possible in the emergency setting is to *be familiar with pre-prepared equipment in each department of your hospital* for:
- gaining access to trachea
- connecting cannula to oxygen supply
- ventilating patient

Since the patient will usually be *in extremis*, vital time is lost by trying to assemble kit at the last moment.

Technique

- Patient in supine position. Clean and extend neck. Fix skin with traction.
- Identify cricothyroid membrane. Stabilize trachea with thumb and forefinger.
- Insert cannula/syringe directing needle 45° caudally, aspirating as cannula advances. Aspiration of air shows entry into trachea.
- Remove syringe and withdraw stylet, advancing cannula downwards.
- Hold cannula securely to patient's neck yourself and avoid kinking.
- Attach oxygen delivery system (see above). Oxygenation achieved by directing oxygen flow through cannula for 1 s and then allowing gas to escape for 3 s. Expiration of gas should occur through the patient's airway—it may be useful to ensure this is possible by inserting an oropharyngeal airway or LMA.
- In emergencies if cricothyroid membrane cannot be felt (e.g. obesity), insert needle in midline below thyroid cartilage. Insertion between tracheal rings is acceptable.
- Resistance to needle insertion is usually due to cartilage of cricoid (or tracheal ring if too low). Withdraw needle 5 mm, and redirect 3 mm caudally.

Complications
Kinking, failure of expiration (occurs via vocal cords if airway patent), inadequate ventilation, bleeding from skin (use pressure—rarely life-threatening), airway soiling (blood), oesophageal laceration, pneumothorax, haematoma, posterior tracheal wall perforation, subcutaneous and mediastinal emphysema (beware use of Sanders injector with cannula misplaced outside trachea), thyroid damage.

Formal cricothyroidotomy (Mini-Trach®)
Description
- Inserted using commercially available kits—usually 4.0 mm ID tube.
- Allows ventilation using Sanders injector or attachment to anaesthetic breathing circuit via its 15 mm connector.
- In an emergency, can be used as first line by anaesthetists familiar with technique and equipment.
- Used to upgrade needle/cannula cricothyroidotomy.
- Used electively to aid bronchial toilet (e.g. Mini-Trach II®, Portex).
- Principal disadvantage is lack of cuff seal (may need to manually occlude upper airway to achieve adequate ventilation of lungs).

Equipment checklists
- Seldinger technique—most sets have cannulae with 15 mm standard connectors, allowing ventilation by connection to breathing circuit, e.g. Cook Melker catheter. In the elective situation, Mini-Trach® kit is usually used.
- QuikTrach® kit—a sharp, curved, conical needle tip allows insertion through the skin without a scalpel incision and immediate connection to breathing circuit.

Technique
- Scalpel incision to skin.
- Passage of Seldinger wire into trachea allows insertion of a wider gauge cannula (4.0 mm ID) mounted on a dilator.
- Shoulder of tube may cause it to catch on the cricothyroid membrane. Try twisting to and fro while inserting, or cut through membrane alongside wire using scalpel.
- Standard 15 mm connector allows oxygenation and ventilation using standard anaesthetic breathing circuit.
- Use local anaesthetic when inserting Mini-Trach® electively.

Surgical tracheostomy
Description
- Mainly used in trauma—allows insertion of a cuffed tube.

Equipment checklist
- Antiseptic solution. Fenestrated drape
- Scalpel
- Gauze swabs
- Size 5 or 6 ET or tracheostomy tube

Technique
- Stabilize cartilages with non-dominant hand.
- Make vertical skin incision over cricothyroid membrane, then carefully incise through membrane transversely.
- Invert scalpel and insert handle into incision and rotate 90° to open airway.
- Insert size 5 or 6 mm cuffed ET or tracheostomy tube through incision into trachea.
- Inflate cuff and ventilate patient.
- Confirm placement as for oroendotracheal tube.

Complications
Aspiration, creation of false passage, tracheal transection, haemorrhage, oesophageal/tracheal laceration, mediastinal emphysema, vocal cord damage, late subglottic stenosis

Paediatric implications
- Needle or cannula cricothyroidotomy is preferred to surgical cricothyroidotomy in children under 12 years of age.
- Use a 20 or 18G cannula for an infant, a 16G cannula for small children, and 14G for children over 12 years.

① Awake fibreoptic intubation

Definition
Topical anaesthesia applied to upper airway allows insertion of endotracheal tube in an awake patient.

Indications
- Known or suspected difficult intubation.
- Known or suspected cervical spine injury (fracture or ligamentous injury).
- Morbid obesity.
- Poor mouth opening (rheumatoid arthritis, TMJ trauma).
- Full stomach, but difficult intubation anticipated or suxamethonium contraindicated (burns, spinal injury).

Contraindications
Absolute
- Uncooperative patient.
- Severe stridor secondary to perilaryngeal obstruction.
- Known mid- or low-tracheal stenosis.
- Allergy to local anaesthetics.
- Fibreoptic intubation is not indicated in the 'can't intubate… can't ventilate' situation.

Relative
- Airway soiling (bloody airway).
- Children.

Preparation
- Full clinical assessment of airway.
- Explanation and consent—cooperation essential. During passage of the endotracheal tube through the vocal cords over the fibrescope, the patient will feel they cannot breathe and should be warned of this.
- Assess nasal passages for patency (on history and unilateral occlusion).
- 1 h pre-procedure—antisialogogue (glycopyrronium 200 µg IM, reduces secretions and optimizes effect of local anaesthetic) and xylometazoline 0.1% nasal spray.
- IV access.
- Oxygen via nasal catheter.

Technique (Table 14.3)
- Use mild sedation—midazolam (1–2 mg) and fentanyl (50–100 µg) or remifentanil infusion (<0.2 µg/kg/min). Verbal contact must be maintained at all times.
- Determine more patent nostril, and spray with cocaine solution (1 mL 5%).
- Dilate nasal passage with warmed 6 mm then 7 mm nasopharyngeal airway lubricated with cocaine or lidocaine gel (cut 7 mm along long axis and insert safety pin to aid grip during manipulation of scope).

- Spray oropharynx with lidocaine 10% and use Forrester spray to topically anaesthetize pharynx using lidocaine 2% (2–4 mL) as far back as possible.
- Instil oxygen (2 L/min) through scope to oxygenate patient, clear secretions from the tip, and aid atomization of injected local anaesthetic.

Table 14.3 Checklist

Decongestant	Xylometazoline—0.1% or phenylephrine 1% nasal spray—administer in advance if possible
Local anaesthetics	Cocaine 5–10%
	Cocaine and lidocaine gel 2%
	Lidocaine spray 10%
	Four syringes of 1.5 mL lidocaine 2%
Drugs	Midazolam, fentanyl/remifentanil
	Induction agents and neuromuscular blockers
Equipment	6.0/6.5 mm nasal endotracheal tube
	6/7 mm nasopharyngeal airways (cut along length)
	Forrester spray
	Safety pin
	Warm water in container
	Nasal oxygen catheter
Equipment checks	Check scope light functions properly, clean tip and focus
	Check oxygen can be delivered down suction port, and lidocaine injected freely

- Pass *lubricated* fibrescope through the nasopharyngeal airway and, having visualized the vocal cords, instil 1.5 mL lidocaine 2% directly onto the cords. Pass through the cords and repeat for tracheal inlet. The trachea can be identified by circular rings of cartilage.
- Load warmed, lubricated ET tube onto scope and re-insert through nasal airway into trachea.
- Remove the 'split' 7 mm nasopharyngeal airway and advance the endotracheal tube over the scope, maintaining the view of the trachea as you advance—be careful not to advance too far or irritation of the carina will cause coughing.
- 90° turn of ETT anticlockwise allows leading edge of bevel to pass between cords (i.e. bevel facing posteriorly).
- Remove scope, carefully visualizing correct tube placement, and confirm with capnography and bag movement. Do not inflate cuff yet as this may cause panic (increased resistance to respiration).
- Induce anaesthesia, inflate cuff, and fix tube securely.

Complications
Poor compliance/coughing, bleeding in airway (from nasal dilatation), excess secretions, laryngospasm, vomiting, and aspiration.

Special considerations

- Where it is not possible to instil oxygen through the scope, administer oxygen 2–4 L/min via nasal cannula.
- *Cricothyroid puncture*—this technique is used by some anaesthetists, but tends to cause vigorous coughing. Identify the cricothyroid membrane (between thyroid cartilage and cricoid ring) and raise a small subcutaneous wheal with 2% lidocaine. Vertically insert a 20/22G cannula attached to a 5 mL syringe containing 2.5 mL lidocaine until air can be freely aspirated. This confirms placement within the trachea. The cannula sheath may not pass easily through the membrane, in which case a 23/25G needle can be used instead. Inject 2–3 mL 2% lidocaine.
- *Choice of ET tube*—the Portex preformed nasal 'Blue Line' ET tube is extremely pliable when warmed. A 6.5 mm tube fits most people, although occasionally a 6 mm may be needed. Shorten proximally by 3 cm to prevent the tube impinging on the nasopharyngeal airway before removal. An alternative would be a 6 or 6.5 mm armoured tube. Standard ET tubes will tend to cause nasal bleeding.
- *Difficulty in visualizing larynx*—ask the patient to protrude their tongue, swallow, or phonate (may improve view).
- 'Red out' indicates too far (oesophagus) or not midline (piriform fossa). Pull back to soft palate and ensure scope is midline. Dimming lights may allow transcutaneous visualization of the tip.
- *'Tube first' technique*—use 6/7 mm nasopharyngeal airways to dilate nasal passage, then insert ET tube 10 cm to back of nasal cavity. Pass scope through ET tube and position with good view of laryngeal inlet. If required, spray further 2% lidocaine onto cords at this stage. Advance scope into trachea (view tracheal rings). Use scope as bougie, advancing tube over scope and into trachea (tip of the scope in neutral position).
- *Considerations for oral route*—use fibrescopic oropharyngeal airway (e.g. Berman airway®, Vital Signs or Ovassapian intubating airway, Hudson; Fig. 14.5) which protects fibrescope, holds tongue forward, and keeps scope in midline. NB Use airway of correct size to ensure tip is just above the laryngeal inlet. Technically much more difficult.
- Contraindications to nasal insertion include coagulopathy, basal skull fracture, CSF leak, and severe nasal disease.
- Positioning depends on preference, either:
  - patient sitting at least 45° upright with operator facing them
  - patient supine with operator facing them or in normal intubating position

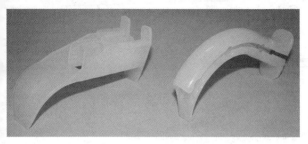

Fig. 14.5 Berman airway and Ovassapian intubating airway.

⑦ Lightwand intubation aids

Definition
A stylet with an end-light to guide intubation by transillumination of the soft tissues of the neck.

Indications
Anticipated or unexpected difficult airway, especially poor mouth opening or neck movement.

Relative contraindications
- Environments with excess ambient light.
- Any facial hair or neck pathology that hinders transillumination.

Complications
As for any attempted oral or nasal intubation.

Equipment
- Lightwands are mouldable fibreoptic stylets with external (Imagica™) or internal (Trachlight™, Laerdal) light sources. They may also be combined with fibreoptic technology and attached to a laryngoscope handle (Levitan FPS, Clarus medical; Fig. 14.6)

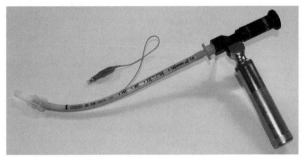

Fig. 14.6 Lightwand.

Preparation

- An ETT should be loaded on to the lubricated stylet with the end of the stylet remaining just inside the tube.
- The tube should be moulded into the 'hockey stick' position by bending it to 90° 3–6 cm from the end.

Technique

- After induction of anaesthesia the patient's head should be slightly extended unless the cervical spine is at risk.
- Ambient light should be kept to a minimum and lights may need to be dimmed.
- Ensure the lightwand is turned on and hold in a pencil grip.
- The non-dominant hand opens the mouth and provides jaw thrust to elevate the epiglottis.
- The stylet is introduced into the oropharynx from the side but rotated into the midline as it passes posterior to the tongue.
- A circle of light in the midline at the level of the hyoid indicates that the tip is lying in the vallecula.
- The light will remain continuously bright as the stylet and tube are advanced successfully into the trachea.
- The stylet is removed and placement confirmed in the usual manner.

Troubleshooting

- Red glow seen off midline—tip in piriform fossa and stylet should be withdrawn and repositioned.
- Briefly losing light and then recovering a dissipated glow indicates oesophageal intubation.

ⓘ **Retrograde intubation**

Definition
Intubation of trachea achieved by passing a guidewire through crico-thyroid membrane and out of the mouth. This acts as a guide for the endotracheal tube.

Indications
- Management of predicted difficult intubation.
- Emergency airway access where laryngoscopy is difficult but mask ventilation is possible.

Contraindications
Relative
- Coagulopathy
- Obscure cricoid or cricothyroid anatomy
- Infection of cricothyroid membrane
- Goitre

Equipment checklist
- Antiseptic solution
- Fenestrated drape
- Gauze swabs
- Scalpel blade
- Retrograde intubation kit
  - commercially available kits avoid difficulties with equipment (e.g. Cook Retrograde Intubation Set®)
  - 16G epidural (Tuohy) needle or 16G cannula, 10 mL syringe containing 3–4 mL sterile saline, guidewire
- Appropriately sized lubricated endotracheal tube—(min. ID 4 mm for Cook set).

Preparation
- In predicted difficult intubation, airway is anaesthetized as described for awake fibreoptic intubation (see pp438–441).
- Relevant anatomy is described on p432.
- Patient supine, neck extended.

Technique (Fig. 14.7)
- Aseptic technique.
- Advance needle or cannula, with 10 mL syringe attached, through crico-thyroid membrane in midline.
- Aim slightly cephalad (compared to caudad for cricothyroidotomy).
- Entry into trachea indicated by aspiration of air into syringe.
- Remove syringe and stylet if using cannula.

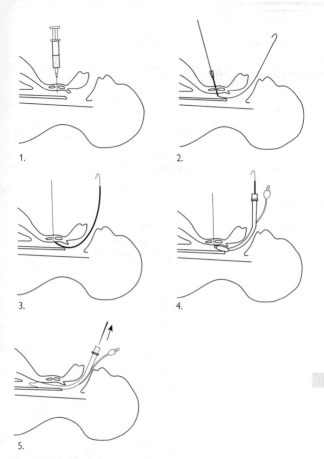

Fig. 14.7 Technique of retrograde intubation.

- Insert J-end of guidewire aiming cephalad, until tip can be retrieved from mouth, using a tongue depressor and Magill forceps. Rolling the wire between your fingers makes it stand away from the mucosa in the oropharynx, aiding retrieval.
- In specialized sets, black mark on wire should be visible at access site, to ensure sufficient length of wire is available in mouth to manipulate the ET tube.
- Remove cannula. (A fibrescope can be placed onto wire at this point, via the suction port, to assess wire placement.)
- Cook set allows anterograde passage of an 11 Fr catheter, which aids subsequent passage of ET tube. Internal diameter of ET tube must be at least 4 mm to use this device.
- The ETT can be mounted on a ureteric or percutaneous nephrostomy dilator (Boston Scientific, MA, USA) to aid passage through the vocal cords. The nephrostomy dilators are shorter (35 cm) and more easily used with a relatively short guidewire. Appropriate sizes are shown in Table 14.4:

Table 14.4 Appropriate dilator sizes for retrograde intubation'

ETT size (ID/mm)	Ureteric/nephrostomy dilator size [French gauge, (OD/mm)]
3.5–4	10F (3.3)
4.5	12F (4.0)
5	14F (4.7)
>5	16F (5.3)

- Pass ETT over wire with 90° turn anticlockwise—allows leading edge of bevel to pass between cords (i.e. bevel facing posterior). Smaller tubes pass more easily through the cords. When tenting is noted at the cricothyroid access site, rotate the tube 180°.
- Maintain control of wire throughout placement.
- Remove guidewire through ETT to avoid soiling neck puncture site. Inflate cuff. Check successful placement in trachea in standard way.

Complications

- As for needle/cannula cricothyroidotomy (see pp432–6).
- Bleeding in airway, difficulties passing the ETT past the vocal cords, epiglottis, or glottic structures.

Paediatric implications

Compliance difficult in younger children. May be possible in children over 12 years.

ⓘ **Chest drain insertion**

Definition
Insertion of catheter into pleural cavity.

Indications
- Pneumothorax
- Traumatic haemothorax or haemopneumothorax
- Pleural effusion
- Empyema
- Postoperative drainage, e.g. thoracotomy, oesophagectomy, cardiac surgery

Contraindications
Absolute (without further investigation)
- Unclear clinical and radiological diagnosis, e.g. bullous lung disease or pneumothorax
- Lung adherent to chest wall

Relative
- Tension pneumothorax should initially be treated by needle thoraco-centesis (see below).
- Coagulopathy, thrombocytopenia, anticoagulation.
- Drainage of postpneumonectomy space is relatively contraindicated.

Note
The National Patient Safety Agency (UK) advises that:
- Chest drains are only inserted by staff with relevant competencies and adequate supervision.
- Ultrasound guidance is strongly advised when inserting a drain for fluid.

Anatomy
- Awake patient 45° head up. Anaesthetized patient may be supine.
- Place ipsilateral arm behind head to expose axillary area.
- Triangle between anterior border of latissimus dorsi, lateral border of pectoralis major, and horizontal line at level of nipple indicates safest area, with minimal risk of damage to underlying structures.
- Insertion site:
  - mid-axillary line, 5th intercostal space
  - pneumothoraces may be treated by catheter inserted apically (mid-clavicular line, 2nd intercostal space). This is also the site for emergency needle thoracocentesis.

Equipment checklist
- Sterile gloves and gown
- Antiseptic solution
- Sterile drapes
- Gauze swabs
- Selection of syringes and needles
- 1% lidocaine with 1:200 000 adrenaline

- Scalpel and blade
- Instrument for blunt dissection, e.g. Spencer–Wells forceps
- Intercostal catheter
  - haemothorax/haemopneumothorax—large-bore catheter (>24 Fr)
  - effusion/empyema—medium-bore catheter (12–24 Fr) unless effusion is known to be transudate, when Pleurocath® sufficient
  - simple pneumothorax—narrow-bore (8–10 Fr) or pigtail catheter, inserted using Seldinger technique (e.g. Pleurocath®)
- Connecting tubing
- Silk suture
- Closed drainage system, including sterile water if underwater seal (ready to attach)
- Clear dressing and strong adhesive tape

Preparation
- Explain procedure and obtain consent when possible.
- IV access.
- Consider sedation and analgesia if appropriate.
- Give prophylactic antibiotics to trauma cases, e.g. cephalosporin.
- For effusions it is advisable to ask a radiologist to label the area of maximal depth of pleural fluid. For larger effusions this can be done prior to the procedure; however, for smaller effusions, it is sensible to use ultrasound during the procedure to ensure the optimal site for chest drain insertion.

Technique
For insertion of a narrow-bore catheter using the Seldinger technique, read instructions provided with set. For insertion of other drains:
- Clean and drape.
- Generously infiltrate 1% lidocaine to skin, muscle, and periosteum in awake patients.
- Make a 2–3 cm horizontal incision through skin and superficial fascia, just superior to rib. Be generous—the incision will need to admit the catheter and one finger.
- From this point, procedure is guided by *blunt dissection* using forceps and avoiding substantial force. If catheter is supplied with a trochar, remove and discard it.
- Bluntly dissect through muscle layers, over top of rib and through parietal pleura.
- Insert finger, confirming access to pleural cavity (by feeling the lung surface). Mount catheter on forceps by passing one arm of forceps through first side hole of catheter, pointing distally. Insert catheter into pleural cavity guided by one finger.
- Ideally direct tube tip *apically* for pneumothorax and *basally* for fluid— difficult in practice!
- Connect to underwater drain.
- Confirm correct placement by fogging in catheter, bubbling of under-water drain, and swinging of fluid in tubing with respiration.
- Secure with two deep 2–0 silk sutures, tied initially at skin and then in multiple knotted loops around catheter.
- Insert wound closure suture to close incision tight around catheter.

- Apply transparent dressing to allow wound inspection. Double clear-dressing fixing of catheter to chest wall, 7–10 cm from skin, increases security.
- Check that catheter is positioned apically on chest X-ray.
- Never apply suction to an intercostal drain inserted following pneumonectomy (causes catastrophic mediastinal shift).
- Remember to send appropriate samples of effusion fluid.

Complications

- Laceration/puncture of intrathoracic or intra-abdominal organs
- Haemorrhage
- Damage to intercostal nerve, vein, artery
- Chest tube malposition, kinking, dislodgement, disconnection
- Air leak around tube at skin, subcutaneous emphysema
- Rapid lung re-expansion leading to pulmonary oedema
- Infection

Needle thoracocentesis

- Indicated when tension pneumothorax is clinically diagnosed (do not wait for a chest X-ray).
- Clean the skin.
- Use at least a 16G cannula (to provide adequate length). Remove the white Luer cap and the 'flash-back' chamber on which the cap sits.
- Advance the open cannula perpendicular to the skin in the second intercostal space, mid-clavicular line of the affected side.
- If the pneumothorax is under pressure ('tension'), a hiss of escaping air may be heard on entry into the pleural cavity—let this air escape.
- Leave the cannula open to air. Avoid kinking and do not remove cannula until intercostal catheter has been inserted.
- Whether or not a pneumothorax was present, you are now obliged to insert an intercostal catheter to formally treat the pneumothorax. The cannula can safely be removed after this.

Further reading

National Patient Safety Agency. Rapid Response Report. Risks of chest drain insertion, 15 May 2008. Available at: http://www.npsa.nhs.uk/patientsafety/alerts-and-directives/rapidrr/risks-of-chest-drain-insertion/

⑦ **One-lung ventilation (OLV)**

Definition
(See also pp230–4)

Term used in thoracic anaesthesia to describe ventilation of one lung, allowing the other to collapse.

Indications for one-lung ventilation (OLV)
- Improving surgical access for lung or oesophageal surgery. Video-assisted thoracoscopic surgery (VATS) is impossible without collapsing a lung.
- Lung protection. OLV is indicated to protect the healthy lung from becoming contaminated by blood or pus in the diseased lung during surgery.
- Intensive care ventilation. Rarely it may be desirable to ventilate a patient's lungs independently using two ventilators so that the normal lung is not subjected to the high pressures required to ventilate the abnormal lung (e.g. after single lung transplant).

Techniques for OLV
There are 3 devices that can be inserted to achieve OLV:
- double-lumen tube
- bronchial blocker
- single-lumen tube inserted beyond the carina.

Double-lumen tubes (DLT)
- Double-lumen tubes have one lumen opening just above the carina and the other opening in a main bronchus.
- Tubes come in sizes 26–41 French gauge—37–39 F is usual for a female and 39–41 F for a male.
- A left-sided tube has its endobronchial portion in the left main bronchus, a right-sided tube in the right main bronchus.
- Either tube can be used for OLV of either lung depending on which lumen is clamped.
- A left-sided DLT is used more commonly as it is easier to position (Fig. 14.8). A right-sided DLT has a Murphy eye (Fig. 14.9), which should be aligned with the entrance to the right upper lobe to allow ventilation. The right upper lobe comes off the right main bronchus at a variable distance from the carina. It may also be anterior, lateral, or posterior.
- A left-sided tube can be used for most operations. For surgery involving the left main bronchus, such as pneumonectomy, it may be preferable to use a right-sided tube, but it may be possible to use a left-sided tube and withdraw it before stapling of the bronchus.

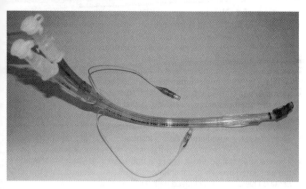

Fig. 14.8 Left-sided DLT.

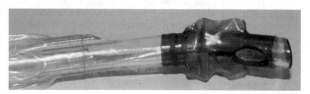

Fig. 14.9 Murphy's eye of a right-sided DLT.

Insertion of a DLT

- Insert tip of tube just through cords and immediately rotate 90° in direction of bronchus you are aiming to intubate. DLTs are bulky and can be awkward to place, particularly in dentulous patients.
- Advance tube until it comes to a halt.
- Inflate tracheal cuff until air leak disappears and check that both lungs ventilate (as for a single-lumen tube).
- Clamp lumen to the lung that you wish to collapse (proximal to the cap) and open cap on clamped side so that air can escape from the lung and collapse can occur. Auscultate the chest to confirm one-lung ventilation. During this process, manual ventilation using high fresh-gas flows allows time for auscultation during inspiration, and also compensates for large air leaks prior to cuff inflation.
- There should still be a leak from the open lumen as gas leaks around the uninflated bronchial cuff. Inflate this in 0.5 mL aliquots until the leak ceases. This is usually achieved with 2 mL air.
- If the patient is positioned in the lateral position the DLT may move. Check for OLV in the new position and that a reasonable tidal volume is possible without excessive pressure (below 35 cmH$_2$O). It is useful to use volume control ventilation while you check—expect the inflation pressure to increase by 5 cmH$_2$O or so. If the airway pressure does not increase, suspect that you have not achieved OLV. Excessive pressures suggest that the DLT has passed too far beyond the carina.
- You may need to increase the FiO$_2$, but SaO$_2$ above 90% is generally acceptable. Increase the respiratory rate to achieve an acceptable end-tidal CO$_2$.

Checking DLT position with a bronchoscope

A check bronchoscopy may be unnecessary for a left-sided tube. However, if inflation pressures are high, if OLV is not achieved, or if oxygenation or CO$_2$ clearance are inadequate, check that the DLT position is correct. Perform bronchoscopy routinely to check the position of a right-sided tube.

Insert scope into tracheal lumen
- Check carina is visible. The carina has the appearance of a sharp line between the main bronchi, whereas other airway divisions have a blunter, gentle curve between them. Check bronchial portion inserts into correct side. You should just see the top of the bronchial cuff, which should not be herniating out of the bronchus.

Now insert into bronchial lumen
- Check that the end of tube is not abutting against the airway wall and that the end of the lumen is therefore patent.
- If the tube is right-sided, look for the Murphy eye in the bronchial lumen. This should open into the right upper lobe lumen.

Troubleshooting

Poor oxygenation
- May result from pulmonary pathology, but first check:
  - position of DLT, particularly that right upper lobe is inflated if a right-sided tube is used
  - other aspects of tube placement with a bronchoscope

- Try to improve oxygenation by:
  - increasing FiO_2
  - applying PEEP to the ventilated lung (as tolerated by inflation pressure)
  - change from volume control to pressure-control ventilation (same tidal volume achieved for lower peak inspiratory pressure)
  - increasing the inspiratory to expiratory ratio (again, as tolerated by inflation pressures)
  - treat hypotension (a low cardiac output may contribute to increased deadspace within the ventilated lung)
  - apply CPAP to the non-ventilated lung if this does not interfere with surgical access

High inflation pressures
- If ventilating the bronchial lumen, check that the tube is not abutting on the endobronchial wall and that the bronchial cuff is just below the carina, not a deeper bronchial division.
- If ventilating the tracheal lumen, check that the bronchial cuff has not herniated into the carina and that the tracheal aperture is well above the carina.
- Suction any secretions from the bronchial tree.

OLV not achieved
- Suction down not-ventilated lumen.
- Check for leak from open lumen (suggests bronchial cuff is malpositioned or underinflated).
- Check bronchial cuff is not herniated.

Bronchial blockers

Definition
A bronchial blocker is essentially a hollow bougie with a cuff that is inserted via a single lumen endotracheal tube to isolate one lung and allow one-lung ventilation (Fig. 14.10).

Indications
- Preference of anaesthetist.
- DLT intubation not possible.
- In situations where the patient has already been intubated with a single-lumen tube, e.g. in ICU.

Insertion of a bronchial blocker (Cook®)

- After intubation with a single-lumen tube, insert the lubricated blocker a short distance into the catheter mount that comes with the set.
- Insert the bronchoscope into the catheter mount passing through the guidewire loop of the blocker.
- Pass the bronchoscope into the main bronchus that you plan to isolate and advance the blocker, following the bronchoscope until it is sitting in a suitable position in the bronchus.
- Inflate the blocker cuff via the pilot tube until the bronchial lumen is filled, checking the cuff remains in position.
- Remove the bronchoscope and extract the guidewire from the blocker—the lung cannot collapse until you have done this. Full collapse takes longer than with a DLT since the lumen of the blocker is narrow.
- Right-sided placement is more difficult because of the proximal origin of the right upper lobe bronchus.

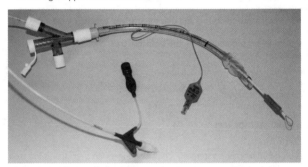

Fig. 14.10 A bronchial blocker.

① In-circuit nebulization

Definition
Administration of nebulized bronchodilator, steroid, or adrenaline to airways of an anaesthetized patient.

Indications
• Bronchospasm in anaesthetized patient.
• Optimization of COPD patient prior to extubation.

Contraindications
Absolute
• Allergy to nebulized drug.

Equipment checklist
• T-piece to fit into circuit (many commercially available) (Fig. 14.11). Various combinations of male–female and female–female 15 mm or 22 mm connectors available, e.g. Cirrus™ series of nebulizers (Intersurgical, New York, USA). Connect nebulizer jar to T-piece.
• Green oxygen tubing.
• External oxygen source with flow regulator.
• Drug to be delivered—optimal volume for adequate delivery is 5 mL (dilute with saline if required).
• Doses (Table 14.5).

Table 14.5 Drug dosages for nebulization

Salbutamol		2.5–5 mg
Ipratropium bromide		250–500 µg
Adrenaline	Adult	5 mL 1:1000
	Paediatric	0.5 mL/kg 1:1000; max 5 mL

Technique
Nebulizer
• Place drug and diluent in nebulizer chamber.
• HME filters absorb nebulized medications. Place nebulizer in circuit between HME filter and patient. A filter can be placed on expiratory limb of circuit to protect flow sensors in ventilator.
• Ensure flow rate of at least 6–10 L/min through nebulizer from oxygen source.
• Deliver continuously or intermittently.
• If possible, increase tidal volume to >500 mL and I:E ratio to 1:1 or 1:1.5.
• Ensure nebulizer functions throughout treatment—chamber should be vertical.

- Remove at termination of treatment and reset ventilator settings.
- With severe bronchospasm, and in children, it may be necessary to ventilate by hand during the therapy.

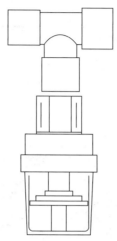

Fig. 14.11 T-piece nebulization chamber.

Troubleshooting

- Addition of driving gas dilutes volatile agent in circuit. Increase inspired vapour concentration and consider supplementing with intravenous anaesthetic agent.
- Agent monitoring may be inaccurate until carrier gas is flushed away.
- Added gas causes over-reading of expired tidal volumes.

! **Connecting a metered dose inhaler (MDI)**

Definition
Connection of standard MDI to anaesthesia circuit to administer bronchodilator to an anaesthetized patient.

Indications
- Mild bronchospasm in anaesthetized patient
- Optimization of COPD patient prior to extubation

Contraindications
Absolute
- Allergy to nebulized drug

Relative
- In severe bronchospasm, IV bronchodilators should be administered

Metered dose inhalers (MDI)
- When used without a specialized connection, most of the drug is deposited in the apparatus.
- In-line devices allow more efficient delivery of metered doses to the patient, e.g. Isothermal Breathing Circuit Accessory® (Allegiance Healthcare Corporation, USA).
- Shake the inhaler before use.
- Place device distal to HME filter in the inspiratory limb.
- Activate device once with inspiration and repeat every 20–30 s.
- Administer 4–10 puffs total.
- As an immediate measure, the bronchodilator can be administered by placing the inhaler into the barrel of a 50 mL syringe. Attach syringe by Luer lock to a 15 cm length of infusion or capnography tubing, which can be fed down an ETT. Discharge 2–6 puffs by downward pressure on syringe plunger. Use of tubing decreases drug deposition in the ETT.
- Alternatively, as an emergency measure, discharge the inhaler directly into the ETT, reconnect the circuit, and ventilate. Repeat 6–10 times. This is a very inefficient method of delivery, as most of the drug does not reach the patient. However, it may be used until a dedicated system is set up.

Troubleshooting
- Only 5% of the dose is delivered in mechanically ventilated patients—be prepared to repeat.
- Flow sensors in certain ventilators may be affected and damaged.

⑦ Vascular access

Large-bore vascular access

- For resuscitation, greatest flow is through a short wide-gauge cannula. Two 14G (orange or brown) cannulae in large forearm or antecubital fossa veins are recommended.
- Devices are available for converting narrow-bore cannulae over a guidewire and dilator to large-bore access (e.g. RIC®—Rapid Infusion Catheter, Arrow International, Reading, USA).
- If a small-bore cannula is already sited, consider injecting 20–50 mL warmed saline to aid identification of larger proximal veins.
- Other potential large-bore vascular access sites are:
  - long saphenous vein
  - external jugular vein—venous valves may prevent full cannulation
  - internal jugular, subclavian, or femoral veins by those experienced at central venepuncture
- Pulmonary artery catheter introducer sheaths are usually 8 Fr gauge:
  - provide best available wide-bore venous access
  - can be inserted into the sites listed above
  - may be difficult to achieve in shocked patients

External jugular venous access (Fig. 14.12)

- This site should be sought early in adults or children where wide-bore venous access is needed urgently.
- Head-down tilt of the patient aids location of the vein. It is often not possible to pass the full length of the cannula due to valves within the vein. This is not a problem as long as the cannula is safely secured in position.

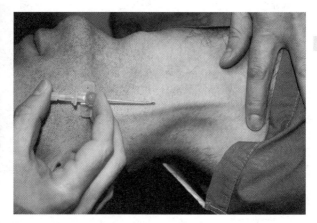

Fig. 14.12 Cannulation of the external jugular vein.

⑦ Internal jugular central venous access

Definition
Placement of a cannula into a central vein.

Indications
- Haemodynamic monitoring (CVP, mixed venous saturation)
- Administration of medications and nutrition
- Haemofiltration and dialysis
- Poor peripheral access

Relative contraindications
- Bleeding disorders
- Infection at site of insertion
- Inability to assume a supine position
- Central vein occlusion

Complications
- Vascular injury (arterial injury, haematoma)
- Pneumothorax
- Arrhythmia
- Air embolism
- Infection
- Catheter-related thrombosis
- Pericardial tamponade

Anatomy
Possible venous access:
- Internal jugular
- Femoral
- Antecubital (for PICC access)
- External jugular
- Subclavian (difficult to place CVC under ultrasound guidance and the vessels are not readily compressible in event of haemorrhage)

Equipment
- CVC kit including: 15 cm 1–5 lumen CVC, 10 mL syringe and needle, dilator, scalpel, guidewire
- Minor procedures' sterile surgical set including: drapes, plastic pot, swabs
- Suture
- 5 mL lidocaine 1%
- Saline
- 2% chlorhexidine
- Tilting bed
- ECG monitoring
- Sterile gown, gloves, hat, and mask

Ultrasound equipment

- Usually linear probe, although curved probe may be adequate.
- Vessels are usually superficial, so most frequencies between 2 and 10 MHz are suitable.
- Sterile sheath for probe, with gel and elastic band (usually included together in a set).

Preparation

- Consent patient.
- Confirm patent vein using ultrasound.
- Scrub for procedure.
- Place the bed in Trendelenburg's position if patient will tolerate it, to prevent air embolism and fill veins.

Technique for right internal jugular CVC insertion under ultrasound guidance

- Clean and drape area. Full aseptic technique.
- Prepare probe:
  - place gel on distal end of sheath and gently roll over probe
  - secure with elastic band
- Place a small amount of gel over site.
- Feel for carotid pulse and place probe transversely across pulse, with non-dominant hand.
- Ensure good contact between skin and probe with gel.
- Aim to view cross-section of carotid artery medially with internal jugular vein laterally (some advocate use of longitudinal view) (Fig. 14.13).
- Confirm identification of internal jugular vein by easy compressibility and distension during a Valsalva manoeuvre. Usually superficial—depth can be estimated using scale on screen (rarely deeper than 3 cm) (Fig. 14.14).
- Using dominant hand, with vein under centre of probe, gently insert needle into anaesthetized skin 1–2 cm above probe at a 60° angle to skin (angle varies depending on depth of vein).
- Scrubbed assistant to hold probe if difficulties encountered with one-handed technique.
- Needle position is visualized by gently agitating needle and syringe along direction of advancement.
- Pass guidewire into vein, confirming position with ultrasound.
- Place central line using Seldinger technique.
- Fix in place (3-point fixation).
- Confirm position with chest X-ray.

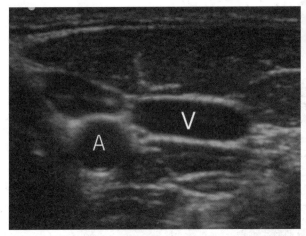

Fig. 14.13 Ultrasound picture of internal jugular vein (v) and carotid artery (a).

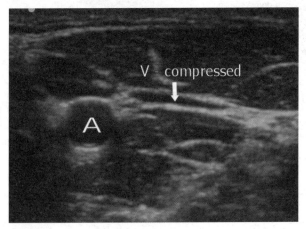

Fig. 14.14 Ultrasound picture of internal jugular vein (v) and carotid artery (a)—note compression of vein on applying pressure.

Technique for right internal jugular CVC insertion using the landmark technique

(Anatomy of the right internal jugular vein is shown in Fig. 14.15)

- Turn the patients head 20° away from the side of insertion (if C-spine cleared).
- Stand on same site as puncture.
- Clean and drape the area. Full aseptic technique.
- Feel for the carotid pulse with your non-dominant index and middle fingers and gently push towards the midline. Do not move these fingers throughout placement.
- Puncture site is at the level of the inferior border of the thyroid cartilage, lateral to the carotid pulse.
- After anaesthetizing the skin, some advocate using a 21G 'seeker' needle to locate the position and depth of the internal jugular vein
- Gently insert needle at 45° to skin, directed to the ipsilateral nipple, aspirating continually.
- Needle often advanced too far and the vein is located as the needle is withdrawn slowly with continued aspiration.
- Pass guidewire into vein.
- Place central line using Seldinger technique.
- Fix in place (3-point fixation).
- Confirm position with chest X-ray.

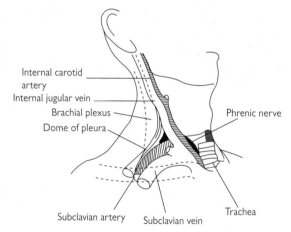

Internal carotid artery
Internal jugular vein
Brachial plexus
Dome of pleura
Phrenic nerve
Subclavian artery
Subclavian vein
Trachea

Fig. 14.15 Anatomy of right internal jugular vein.

Ultrasound

- Reflection of sound occurs at interfaces between tissues of different impedance and is shown as an echo of varying brightness:
  - fluid appears black
  - bone and air appear white
- Veins are non-pulsatile, easily compressible, and distend, when patient head-down or performs a Valsalva manoeuvre. Arteries are pulsatile and are non-compressible with moderate probe pressure.
- Two-dimensional (2D) ultrasound guidance allows:
  - real-time visualization of veins and neighbouring structures prior to and during needle insertion
  - detection of anatomical variants and thrombus within veins
  - possible reduction in rate of haematoma, carotid puncture, nerve injury, pneumothorax, catheter misplacement, number of needle passes
  - advisable in presence of: abnormal anatomy, coagulopathy, previous line insertions, bullous emphysema, orthopnoea

Correct placement

- The tip of the catheter should be in the superior vena cava (SVC) just above the pericardial reflection. Too low and there is a risk of erosion through the vessel wall causing pericardial tamponade, arrhythmias, or tricuspid valve damage.
- Perforation of the SVC above the pericardial reflection is probably greater if the angle of the catheter tip to the wall is >40° (more likely in the upper SVC and innominate veins).
- It is generally accepted that the catheter tip should be located at the level of the carina on CXR, in a vertical position (parallel to the walls of the SVC). Length is variable, but 11–14 cm is usually adequate for a right internal jugular, slightly longer for a left internal jugular.

⚙️ Femoral venous access

Definition
Central venous access via femoral vein at groin.

Indications
- Difficult peripheral venous access.
- Central access for:
  - fluid resuscitation (e.g. pulmonary artery catheter introducer sheath)
  - drug administration (vasopressors, inotropes)
  - transvenous pacing
  - pulmonary artery catheter
  - haemofiltration
- Patients in whom jugular or subclavian venous access is prohibited or unsuccessful.

Contraindications
Relative
- Pelvic or abdominal trauma.
- Trauma in limb in which catheter is to be placed.

Anatomy
- Femoral vein is located immediately medial to femoral artery (from lateral to medial, NAVY: Nerve, Artery, Vein, Y-fronts).
- Vein should be approached below inguinal ligament, to avoid risk of intra-abdominal placement.

Equipment checklist
See 'Internal jugular access', p462.
As with internal jugular vein cannulation it is advisable to use ultrasound to locate and cannulate the femoral vein.

Preparation
- Patient in supine position.
- Sand/saline bag under buttock extends hip to improve access.
- Obese patients may require abdomen retraction by assistant.
- Right-handed operators may find it easier to stand on patient's right (both for left- and right-sided insertions).

Technique
- Aseptic technique. Clean and drape.
- Position guidewire in holder with the tip just showing and leave within reach of your dominant hand.
- Palpate femoral artery distal to inguinal ligament.
- Keep your finger gently over the artery and introduce the needle with mounted 5 mL syringe 1 cm medial to artery, at 45° to skin, heading towards the umbilicus. Too firm pressure will occlude the vein.
- Gently aspirate on syringe as needle is advanced.

- When blood is aspirated, anchor needle securely in exact position and check that blood still flows freely into syringe. If any resistance felt, stop advancing, gently withdraw needle whilst aspirating. It is not uncommon to locate vein on withdrawal.
- Remove syringe, checking puncture is not arterial (bright red, pulsatile), and insert guidewire through needle.
- If guidewire will not pass freely, remove it, recheck for free aspiration of blood, and repeat wire insertion.
- Continue as for CVC insertion.

Complications

Arterial puncture, intra-abdominal bleeding if approach too proximal, infection (higher incidence than subclavian or jugular access).

Paediatric implications

- Ensure that site of skin puncture is well below the inguinal ligament to avoid inadvertent intra-abdominal puncture.
- Appropriate sizes of central venous catheter are shown in Table 14.6:

Table 14.6 Paediatric femoral venous catheter sizes

Patient weight (kg)	Catheter size (French gauge)
<5	3 or 4
5–15	5 or 7
>15	7–11

⚙ Intraosseous cannulation

Definition
Cannulation of marrow cavity of long bone allowing rapid emergency vascular access for critically ill child or adult.

Indications
- Emergency vascular access. Use when venous cannulation is likely to take >90s or after two failures to achieve access.
- Allows blood sampling and administration of fluids/drugs. Onset of drug action and plasma concentration similar to intravenous route.

Contraindications
Absolute
- Fracture proximal to site (can site in femur, proximal to fractured tibia)
- Osteomyelitis
- Fracture at site

Relative
- Although previously not advised for children >6 years old, intraosseous cannulation is increasingly used in the armed forces and emergency departments for rapid vascular access in adults.

Anatomy
- Tibial site most commonly used (Fig. 14.16).
- Palpate tibial tuberosity.
- Site of insertion is 2–3 cm inferior and medial to the tibial tuberosity on flat anteromedial aspect of tibia.
- Femoral site—anterolateral surface of femur 3 cm above lateral condyle of femur.

Equipment checklist
- Antiseptic solution
- 18G intraosseous needle (14G, 16G also available). A standard 19G (white) needle can be used where facilities are limited, but the needle is more likely to become blocked with a core of bone.
- Sterile gloves. Fenestrated drape
- Local anaesthetic (if indicated)—1% lidocaine
- 5 mL syringe, 50 mL syringe
- Fluids with giving set, 3-way tap and extension
- Blood sample tubes (crossmatch, electrolytes)

Preparation
Flex patient's knee and place sandbag behind it as support.

Technique
- Use aseptic technique when inserting needle.
- Identify site as above.

- If child conscious, infiltrate with local anaesthetic, including periosteum.
- Grasp knee above site of insertion to brace leg.
- Insert intraosseous needle at 90° to skin.
- Advance needle with drilling, rotatory motion.
- Stop when 'give' is felt as needle penetrates cortex and enters bone medulla.
- Remove trochar.
- Correct position in marrow is suggested by:
  - convincing 'give' on entering marrow cavity
  - needle remaining upright without support
  - aspiration of blood with 5 mL syringe
- Send blood for crossmatch, electrolytes, and measure glucose at the bedside (FBC is unreliable using marrow samples).
- If no blood is aspirated, flush with saline and repeat aspiration.
- Secure with sterile gauze and strapping. Cardboard tube from roll of tape placed over needle and taped in place provides secure positioning.
- Infusion of fluids:
  - appropriate for infusion of blood products, synthetic colloids, and crystalloid solutions
  - fluids will not flow passively into marrow—use 50 mL syringe attached by 3-way tap to giving set
  - watch for local soft-tissue swelling, suggesting cannula misplacement
- Administration of drugs:
  - all resuscitation drugs (except bretylium) can be given by this route
  - each drug should be followed by a 5–10 mL saline flush
  - doses are as recommended for IV administration
- Should be replaced by venous access and removed within 6 h.

Complications

Infection/osteomyelitis, compartment syndrome, skin necrosis, tibial fracture in neonates.

Intraosseous access in adults

- Intraosseous access is increasingly used for rapid intravascular access in adults, particularly in the armed forces, and increasingly in emergency departments.
- Available sterile, disposable kits include the F.A.S.T.1™, a manual device and the EZ-IO®, which uses a battery-powered drill for intraosseous cannulation. The EZ-IO® comes with an over-40 kg needle for adults and a 3–39 kg needle for paediatric use.
- Recommended sites for access are the tibial plateau (Fig. 14.16), the anterior superior iliac spine, the humeral head, and the sternum.

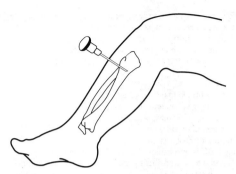

Fig. 14.16 Tibial technique for intraosseous cannulation.

⚙ Cut-down vascular access

Description
Insertion of large-bore cannula into long saphenous/basilic vein under
direct vision after dissection.

Indications
• For resuscitation of patients in whom venous access is difficult
  because of injuries or hypovolaemia.

Contraindications
Relative
• Local infection
• Previous cut-down at same site

Anatomy
• Usual site is long saphenous vein:
  • lies 2 cm anterior and superior to medial malleolus of ankle
• Alternative is basilic vein in antecubital fossa:
  • 2 cm anterior and superior to medial epicondyle at the elbow

Equipment checklist
• Antiseptic solution
• Fenestrated drape
• Sterile gloves
• Arterial forceps
• Scalpel
• Sutures
• Two silk ligatures
• 14G cannula

Preparation
Patient supine

Technique (Fig. 14.17)
• Aseptic technique.
• Infiltrate with 1% lidocaine, careful to avoid venepuncture.
• Make 2.5 cm transverse incision through full thickness of skin over vein.
• Blunt-dissect using curved arterial forceps to identify vein and dissect
  2 cm length free from surrounding tissues.
• Ligate distal mobilized vein, leaving suture in place for traction.
• Pass tie around proximal end of vein.
• Make small transverse incision through vein wall (venotomy) and dilate
  hole with arterial forceps.
• Introduce wide-bore cannula (with needle/stylet removed) through
  venotomy and secure in place by tightening proximal ligature around
  vein and cannula. Take any samples needed (e.g. crossmatch, FBC, electrolytes, and blood sugar).

- Connect to giving set.
- Close incision with suture.
- Apply sterile dressing.

Complications

Cellulitis, haematoma, phlebitis (consider removal within 48h of insertion), perforation of posterior wall of vein, thrombosis, nerve damage, arterial damage.

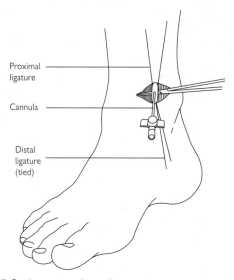

Proximal ligature

Cannula

Distal ligature (tied)

Fig. 14.17 Cut-down access to long saphenous vein.

⑦ Intra-arterial blood pressure monitoring (IBP)

Definition
- Invasive (intra-arterial) blood pressure (IBP) monitoring involves inserting a catheter into a suitable artery and displaying the measured pressure wave as a 'beat-to-beat' record of the patient's blood pressure.

Indications
- Sudden changes in BP anticipated (e.g. vascular surgery).
- Close control of BP required (e.g. head injury).
- Inotropic support..
- As part of a pulse contour analysis system to estimate intravascular volume status.
- Unsuitability of non-invasive blood pressure monitoring (e.g. morbid obesity, atrial fibrillation).
- Repeated arterial blood sampling.

Contraindications
- Local thrombosis and embolization. Avoid arteries with no collateral supply (e.g. brachial artery).
- Inadvertent intra-arterial drug administration possible. Careful labelling is important

Equipment checklist
- Components of an IBP system can be considered in three parts (Fig. 14.18):
  - measuring apparatus
  - transducer
  - display
- The measuring apparatus consists of:
  - a short, stiff-walled arterial cannula (20G in adults, 22G in children)
  - stiff-walled tubing containing a continuous column of saline which conducts the pressure wave to the transducer
  - a flushing system consisting of a 500 mL bag of saline pressurized to 300 mmHg via a flushing device. The flush system provides a slow but continual flushing of the system at approximately 4–5 mL/h. There is also a 3-way tap to allow arterial blood sampling and the removal of air if necessary.

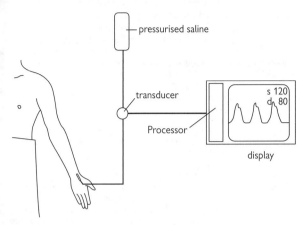

Fig. 14.18 Components of an IBP system.

Preparation

- The usual location for insertion of the arterial catheter is the radial artery. It is advisable to perform Allen's test to detect adequacy of collateral supply to the hand via the ulnar artery (Fig. 14.19). The test is not infallible and can only be performed in conscious patients. The femoral artery, ulnar artery, arteries of the foot and ankle, and even the axillary artery may also be used.

Insertion of a radial arterial line

- Should be performed as an aseptic technique.
- Infiltrate the skin with 1% plain lidocaine.
- Abduct the arm to the anatomical position and hyperextend the wrist—this is most conveniently done by an assistant, if not use tape to secure the patient's hand extended over a bag of fluid (Fig. 14.20)
- Use a cannula with which you are comfortable. Some incorporate a guidewire as part of a Seldinger technique (Fig. 14.21). Do not use a cannula with an injection port.
- Palpate the artery with the fingers of one hand and insert the cannula at an angle of about 30° (Fig. 14.22). Once 'flashback' has been obtained bring the cannula level with the skin and advance 2–3 mm to ensure the tip is in the arterial lumen. At this stage the cannula can be advanced over the needle or the guidewire can be introduced.
- Tape the cannula securely in position, taking care not to kink it.
- Connect the arterial catheter to the tubing and transducer, checking for a clear arterial waveform.
- 'Zero' the transducer and secure approximately level with the heart.

Practical tips and troubleshooting

- The radial artery is very superficial at the wrist and easy to inadvertently transfix. Remove the needle and then slowly withdraw the cannula, aspirating using a 5 mL syringe. As the tip of the cannula re-enters the artery, blood will flow into the syringe briskly. From this point, slowly advance the cannula whilst rotating the cannula in a twisting motion about its long axis.
- If you enter but fail to cannulate the artery it may go into spasm, making cannulation progressively more difficult.
- If locating the artery is difficult, an alternative method is to position your thumb so that the radial pulse is running directly under the centre of your thumb. Then advance the cannula at 30° under the centre point of your thumb (Fig. 14.23).
- After attaching the catheter to the saline column take great care to ensure there are no air bubbles in the system before flushing.
- If the blood pressure reading increases suddenly, check the position of the transducer—it may have fallen on the floor.
- If the waveform disappears or decreases in amplitude, the catheter may be kinked, blocked with clot, or an air bubble may be damping the trace. Try extending the wrist, aspirate any air, and then flush the catheter, or withdraw it slightly to check it is not kinked.
- Note that over- or under-damped traces will give false blood pressure values. An under-damped trace will overestimate systolic pressure and underestimate diastolic pressure as the system 'over oscillates'. A low amplitude, over-damped trace will underestimate the systolic blood pressure and overestimate the diastolic blood pressure. Fortunately, the value for the mean arterial blood pressure is little affected and can usually be taken as accurate.

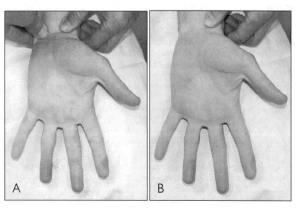

Fig. 14.19 Allen's test: Ask the patient to make a fist and use your thumbs to occlude the patient's radial and ulnar arteries. Ask the patient to unclench their fist—the palm will remain pale whilst the blood supply is still occluded. When you stop occluding the ulnar artery, the palm will flush red if the ulnar artery is patent.

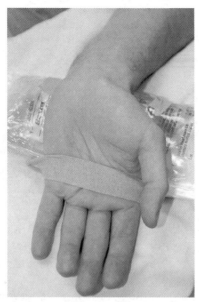

Fig. 14.20 A technique for extending the patient's wrist using adhesive tape and a fluid bag.

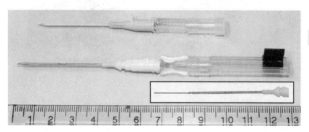

Fig. 14.21 Two 20G arterial cannulae—the lower cannula has a guidewire that can be slid into the artery through the needle to allow smooth placement of the cannula (inset).

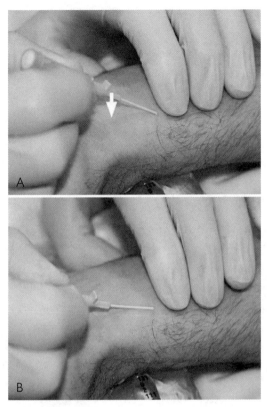

Fig. 14.22 Arterial cannulation.

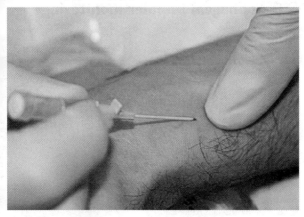

Fig. 14.23 An alternative means of locating the radial artery.

ⓘ **Oesophageal Doppler monitoring**

Definition
Ultrasonic Doppler measurement of blood velocity in descending thoracic aorta, from which cardiac output and haemodynamic status can be estimated.

Indications
Minimally invasive system of monitoring cardiac output, haemodynamic status, and response to therapy in patients with critical illness and patients undergoing surgery.

Contraindications
Absolute
- Known or suspected oesophageal varices
- Oesophagectomy

Relative
- Difficult in conscious patients
- Care needed in severe coagulopathy

Anatomy and theory
- The oesophageal Doppler probe is positioned to measure velocity of blood flow in the descending aorta (Fig. 14.24).
- Characteristics of velocity versus time waveform allow further estimations of patient's haemodynamic status.
- Cardiac output is calculated using aortic diameter (either measured or using data appropriate to the age, weight, and height of the patient).
- Measured values (Fig. 14.25; Table 14.7):
  - heart rate (HR)
  - stroke distance (SD)
  - peak velocity (PV)
  - mean acceleration (MA)
  - corrected flow time (FT_c)
- Derived values:
  - cardiac output and cardiac index (CO, CI)
  - stroke volume and stroke volume index (SV, SVI)
  - systemic vascular resistance (SVR)

In patients undergoing surgery, oesophageal Doppler is particularly useful for assessing the requirement for fluid therapy guided by PV, FT_c, and SV. Cardiac output values are less useful and vary greatly with heart rate.

Comparison of measured to normal values and estimation of cardiac output are more useful in critically ill patients, and in this setting it can be seen more as a cardiac output monitor.

Advantages
- Easy and non-traumatic to insert.
- Avoids vascular puncture.
- Continuous output.

- Transportable.
- Calculated CO correlates well with CO measured with pulmonary catheter thermodilution method.
- Newer probes (12n series from Deltex) allow use in awake or sedated patients.

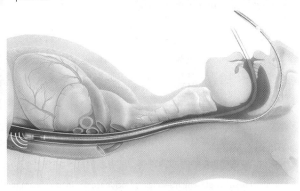

Fig. 14.24 Position of oesophageal Doppler probe (35–40 cm at incisors).

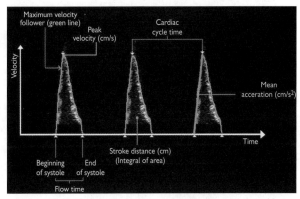

Fig. 14.25 Anatomy of a waveform (Cardio Q®).[1]

Table 14.7 Normal values

Parameter	Normal range	Interpretation	
		Low	High
Corrected flow time (FT_c)	330–360 ms	FT_c <330 ms • Low LV filling—hypovolaemia • High afterload—vasoconstriction, obstructed circulation	FT_c >350 ms • Conditions with low SVR—sepsis, pregnancy
Peak velocity (PV)	20 yr 90–120 cm/s 50 yr 70–100 cm/s 70 yr 50–80 cm/s	• Decreases with decreased LV contractility • Decreases with increased afterload	• Increases with LV contractility

Disadvantages
- Isolated measurements are misleading. Trends and response to therapy are more useful.
- Learning curve for placement—angle of incidence of Doppler beam to descending aortic blood flow is critical and it may be difficult to achieve a satisfactory trace.
- Less useful for patients in lateral position (e.g. fractured neck of femur surgery, thoracic surgery), since mediastinal movement with respiration makes probe placement difficult.
- Nasogastric tube may interfere with trace.
- Errors resulting from drift and repositioning.
- Cardiac output and SVR are inferred.

Equipment
Monitors
- First generation machines:
  - e.g. CardioQ® (Deltex Medical)
  - cardiac output is calculated using aortic diameter from population average for given age, weight, and height
- Second-generation machines:
  - e.g. Haemosonic 100® (Arrow International)
  - uses continuous M-mode ultrasound for orientation of probe to achieve optimal measurements of peak velocity
  - M-mode is used during set-up of machine and displayed continuously in a second window on screen. Reduces operator dependence
  - CO is calculated using beat-to-beat aortic diameter measurements

Oesophageal probes
Probes are narrow gauge, similar to large-bore NG tube:
- CardioQ®
  - probes are single-patient use. Function ceases after a set time (time depending on cost of probe)

- paediatric probes (KDP72) are of similar construction to the adult probes, but shorter and with 7 depth markers (rather than 3) to cover patients from 3 kg to 16 years
- 'awake' (narrow gauge, flexible) probes for unsedated patients are designed to have enhanced flexibility whilst maintaining rotational torque
- The Haemosonic 100®:
  - reusable probe with disposable sheaths
  - applying sheath with ultrasound gel (and excluding air which is critical for obtaining good data) can be difficult and time-consuming
  - can be left in as long as an NG tube. Gel in sheath tends to dry out and affect performance after prolonged use

Preparation

Preparation and technique are described for CardioQ® monitor:
- Easiest in unconscious patients.
- Connect probe to Patient Interface Cable.
- Dial in patient's age, weight, and height. Press 'accept data'.
- Apply water-based lubricant to lower part of probe.

Technique

Location of descending aortic waveform

- Insert the probe 35–40 cm from incisors (in adults) (see Fig. 14.24). Avoid excessive force.
- Rotate the detector head and adjust the insertion depth to achieve the best waveform of descending aortic velocity.
- Use 'audio' and adjust volume output to assist location.

Optimizing waveform

- Activate 'peak velocity display'. Adjust probe to achieve highest 'blue line' on screen and sharpest audible signal quality.
- Activate 'auto gain' (yellow line tracing around waveform confirms this).
- Begin monitoring. Green trace line replaces yellow line. (Fig. 14.26 shows some examples of typical waveforms.)

Complications

Oesophageal injury, damage to probe

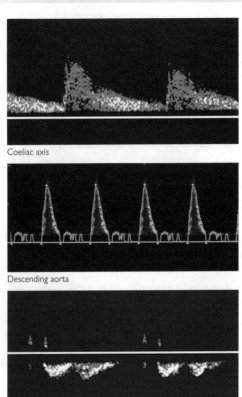

Coeliac axis

Descending aorta

Intracardiac

Fig. 14.26 Typical CardioQ® waveforms.[1]

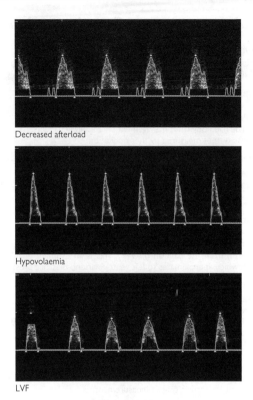

Decreased afterload

Hypovolaemia

LVF

Fig. 14.26 (cont.) Typical CardioQ® waveforms.[1]

1 With permission of Deltex Medical.

① Pulmonary artery flotation catheter

Definition
Flexible catheter inserted into pulmonary artery by flotation through right atrium and ventricle (Swan–Ganz catheter).

Indications
- Allows measurement of the pulmonary artery wedge pressure (PAWP), an estimate of left atrial filling pressure.
- To guide haemodynamic management of critically ill patients.
- Cardiac output measured by thermodilution.

Contraindications
Relative
- As for CVC insertion
- Tricuspid valve stenosis or replacement

Anatomy
Figure 14.27 shows the route of insertion of a pulmonary arterial catheter (PAC). In the 'wedged' position, the tip of the PAC measures pressure downstream from the balloon (PAWP). This is an estimate of left atrial pressure, which approximates to left ventricular end-diastolic pressure.

Equipment checklist
- Antiseptic solution. Sterile gown and gloves
- 4 Sterile drapes. Basic procedure kit
- Line kit. Separate introducer sheath, insertion kit, and catheter set
- Local anaesthetic: 10 mL 1% lidocaine
- Two 3-way taps. 10 mL sterile saline. Scalpel blade
- Non-absorbable monofilament suture. Suture holder
- Non-occlusive dressing
- Primed pressure transducer line, connected to monitor
- Equipment for cardiac output measurement

Preparation
- Choice of site:
  - for ease of flotation: right internal jugular > left internal jugular = left subclavian > right subclavian
  - femoral and basilic veins can be used
- Have pressure transducer prepared (needed to guide insertion of catheter). Keep distal 30 cm of tubing sterile.
- Do not open PAC until PAC sheath safely inserted.
- Patient supine and slightly head down.

Technique
- Clean skin
- Four large drapes to cover entire patient

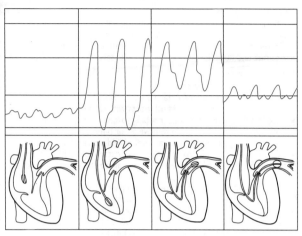

Fig. 14.27 Pulmonary artery catheter pressure waveforms.

Insert sheath as for any central catheter
- Check for free aspiration of venous blood—if not, tip of sheath may be abutting on wall of major vein. Withdraw 1 cm if necessary.
- On removal of wire and dilator, cap of sheath is self-sealing.
- Aspirate and flush side port and sheath with saline and suture in position.

Preparation of PAC
- Open PAC set. Leave in tray.
- Most PACs have 4 lumens. Attach 3-way taps to CVC/proximal lumen and 'medications' lumen, and flush ports with saline.
- Attach sterile end of transducer tubing to 'distal' lumen, which exits at PAC tip, and flush through to remove all air bubbles.
- Zero the transducer and place at level of mid-axillary line.
- Remove balloon from protective housing. Attach lockable 2 mL syringe to balloon port and inflate with 1–1.5 mL air to check function (do not over-distend).
- If PAC measures SvO_2, calibrate before tip of PAC is removed from housing—follow manufacturer's instructions.
- If PAC set contains a safety chamber, insert this between the inflation syringe and balloon port. Chamber contains a balloon whose inflation indicates that distal balloon is being inflated in too small a cavity (usually distal pulmonary vessel or still in introducer sheath).
- Mount sterile cover on catheter prior to insertion.

Flotation of catheter
- With natural curve of PAC orientated to suit insertion site, insert tip of catheter into sheath.
- Advance PAC 10–12 cm, at which point the tip and balloon exit sheath. Inflate balloon, confirming SVC waveform on monitor (see Fig. 14.27).
- Slowly advance catheter, watching transduced waveform to indicate its position.
- ***Never withdraw catheter with balloon inflated*** (risks damage to tricuspid and pulmonary valves).
- Straightforward insertion will show progression from SVC/RA, through tricuspid valve (often accompanied by a run of ventricular ectopics) to RV (pressures in normal patient of 25/3 mmHg) and then into pulmonary trunk (identical systolic pressure to RV with higher diastolic pressure, 25/12 mmHg).
- Slow further advancement into one or other pulmonary artery results in 'wedging' of balloon in artery—CVP waveform but 5–7 mmHg higher. Note length of PAC insertion to achieve wedging.
- Do not leave catheter wedged for more than 20 s (risk of pulmonary ischaemia).
- Deflate balloon and ensure trace returns to pulmonary artery waveform.

Troubleshooting
- May take several attempts.
- If, during insertion, catheter cannot be inserted past a certain point (e.g. still RA waveform at 40 cm) it is likely to be coiled. Average distances to each chamber in a 70 kg adult are shown in Table 14.8.
- Deflate balloon and withdraw back to 10 cm.

Table 14.8 Choice of insertion site for PAC

Insertion site		Distance to: (cm)			Disadvantages
		RA	RV	PA	
Internal jugular		15–20	30	40	Pneumothorax, carotid puncture
Subclavian		15–20	30	40	Pneumothorax, haemothorax
Femoral		30	40	50	Difficult to float, higher risk of infection, DVT
Antecubital	Right	40	50	60	Difficult to float, lower success rate, high risk of phlebitis and infection
	Left	50	60	70	

- Try different speeds of insertion and different orientations of catheter to navigate curves of heart.
- Insertion is more difficult in patients with low cardiac output states, and inotropic support may ease insertion.

Complications

Complications of CVC placement: arrhythmias, infection/endocarditis, pulmonary artery rupture/infarction, valvular/myocardial injury

Using a pulmonary artery catheter

Measured values

- Pulmonary capillary wedge pressure (PCWP):
  - an estimate of left atrial pressure, which is an estimate of left ventricular end-diastolic pressure—an indication of filling of left side of heart (i.e. an estimate of the left ventricular end-diastolic volume and preload)
  - takes no account of ventricular compliance, which greatly influences the relationship between ventricular pressure and volume
  - measurement should be taken at end-expiration whether spontaneously breathing or mechanically ventilated (Fig. 14.28)
- Cardiac output (CO):
  - measured by thermodilution
  - 10 mL iced water is injected into proximal port (right atrial port) of the catheter and temperature is recorded from the pulmonary artery (PA)
  - CO is calculated from the area under the curve of graph of temperature change plotted against time.
  - average at least 3 readings
- Mixed venous oxygen saturation:
  - saturation measured on blood taken from the PA
  - slowly withdraw 2 mL of 'deadspace' fluid from the distal (monitoring) lumen and then withdraw 1 mL mixed venous blood to be analysed in blood gas machine

Interpreting measured and derived values from a PAC

- Use of PAC has not been proven to be beneficial.
- Use varies dramatically throughout the world, and methods of interpretation of the measured values vary greatly.

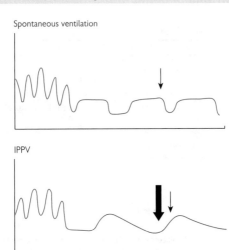

Spontaneous ventilation

IPPV

Assisted spontaneous ventilation

Fig. 14.28 Wedging procedure during different modes of ventilation (arrows show end-expiration where PAWP should be measured).

General considerations

- Most reliable information is available from the measured values, with less emphasis on derived values. Many clinicians ignore derived values such as SVRI and LVSWI.
- Don't just treat the numbers—be dubious of the measurements if they do not support what you find clinically.
- Confirm findings with another method if possible ('Oesophageal Doppler monitoring', see pp482–7).
- Table 14.9 gives normal haemodynamic values.

Table 14.9 Normal haemodynamic values

	Measured values	
	Normal value	Units
Pulmonary artery pressure (PAP)	Systolic: 15–30 Diastolic: 5–12	mmHg
Pulmonary capillary wedge pressure (PCWP)	5–15	mmHg
Cardiac output (CO)	4.5–8	L/min
Mixed venous oxygen tension or saturation (PvO_2 or SvO_2)	5.3 (40) 70–75	kPa (mmHg) %

	Derived values		
	Formula	Normal value	Units
Cardiac Index (CI)	CO/BSA	2.7–4	$L/min/m^2$
Stroke volume (SV)	(CO/HR) 1000	60–130	mL
Stroke volume index (SVI)	SV/BSA	38–60	mL/m^2
Systemic vascular resistance (SVR)	$80 \times$ (MAP – CVP)/CO	770–1500	$dyn.s/cm^5$
Systemic vascular resistance index (SVRI)	$80 \times$ (MAP – CVP)/CI	1860–2500	$dyn.s/cm^5/m^2$
Pulmonary vascular resistance (PVR)	$80 \times$ (PAP – PCWP)/CO	100–250	$dyn.s/cm^5$
Pulmonary vascular resistance index (PVRI)	$80 \times$ (PAP – PCWP)/CI	225–315	$dyn.s/cm^5/m^2$
Left ventricular stroke work index (LVSWI)	$SVI \times MAP \times 0.0144$	50–62	$g.m/m^2$

BSA, body surface area; HR, heart rate; CVP, central venous pressure, MAP, mean arterial pressure.

☠ Emergency pacing

Definition

Repetitive extrinsic electrical stimulation of cardiac activity as treatment of acute cardiovascular compromise related to cardiac arrhythmia.
Temporary pacing can be:

- Internal:
  - transvenous/endocardial (electrodes placed via a central vein)
  - epicardial (electrodes placed on the external surface of the heart at thoracotomy)
- External (transcutaneous) pacing:
  - used as a bridge to temporary internal pacing during acute haemodynamic compromise
  - two pad electrodes are placed on anterior and posterior chest wall

Indications

Emergency surgery

Emergency pacing may be required if symptomatic or major surgery is planned in the presence of:

- second- or third-degree AV block
- intermittent AV block
- first-degree AV block with LBBB

(Bundle branch block, bi-/trifascicular block, and Wenckebach are unlikely to progress to higher block under anaesthesia)

Patients requiring resuscitation

Temporary transvenous pacing required with following conditions if contributing to low BP or cardiac output:

- ventricular asystole with atrial ECG activity
- sinus bradycardia
- complete (third-degree) heart block
- Möbitz type II second-degree AV block (high risk of progression to complete heart block)
- ventricular tachyarrhythmias requiring overdrive pacing

External pacing should be used pending transvenous insertion of pacing wire.

Cardiac surgery

The cardiac surgeon will place epicardial leads (atrial, ventricular, or both) if:

- procedure with risk of bradyarrhythmia or conduction abnormality, e.g. aortic valve surgery
- conduction abnormality during procedure or coming off cardiopulmonary bypass

Contraindications

Relative

- Consider contraindications to central venous access.
- External pacing poorly tolerated in conscious patients.

External pacing (transcutaneous)
- Indicated as bridging treatment during resuscitation.
- Causes considerable discomfort to patients if conscious, causing jerking and interference with respiration.

Equipment checklist
- External pacemaker is usually available as plug-in unit of some defibrillators (ask Emergency Department or CCU)
- 2 pacing electrode pads
- Assistants to roll patient

Preparation
- If conscious, inform patient and explain likely discomfort.
- Judicious sedation may be necessary, as tolerated by haemodynamic status. Patient may regain consciousness with improved cardiac output and require sedation to continue pacing.
- Inform cardiology team of likely need for transvenous pacing.

Technique
- Place black (negative) electrode on anterior chest wall to the left of the lower sternum. Roll patient to right side and place red (positive) electrode in corresponding position on posterior chest wall.
- Connect gel electrode pads to machine.
- Set required pacing rate on pacing device/defibrillator and set the current output to 70 mA.
- Commence pacing and increase current in increments of 5 mA until capture is seen on ECG monitor (regular association between pacing spike and subsequent QRS complex).
- Once pacing captured, set at 5–10 mA above threshold.
- If no capture at 120 mA, re-site electrodes.

Epicardial pacing
While working in a cardiac theatre the surgeon may hand you the pacing wires and ask you to connect them to a pacing box and commence pacing.
- Leads are placed and secured on epicardium during surgery.
- Used in cardiac theatre and during recovery period.
- Usually two ventricular leads ± two atrial leads.
- Leads leave body through skin just below xiphisternum. By convention, atrial are to right side of patient and ventricular to left.

Ventricular pacing
- Place one ventricular lead in each ventricular port on pacing box and screw tight to secure.
- Surgeon may wish to check threshold as above.
- After discussion with surgeon, pace on VVI mode at a set ventricular rate (usually 70–80 bpm for adults).

Atrial pacing
- In addition to ventricular leads, place one atrial lead in each atrial port on pacing box and screw tight to secure.
- Set desired atrial rate and a voltage of 2–3 times the atrial threshold. In the presence of normal AV conduction, setting ventricular output at zero will allow atrial pacing.
- If AV conduction block present, set ventricular output voltage to 2–3 times threshold and required AV delay (about 120 ms). This will achieve sequential AV pacing.
- Remove wires by gentle traction when no longer required.

! Anaesthesia for patients with pacemakers

Generic code for description of pacemakers

- The code consists of five letters.
- The first three describe anti-bradycardia functions and are always stated.
- The fourth and fifth letters relate to additional functions and are omitted if these functions are not available.

1st letter	Chamber paced	V, ventricle A, atrium D, dual O, none
2nd letter	Chamber sensed	2nd letter V, ventricle A, atrium D, dual O, none
3rd letter	Response to sensing	T, triggered I, inhibited D, dual O, none
4th letter	Programmability or rate modulation	P, simple programmable M, multi-programmable R, rate modulation
5th letter	Anti-tachycardia functions	P, pacing S, shock

Examples

VVI   Ventricular demand pacing. Ventricle sensed and paced if no spontaneous rhythm.

DDD   Pacing and sensing in both chambers. Atrial impulse inhibits atrial output. Subsequent ventricular impulse inhibits ventricular output. Paces ventricle in absence of AV conduction.

Preparation for surgery

- Patient should attend cardiac clinic regularly for pacemaker check. Ensure latest check is within 1 year and satisfactory.
- Preoperative ECG will not identify all problems. Pacing spikes may not be present if sensing appropriately above threshold rate for pacing.
- Where appropriate, the back-up pacing rate can be increased to increase the cardiac output in preparation for surgery.

Cardiovascular considerations

- Pacemakers set to treat underlying bradycardia (e.g. VVI) produce a fixed cardiac output. Any fall in preload or afterload leads to little or no compensatory tachycardia.

- Preload with 500–1000 mL crystalloid. Use a careful, slow IV or gaseous induction for GA. Spinal anaesthesia is not precluded and may be well tolerated, but be prepared to treat hypotension.
- The response to beta-agonists such as ephedrine may be minimal, and BP is better maintained with alpha-agonists such as metaraminol (0.5–1.0 mg IV).

Use of diathermy

- Bipolar diathermy is safe with pacemakers.
- Conventional (unipolar) diathermy may be used; however, sustained current conduction in the pacing wires will cause heating and myocardial damage. In addition, the pacemaker may detect the diathermy as ventricular activity and inhibit its output (only for the duration of diathermy usage).
- The plate should be positioned so that the current flow is away from the pacemaker site and the diathermy is used in short bursts.
- The use of a magnet to convert a pacemaker to VOO (and so pace at a fixed background rate) is not recommended by cardiac technicians, although some still recommend it as a last resort in severe haemodynamic compromise.

Anaesthesia for patients with implantable cardioverter defibrillators (ICD)

- ICDs are inserted to prevent sudden cardiac death in patients suffering from, or at risk of, ventricular arrhythmias.
- Surgical or endoscopic diathermy may activate the ICD, and so the device should be inactivated by a cardiac technician if surgery is required.
- An external defibrillator should be immediately available in theatre and recovery.
- The ICD should be reactivated before the patient leaves the theatre area.
- ICDs may also be activated by magnetic resonance imaging and extracorporeal shock wave lithotripsy.
- Use of a peripheral nerve stimulator should also be avoided.
- The same practice applies to pacemakers with overdrive pacing capabilities.

ⓘ **Transport of the critically ill**

Definition
Transport of patients with critical illness or injury, who require ongoing resuscitation, monitoring, and treatment.
- intrahospital transport, e.g. from emergency department to operating theatre, radiology, or ICU
- interhospital transport, e.g. local or district general hospital to neurosurgery, burns, or paediatric ICU for specialist therapy or investigation

Principles of safe transport
- Staff experienced in intensive care and transfer (specialist registrar or consultant with experienced nurse).
- Specialist transport team (e.g. paediatric retrieval team)—may improve outcome but can cause delay.
- Appropriate equipment and vehicle.
- Extensive monitoring.
- Stabilization before departure.
- Continuing reassessment.
- Direct handover.
- Thorough documentation and audit of performance.

Hazards of transport (Table 14.10)
- Deranged physiology, worsened by movement—acceleration/deceleration/vibration affecting cardiovascular status and intracranial pressure.
- Isolated situation.
- Limited space (especially helicopters).
- Temperature and pressure changes.
- Failure of monitoring, noise interference.
- Vehicular accidents.

Equipment
Transfer vehicle
- Customized with adequate space, light, gases, electrical power, and communications.
- Mode—consider urgency, mobilization time, geography, weather, traffic, and costs.
- Consider air transfer if over 50 miles (80 km).

Aeromedical transfer
- With increasing altitude, PaO_2 decreases and air spaces expand.
- Most aircraft are pressurized to 1500–2000 m altitude (PaO_2 at 1500 m is about 10 kPa or 75 mmHg).
- Insert naso/orogastric tube and consider intercostal catheter in chest trauma.
- Replace air in endotracheal tube cuff with saline.

- Problems with temperature control, noise, and vibration.
- Helicopters fly at relatively low altitude and avoid some of these problems. However, transportation in a helicopter is cramped with poor access to the patient.

Table 14.10 Transfer vehicle options

	Road	Helicopter	Aeroplane
Distance	<50 miles (80 km)	50–150 miles (80–240 km)	>150 miles (240 km)
Speed	Slow	Fast, particularly if direct	Fast—may be slowed by number of transfers
Cost	Low	Expensive	Very expensive
Patient access	Good	Usually poor	Good
Noise and vibration	Moderate	Poor	Moderate—poor on take-off and landing
Altitude	None	Low	High

Specific equipment

- Must be robust, light, and battery operated
- Portable ventilator with disconnection and high-pressure alarms. Ability to alter minute volume, FiO_2, I:E ratio, and PEEP
- Oxygen supply sufficient for duration of trip and reserve of 2 h (Table 14.11).
- Portable monitor for ECG, invasive pressures, non-invasive blood pressures, oxygen saturation, end-tidal CO_2, temperature
- Adequate battery supplies for monitor and infusion pumps Some ambulances have a transformer to allow use of electrical power
- Defibrillator (**do not** use in the air unless designed for this purpose: risk of catastrophic damage to electrical systems of helicopters) and suction source
- Pre-prepared transfer drug box and airway/intubation box
- Warming blanket
- Observation chart and pen

Table 14.11 Calculating oxygen reserves

Size of oxygen cylinder (volume, litres)	Operation time (min) for different minute volumes (FiO_2 1.0)		
	Minute volume 5 L/min	Minute volume 7 L/min	Minute volume 10 L/min
D (340)	56	42	30
E (680)	113	85	61
F (1360)	226	170	123

Equipment problems
- Multiple leads can be neatly enclosed in a length of 22 cm diameter corrugated tubing cut down one side of its entire length.
- Vibration makes non-invasive blood pressure monitoring inoperable or inaccurate. Use invasive BP if possible.
- Unreliable pulse oximetry in cold, moving patients (consider ear probe).
- Battery life for monitors and infusion pumps varies greatly, depending on manufacturer, but must be known. Take spare battery packs.
- Battery life of infusion pumps varies with the rate of infusion.

Preparation
- Ensure meticulous stabilization prior to departure.
- Familiarize yourself with the patient's history by examining the notes and receiving a full handover.
- Examine the patient thoroughly.
- Introduce yourself to the patient (if conscious) and their family, explaining your role.

Preparation checklist
Predict what could go wrong and check you have the means to deal with any likely occurrences. For example: BP increases, BP decreases, high ventilator pressure, ventilator fails, endotracheal tube displaced, oxygen saturation falls.

A: airway
- Is the airway safe? If in any doubt or high risk of deterioration (e.g. burn around mouth with risk of burn to airway) anaesthetize, paralyse, and intubate.
- Cervical control throughout transport if any history of trauma.
- Secure endotracheal tube—check length at teeth.

B: breathing
- Portable ventilator—check familiarity with controls. Check arterial blood gas whilst on transport ventilator prior to departure. Compare to end-tidal CO_2 at time of sampling—end-tidal is usually (but not reliably) 0.4–0.6 kPa (3–4.5 mmHg) lower than the arterial level.
- Auscultate chest—good equal air entry.
- Self-inflating (AMBU®) bag in the event of ventilator or oxygen failure.
- Suction (ambulance may have this).
- Adequate sedation, analgesia, muscle relaxation.
- Adequate reserves of oxygen.
- Intercostal catheter inserted if any chance of pneumothorax.

C: circulation
- Continuous access to a part of the patient required (e.g. finger for capillary refill time).
- Two large-bore intravenous cannulae. Restored blood volume.
- External bleeding controlled.
- Invasive BP and CVP when indicated.

- Inotropes and vasopressors—for infusions, have syringes mixed if their use is at all likely. Prepare other vasoactive drugs to dilutions with which you are familiar.
- Several syringes of saline flush.
- Urinary catheter to monitor urine output.

D: disability
- Consider intubation in every patient who is not fully conscious or is at risk of deterioration.
- Monitor GCS, pupillary signs.
- Mannitol (0.5 g/kg) available in head-injured patients.
- NG/orogastric tube.

E: exposure
- Temperature loss.
- Splint long bones.
- Pumps and batteries.

F: forgotten?
- Inform senior colleague and ensure adequate cover of ICU/theatres at base hospital.
- All notes (photocopied), referral letter, results of investigations, X-rays, CT scans, blood products available.
- Clarify destination hospital, receiving doctor, department (e.g. straight to neuro-theatres or to ICU). Take contact numbers.
- Inform receiving unit/hospital on departure from base hospital.
- Inform relatives.
- Mobile phone, warm clothes, money, credit card needed.
- Plan return journey.
- Medical indemnity and insurance for death, disability of transfer staff.

Paediatric implications
- Risk of hypothermia, especially in infants. Monitor core temperature and use hot-air blankets, hats, and bubble wrap to minimize heat loss.
- Ensure secure IV access.
- Specialized monitoring (e.g. saturation probes).
- Dedicated paediatric drug and intubation boxes.
- Often greater input from receiving unit (e.g. pre-calculated drug doses and infusion details can be faxed or e-mailed).
- Paediatric or neonatal retrieval services.

Appendix 1: Drugs

Emergency drug formulary

(Adapted from the Oxford Handbook of Anaesthesia. Note: many drugs are unlicensed in children but are in routine use.)

Drug	Description and perioperative indications	Cautions and contraindications	Side-effects	Dose (paediatric)	Dose (adult)
Adenosine	Endogenous nucleoside with anti-arrhythmic activity. Slows conduction through AV node. Treatment of acute paroxysmal SVT (including WPW) or differentiation of SVT from VT. Duration 10s	Second- or third-degree heart block. Asthma. Reduce dose in heart transplant or dipyridamole treatment	Flushing, dyspnoea, headache—all transient	0.1 mg/kg, increasing by 0.05 mg/kg to max. 0.5 mg/kg	6 mg fast IV bolus, increasing to 12 mg at 2 min intervals as necessary
Adrenaline	Endogenous catecholamine with alpha and beta action: 1. Treatment of anaphylaxis 2. Bronchodilator 3. Positive inotrope 4. Given by nebulizer for croup 5. Prolongation of local anaesthetic action 1:1000 contains 1 mg/mL, 1:10000 contains 100 µg/mL, 1:200000 contains 5 µg/mL	Arrhythmias, especially with halothane. Caution in elderly. Via central catheter whenever possible	Hypertension, tachycardia, anxiety, hyperglycaemia, arrhythmias. Reduces uterine blood flow	Indications 1–3: IV/IM/IO 0.1 mL/kg of 1:10000 (10 µg/kg). ET 0.1 mL/kg of 1:1000 (100 µg/kg). Infusion 0.05–0.5 µg/kg/min 4: Nebulization 0.5 mL/kg (up to 5 mL) 1:1000	Indications 1–3: IV/IM/ET 1 mL aliquots of 1:10000 up to 5–10 mL (0.5–1 mg). Infusion 2–20 µg/min (0.04–0.4 µg/kg/min) 4: Nebulization 5 mL 1:1000 5: Maximum dose for infiltration 2 µg/kg

Drug	Description	Cautions/Contraindications	Side effects	Dose
Aminophylline	Methylxanthine bronchodilator used in prevention and treatment of asthma. Converted to theophylline, a phosphodiesterase inhibitor: Serum levels 10–20 mg/L(55–110 µmol/L)	Caution in patients already receiving oral or IV theophyllines. Where serum level known aminophylline 0.6 mg/kg should increase level by 1 mg/L	Palpitations, tachycardia, tachypnoea, seizures, nausea, arrhythmias	5 mg/kg over 30 min, then infusion 0.5–1 mg/kg/h 1 month–9 yrs 1 mg/kg/hr; 9–16 yrs 0.8 mg/kg/hr	5 mg/kg over 30 min, then infusion 0.5 mg/kg/h
Amiodarone	Mixed class 1C and III anti-arrhythmic useful in treatment of supraventricular and ventricular arrhythmias	Via central catheter. Sinoatrial heart block, thyroid dysfunction, pregnancy, porphyria	Commonly causes thyroid dysfunction and reversible corneal deposits	5 mg/kg over 30 min, then 300 µg/kg/hr to max 1.5mg/kg/hr. Maximum 1.2g in 24 hr. For drug resistant VF bolus over 3 min	5 mg/kg over 1–2 h. Maximum 1.2g in 24 h 300mg slow IV bolus for defib.-resistant VF
Atenolol	Cardioselective β-blocker. Long acting	Asthma, heart failure, AV block, verapamil treatment	Bradycardia, hypotension, and decreased contractility	0.05 mg/kg every 5 min—max. four doses	5–10 mg over 10 min. PO: 50 mg od
Atropine	Muscarinic acetylcholine antagonist. Vagal blockade at AV and sinus node increases heart rate (transient decrease at low doses due to weak agonist effect). Tertiary amine, therefore crosses blood–brain barrier	Obstructive uropathy and cardiovascular disease. Glaucoma, myasthenia gravis	Decreases secretions, and lower oesophageal sphincter tone, relaxes bronchial smooth muscle. Confusion in elderly	IV: 10–20 µg/kg. Control of muscarinic effects of neostigmine: 10–20 µg/kg. IM/SC: 10–30 µg/kg. PO: 40 µg/kg	300–600 µg. Prevention of muscarinic effects of neostigmine: 600–1200 µg. Cardiac arrest: 3 mg

IV = intravenous. IM = intramuscular. SC = subcutaneous. PO = per os (oral). SL = sublingual. ET = endotracheal. od = once daily, bd = twice daily, tds = three times daily. qds = four times daily. NR = not recommended. Doses are intravenous and dilutions in 0.9% saline unless otherwise stated.

Drug	Description and perioperative indications	Cautions and contraindications	Side-effects	Dose (paediatric)	Dose (adult)
Bicarbonate (sodium)	Alkaline salt used for correction of acidosis and to enhance onset of action of local anaesthetics. 8.4% = 1000mmol/L. Dose (mmol) in acidosis: weight (kg) × base deficit × 0.3	Precipitation with calcium-containing solutions, increased CO_2 production, necrosis on extravasation. Via central catheter if possible	Alkalosis, hypokalaemia, hypernatraemia, hypocalcaemia	1mL/kg 8.4% solution (1mmol/kg)	Dependent on degree of acidosis. Resuscitation: 50mL of 8.4% then recheck blood gases
Calcium chloride	Electrolyte replacement, positive inotrope. hyperkalaemia, hypermagnesaemia. Calcium chloride 10% contains Ca^{2+} 680 μmol/mL	Necrosis on extravasation. Incompatible with bicarbonate	Arrhythmias, hypertension, hypercalcaemia	0.1–0.2mL/kg 10% solution	2–5mL 10% solution (10mg/kg, 0.07mmol/kg)
Calcium gluconate	As calcium chloride. Calcium gluconate 10% contains Ca^{2+} 220 μmol/mL	Less phlebitis than calcium chloride	As calcium chloride	0.3–0.5mL/kg 10% solution (max. 20mL)	6–15mL of 10% solution (30mg/kg, 0.07mmol/kg)
Chlorpromazine	Phenothiazine, antipsychotic. Mild α-blocking action. Potent anti-emetic and used for chronic hiccups	Hypotension	Extrapyramidal and anticholinergic symptoms, sedation, hypotension	0.1–1mg/kg over 20 min	Up to 25 mg (at 1 mg/min diluted in saline to 1mg/mL). Deep IM: 25–50 mg 6–8hourly
Clomethiazole	Hypnotic sedative used in alcohol withdrawal and status epilepticus. IV preparation no longer available	Caution in elderly	Nasal congestion, confusion, phlebitis, hypotension, coma		PO: 1–2 capsules at night
Dantrolene	Direct-acting skeletal muscle relaxant used in treatment of malignant hyperpyrexia and neuroleptic malignant syndrome. 20mg vial—reconstitute in 60mL warm water and give via blood set	Avoid combination with calcium-channel blockers (verapamil) as may cause hyperkalaemia and cardiovascular collapse. Crosses placenta	Skeletal muscle weakness (22%), phlebitis (10%)	1mg/kg repeated every 5 min to a maximum of 10mg/kg	1mg/kg repeated every 5 min to a maximum of 10mg/kg. Usually 2.5mg/kg

Drug					
Dexamethasone	Prednisolone derivative corticosteroid. Less sodium retention than hydrocortisone. Cerebral oedema, oedema prevention, anti-emetic	Interacts with anticholinesterase agents to increase weakness in myasthenia gravis	See Prednisolone	IV/IM/SC: 100–400 µg/kg daily. Cerebral oedema: loading dose 20 mg then 4 mg 2–3 hourly reducing after 3 days. Croup: 250 µg/kg, then 125 µg/kg qds for 24 h	IV/IM/SC: 4–8 mg. Cerebral oedema: loading dose 10 mg then 4 mg qds reducing after 3 days (dexamethasone 0.75 mg = prednisolone 5 mg)
Diazepam	Long-acting benzodiazepine. Sedation or termination of status epilepticus. Alcohol withdrawal	Thrombophlebitis: emulsion (Diazemuls®) less irritant to veins	Sedation, circulatory depression	0.2–0.4 mg/kg. Rectal: 0.5 mg/kg as Stesolid® or may use IV preparation	2–10 mg, repeat if required
Digoxin	Cardiac glycoside. Weak inotrope and control of ventricular response in supraventricular arrhythmia. Therapeutic levels 0.5–2 µg/L	Reduce dose in elderly. Enhanced effect/toxicity in hypokalaemia. Avoid cardioversion in toxicity	Anorexia, nausea, fatigue, arrhythmias	Loading dose 10 µg/kg tds for 24 h.	Rapid IV loading: 250–500 µg over 30min. Maximum 1mg/24h. PO loading: 1–1.5 mg in divided doses over 24h. PO maintenance: 125–250 µg/day
Dobutamine	β$_1$-adrenergic agonist, positive inotrope and chronotrope. Cardiac failure	Arrhythmias and hypertension. Phlebitis, but can be administered peripherally	Tachycardia. Decreased peripheral and pulmonary vascular resistance	Infusion: 2–20 µg/kg/min	Infusion: 2.5–10 µg/kg/min
Dopamine	Naturally occurring catecholamine with α, β$_1$, and dopaminergic activity. Inotropic agent	Via central catheter. Phaeochromocytoma (due to noradrenaline release)	Tachycardia, dysrhythmias	Infusion: 2–20 µg/kg/min	Infusion: 2–10 µg/kg/min

IV = intravenous. IM = intramuscular. SC = subcutaneous. PO = per os (oral). SL = sublingual. ET = endotracheal. od = once daily. bd = twice daily. tds = three times daily. qds = four times daily. NR = not recommended. Doses are intravenous and dilutions in 0.9% saline unless otherwise stated.

Drug	Description and perioperative indications	Cautions and contraindications	Side-effects	Dose (paediatric)	Dose (adult)
Dopexamine	Catecholamine with β₂ and dopaminergic activity. Inotropic agent	Via central catheter. Phaeochromocytoma, hypokalaemia	Tachycardia	Infusion: 0.5–6 µg/kg/min	Infusion: 0.5–6 µg/kg/min
Doxapram	Respiratory stimulant acting through carotid chemoreceptors and medulla. Duration 12 min	Epilepsy, airway obstruction, acute asthma, severe CVS disease	Risk of arrhythmia. Hypertension	1 mg/kg slowly.	1–1.5 mg/kg over >30 s. Infusion: 2–4 mg/min
Enoximone	Type III phosphodiesterase inhibitor used in cardiac failure with increased filling pressures. Inodilator	Stenotic valvular disease, cardiomyopathy	Arrhythmias, hypotension, nausea	Infusion: 5–20 µg/kg/min	Infusion: 90 µg/kg/min for 10–30 min, then 5–20 µg/kg/min (max 24 mg/kg/day)
Ephedrine	Direct and indirect sympathomimetic. Vasopressor. safe in pregnancy. Duration 10–60 min	Caution in elderly, hypertension and CVS disease. Tachyphylaxis. Avoid with MAOI	Tachycardia, hypertension		3–6 mg repeated (dilute 30 mg in 10 mL saline, 1 mL increments). IM: 30 mg
Ergometrine	Ergot alkaloid used to control uterine hypotony or bleeding Syntometrine® = ergometrine 500 µg/mL and oxytocin 5 Un/mL	Severe cardiac disease or hypertension	Vasoconstriction, hypertension, vomiting		IM: 1 mL as Syntometrine®. Not recommended IV

Drug	Description	Cautions	Side effects	Dose	Dose
Esmolol	Short-acting cardioselective β-blocker. Metabolized by red cell esterases. Treatment of supraventricular tachycardia or intraoperative hypertension. Duration 10 min.	Asthma, heart failure, AV block, verapamil treatment	Hypotension, bradycardia. May prolong action of suxamethonium	SVT: 0.5 mg/kg over 1 min, then 50–200 µg/kg/min	SVT: 0.5 mg/kg over 1 min, then 50–200 µg/kg/min. Hypertension: 25–100 mg, then 50–300 µg/kg/min
Flumazenil	Benzodiazepine receptor antagonist. Duration 45–90 min	Benzodiazepine dependence (acute withdrawal), resedation if long-acting benzodiazepine	Arrhythmia, seizures	10 µg/kg, then repeat up to 40 µg/kg, max single dose 200 µg. Infusion: 2–10 µg/kg/h	200 µg then 100 µg at 60s intervals (up to maximum 1 mg). Infusion: 100–400 µg/h
Fosphenytoin	Prodrug of phenytoin. Can be administered more rapidly. Dosages in phenytoin equivalents (PE): fosphenytoin 1.5 mg = phenytoin 1 mg	See Phenytoin Monitor ECG/BP. Infusion rate: 50–100 mg(PE)/min (status 100–150 mg(PE)/min)	See Phenytoin	>5 years: 20 mg(PE)/kg then 4–5 mg(PE)/kg daily Infusion rate: 1–2 mg(PE)/kg/min	Infusion: 20 mg(PE)/kg then 4–5 mg(PE)/kg daily. Status: 15 mg(PE)/kg Can also be administered IM
Furosemide (frusemide)	Loop diuretic used in treatment of hypertension, congestive cardiac failure, renal failure, fluid overload		Hypotension, tinnitus, ototoxicity, hypokalaemia	0.5–1.5 mg/kg bd	10–40 mg slowly.
Glucagon	Polypeptide hormone used in treatment of hypoglycaemia and overdose of β-blocker. Hyperglycaemic action lasts 10–30 min	Glucose must be administered as soon as possible. Phaeochromocytoma	Hypertension, hypotension, nausea, vomiting	β blocker overdose 50–150 µg/kg followed by infusion 50 µg/kg/h in 5% glucose	SC/IM/IV: 1 U (1 mg). β-blocker overdose 2–10 mg followed by infusion 50 µg/kg/h in 5% glucose

IV = intravenous. IM = intramuscular. SC = subcutaneous. PO = per os (oral). SL = sublingual. ET = endotracheal. od = once daily. bd = twice daily. tds = three times daily. qds = four times daily. NR = not recommended. Doses are intravenous and dilutions in 0.9% saline unless otherwise stated.

Drug	Description and perioperative indications	Cautions and contraindications	Side-effects	Dose (paediatric)	Dose (adult)
Glucose	Treatment of hypoglycaemia in unconscious patient	50% solution irritant therefore flush after administration		5 mL/kg of glucose 10%	25 mLs of 50% glucose. Can use more dilute solutions
Glyceryl trinitrate	Organic nitrate vasodilator. Controlled hypotension, angina, congestive cardiac failure	Remove patches before defibrillation to avoid electrical arcing	Tachycardia, hypotension, headache, nausea, flushing, methaemoglobinaemia	1–3 μg/kg/min; max 10 μg/kg/min.	Infusion: 0.5–10 mg/h. SL tabs: 0.3–1 mg prn. SL spray: 400 μg prn. Patch: 5–10 mg/24h
Glycopyrronium bromide	Quaternary ammonium anticholinergic agent. Bradycardia, blockade of muscarinic effects of anticholinesterases, antisialogogue	Caution in glaucoma, cardiovascular disease. Unlike atropine does not cross blood–brain barrier	Paradoxical bradycardia in small doses. Reduces lower oesophageal sphincter tone	4–8 μg/kg. Control of muscarinic effects of neostigmine: 10 μg/kg	200–400 μg. Control of muscarinic effects of neostigmine: 10–15 μg/kg (or 200 μg for each 1 mg neostigmine)
Haloperidol	Butyrophenone derivative antipsychotic. Useful anti-emetic	Neuroleptic malignant syndrome	Extrapyramidal reactions	NR	IM/IV: 2–10 mg 4–8 hourly (max. 18 mg/day) Antiemetic: 0.5–2 mg IV
Hyaluronidase	Enzyme used to enhance permeation of injected fluids or local anaesthetics. Treatment of extravasation. Hyperdermoclysis: 150 U/L	Not for intravenous administration	Occasional severe allergy	Local anaesthetic: 15 U/mL	Ophthalmology: 10–15 U/mL local Extravasation: 1500 U in 1 mL saline infiltrated to affected area

Drug	Description	Notes	Dose	Dose 2
Hydralazine	Direct-acting arteriolar vasodilator used to control arterial pressure. Duration 2–4 h	Higher doses required in rapid acetylators. SLE	Increased heart rate, cardiac output, stroke volume	0.1–0.5 mg/kg	5 mg every 5 min to a maximum of 20 mg
Hydrocortisone (cortisol)	Endogenous steroid with anti-inflammatory and potent mineralocorticoid action (steroid of choice in replacement therapy—active form of cortisone). Treatment of allergy	(Hydrocortisone 20 mg = prednisolone 5 mg)	Hyperglycaemia, hypertension, psychic disturbance, muscle weakness, fluid retention	4 mg/kg then 2–4 mg/kg qds	IV/IM: 50–200 mg qds. Adrenal suppression and surgery: 25–50 mg at induction then 25 mg qds PO: 10–20 mg/day
Imipenem	Carbapenem broad-spectrum antibiotic. Administered with cilastatin to reduce renal metabolism	Caution in renal failure and pregnancy	Nausea, vomiting, diarrhoea, convulsions, thrombophlebitis	>3 months: 15 mg/kg over 30 min qds (25 mg/kg severe infections)	Slow IV (1 h): 250–500 mg qds. Surgical prophylaxis: 1 g at induction, repeated after 3 h
Insulin (Actrapid®)	Human soluble pancreatic hormone facilitating intra-cellular transport of glucose and anabolism. Diabetes mellitus, ketoacidosis, and hyperkalaemia	Monitor blood glucose and serum potassium. Store at 2–8°C	Hypoglycaemia, hypokalaemia	Ketoacidosis: 0.1–0.2 U/kg then 0.1 U/kg/h	Ketoacidosis: 10–20 U then 5–10 U/h. Hyperkalaemia (pp296–7)
Intralipid 20%	Intralipid® 20% lipid emulsion used in the treatment of LA. Induced cardiate arrest	Continue CPR throughout treatment. Propofol is **NOT** a suitable substitute			Initial bolus: 1.5 mL/kg (100 mL for 70 kg man). Repeat twice at 5 min intervals if necessary. Infusion: 0.25 mL/kg/min for 70 kg man)

IV = intravenous. IM = intramuscular. SC = subcutaneous. PO = per os (oral). SL = sublingual. ET = endotracheal. od = once daily. bd = twice daily. tds = three times daily. qds = four times daily. NR = not recommended. Doses are intravenous and dilutions in 0.9% saline unless otherwise stated.

Drug	Description and perioperative indications	Cautions and contraindications	Side-effects	Dose (paediatric)	Dose (adult)
Isoprenaline	Synthetic catecholamine with potent β-adrenergic agonist activity. Emergency treatment of heart block or bradycardia unresponsive to atropine. β-Blocker overdose	Ischaemic heart disease, hyperthyroidism, diabetes mellitus	Tachycardia, arrhythmias, sweating, tremor	Infusion: 1–10 μg/kg/h	Infusion: 0.5–10 μg/min (2 mg in 500 mL 5% glucose at 7–150 mL/h or 1 mg in 50 mL at 1.5–30 mL/h)
Ketamine	Phencyclidine derivative producing dissociative anaesthesia. Induction/ maintenance of anaesthesia in high-risk or hypovolaemic patients	Emergence delirium reduced by benzodiazepines. Caution in hypertension. Control excess salivation with antimuscarinic agent	Bronchodilatation. Increased ICP, blood pressure, uterine tone, salivation. Respiratory depression if given rapidly	Induction: 1–2 mg/ kg IV, 5–10 mg/kg IM. Infusion: 1–3 mg/kg/h	Induction: 1–2 mg/kg IV, 5–10 mg/kg IM. Infusion: 1–3 mg/kg/h (analgesia only 0.25 mg/ kg/h)
Labetalol	Combined α- (mild) and β-adrenergic receptor antagonist. Blood pressure control without reflex tachycardia. Duration 2–4 h	Asthma, heart failure, AV block, verapamil treatment	Hypotension, bradycardia, bronchospasm, liver damage	1 month–12 yrs 0.25–0.5 mg/kg; max 20 mg; 12–18 yrs 50 mg over 1 min, repeated after 5 min; max 200 mg	5 mg increments up to 100 mg. Infusion: 20–160 mg/h (in glucose)
Lorazepam	Benzodiazepine: 1. Sedation or premedication. 2. Status epilepticus. Duration 6–10 h	Decreased requirement for anaesthetic agents	Respiratory depression in combination with opioids. Amnesia		1. PO: 2–4 mg 1–2 h preop. IV/IM: 1.5–2.5 mg 2. Status: 4 mg IV
Lormetazepam	Benzodiazepine hypnotic sedative premed.	Decreased requirement for anaesthetic agents	Respiratory depression in combination with opioids. Amnesia	NR	0.5–1.5 mg 1–2 h preop. (elderly 0.5 mg)

Drug	Description	Cautions/Effects	Dose	Notes
Magnesium sulphate	Essential mineral used to treat: 1. Hypomagnesaemia 2. Arrhythmias 3. Eclamptic seizures 4. Severe asthma	Potentiates muscle relaxants. Monitoring of serum level essential during treatment. Myasthenia and muscular dystrophy. Heart block	40 mg/kg; max 2 g	1. Hypomagnesaemia: 2 g over 10 min then 1 g/h. 2. Arrhythmias: 2 g (8 mmol) over 10 min. 3. Eclampsia: 4 g (16 mmol) over 10 min then 1 g/h for 24 h (see pp156–9)
Mannitol	Osmotic diuretic used for renal protection and reduction of intracranial pressure. 20% solution = 20 g/100 mL	Extracellular volume expansion, especially in severe renal or cardiovascular disease	0.25–0.5 g/kg	0.25–1 g/kg (typically 0.5 g/kg of 20% solution)
Metaraminol	Potent direct/indirect acting α-adrenergic sympathomimetic. Treatment of hypotension. Duration 20–60 min	MAOIs, pregnancy. Caution in elderly and hypertensives. Extravasation can cause necrosis	10 µg/kg then 0.1–1 µg/kg/min	0.5–2 mg. Dilute 10 mg in 20 mL saline and give 0.5–1 mL increments (increase dilution in elderly)
Methoxamine	Potent direct-acting α₁- adrenergic sympathomimetic. Treatment of hypotension. Duration 15–60 min	Pregnancy. Caution in elderly and hypertensives. Extravasation can cause and decreased renal perfusion necrosis	10 µg/kg increment	1–2 mg. Dilute 20 mg in 20 mL saline and give 0.5–1 mL increments (increase dilution in elderly)

IV = intravenous. IM = intramuscular. SC = subcutaneous. PO = per os (oral). SL = sublingual. ET = endotracheal. od = once daily. bd = twice daily. tds = three times daily. qds = four times daily. NR = not recommended. Doses are intravenous and dilutions in 0.9% saline unless otherwise stated.

Drug	Description and perioperative indications	Cautions and contraindications	Side-effects	Dose (paediatric)	Dose (adult)
Methyl-thioninium chloride (Methylene blue)	1. Treatment of methaemoglobinaemia. 2. Ureteric identification during surgery (renally excreted). 3. Identification of parathyroid glands during surgery	G-6-PD deficiency. Blue coloration causes acute changes in pulse oximetry readings	Tachycardia, nausea, stains skin	1 mg/kg slow IV	1 mg/kg slow IV
Metoprolol	Cardioselective β–blocker	Asthma, heart failure, AV block, verapamil treatment	Causes bradycardia, hypotension, and decreased cardiac contractility		1–5 mg over 10 min
Midazolam	Short-acting benzodiazepine. Sedative, anxiolytic, amnesic, anticonvulsant. Duration 20–60 min. Oral administration of IV preparation effective though larger dose required	Reduce dose in elderly (very sensitive)	Hypotension, respiratory depression, apnoea	Sedation: IV 50 μg/kg (max 6 mg under 6 years; max 10 mg over 6 yrs); PO: 0.5 mg/kg (use IV preparation in orange juice); max 20 mg. Buccal 0.2 mg/kg 6 months–10 years; max 5 mg; >10 yrs 6–8 mg)	Sedation: 0.5–5 mg, titrate to effect. PO: 0.5 mg/kg (use IV preparation in orange juice). IM: 2.5–10 mg (0.1 mg/kg)
Milrinone	Selective phosphodiesterase inhibitor used in cardiac failure with increased filling pressures. Inodilator used after cardiac surgery	Stenotic valvular disease, cardiomyopathy	Arrhythmias, hypotension, nausea	50 μg/kg over 10 min, then 0.375–0.75 μg/kg/min. Maximum 1.13 mg/kg/day	50 μg/kg over 10 min, then 0.375–0.75 μg/kg/min. Maximum 1.13 mg/kg/day

Drug	Notes	Adverse effects	Dose
Naloxone	Pure opioid antagonist. Can be used in low doses to reverse pruritus associated with epidural opiates and as depot IM injection in newborn of mothers given opioids	Beware re-narcotization if reversing long-acting opioid. Caution in opioid addicts—may precipitate acute withdrawal. Duration of action 30 min	5–10 µg/kg. Infusion: 5–20 µg/kg/h. IM depot in newborn: 200 µg. Pruritus: 0.5 µg/kg	200–400 µg titrated to desired effect. Treatment of opioid/epidural pruritus: 100 µg bolus plus 300 µg added to IV fluids
Neostigmine	Anticholinesterase used for: 1. Reversal of non-depolarizing muscle relaxant. 2. Treatment of myasthenia gravis. Duration 60 min IV (2–4 h PO)	Bradycardia, nausea excessive salivation (muscarinic effects)	Administer with antimuscarinic agent	50 µg/kg with atropine 20 µg/kg or glycopyrronium 10 µg/kg	1. 50–70 µg/kg (max. 5 mg) with atropine 10–20 µg/kg or glycopyrronium 10–15 µg/kg. 2. PO: 15–30 mg at suitable intervals
Neostigmine and glycopyrronium	Combination of neostigmine methylsulphate (2.5 mg) and glycopyrronium (500 µg) per 1 mL	See Neostigmine	See Neostigmine	0.02 mL/kg (dilute 1 mL with 4 mL saline, give 0.1 mL/kg)	1 mL over 30 s; repeated once if necessary
Nimodipine	Calcium channel blocker used to prevent vascular spasm after subarachnoid haemorrhage	Via central catheter. Cerebral oedema, raised intracranial pressure, grapefruit juice. Incompatible with PVC	Hypotension, flushing, headache	Infusion: 15–30 µg/kg/ hr; max 2 mg/hr	PO: 60 mg 4-hourly (maximum 360 mg/day). Infusion: 1 mg/h increasing after 2 h to 2 mg/h
Nitroprusside (sodium—SNP)	Nitric oxide generating potent peripheral vasodilator. Controlled hypotension	Protect solution from light. Metabolism yields cyanide which is then converted to thiocyanate	Methaemoglobin-aemia, hypotension, tachycardia. Cyanide causes tachycardia, sweating, acidosis	Infusion: 0.5–8 µg/kg/ min. Maximum 4 µg/ kg/min >24 h	Infusion: 0.5–8 µg/kg/min (up to 6 µg/kg/min). Maximum dose: 1.5 mg/kg (acutely)

IV = intravenous. IM = intramuscular. SC = subcutaneous. PO = per os (oral). SL = sublingual. ET = endotracheal. od = once daily. bd = twice daily. tds = three times daily. qds = four times daily. NR = not recommended. Doses are intravenous and dilutions in 0.9% saline unless otherwise stated.

Drug	Description and perioperative indications	Cautions and contraindications	Side-effects	Dose (paediatric)	Dose (adult)
Noradrenaline	Potent catecholamine α adrenergic agonist. Vasoconstriction	Via central catheter only. Potentiated by MAOI and TCA	Reflex bradycardia, arrhythmia, hypertension	Infusion: 0.02–1 µg/kg/min	Infusion: 2–20 µg/min (0.04–0.4 µg/kg/min)
Octreotide	Somatostatin analogue used in treatment of carcinoid, acromegaly, and variceal bleeding (unlicensed use)	Pituitary tumour expansion, reduced need for anti-diabetic treatments	GI disturbance, gallstones, hyper- and hypoglycaemia	SC: 1–2 µg/kg 4–6 hourly	SC: 50 µg od/bd increased up to 200 µg tds. IV: 50 µg diluted in saline (ECG monitoring)
Oxytocin	Nonapeptide hormone which stimulates uterine contraction. Induction of labour and prevention of postpartum haemorrhage		Vasodilatation, hypotension, flushing, tachycardia		Postpartum slow IV: 5 U, followed if required by infusion (5–30 U in 500 mL glucose at 0.02–0.04 U/min)
Paraldehyde	Status epilepticus			PR: 0.3 mL/kg	Deep IM: 5–10 mL. PR: 10–20 mL
Phentolamine	α₁- and α₂-adrenergic antagonist. Peripheral vasodilatation and controlled hypotension. Treatment of extravasation. Duration 10 min	Treat excessive hypotension with noradrenaline or methoxamine (not adrenaline/ephedrine due to β-effects)	Hypotension, tachycardia, flushing	50–100 µg/kg	2–5 mg (10 mg in 10 mL saline, 1 mL aliquots)
Phenylephrine	Selective direct-acting α-adrenergic agonist. Peripheral vasoconstriction and treatment of hypotension. Duration 20 min	Caution in elderly or cardiovascular disease. Hyperthyroidism	Reflex bradycardia, arrhythmias	2–20 µg/kg repeated as required	20–100 µg increments (10 mg in 500 mL saline, 1 mL aliquots.) IM: 2–5 mg. Infusion: 30–60 µg/min

Drug	Indication/Notes	Cautions	Side effects	Paediatric dose	Adult dose
Phenytoin	Anticonvulsant and treatment of digoxin toxicity. Serum levels 10–20 mg/L (40–80 μmol/L)	Avoid in AV heart block and pregnancy. Monitor ECG/ BP. Porphyria	Hypotension, AV conduction defects, ataxia. Enzyme induction	Loading dose: 18 mg/kg over 1 h	18 mg/kg over 1 h (dilute to 10 mg/mL in saline), then 100 mg tds. Arrhythmia: 3.5–5 mg/kg (rate <50 mg/min)
Potassium chloride	Electrolyte replacement (see pp298–9)	Dilute solution before administration	Rapid infusion can cause cardiac arrest. High concentration causes phlebitis	0.2 mmol/kg over 1 h. Maintenance: 1–2 mmol/kg/day	10–20 mmol/h (max. concentration 40 mmol/L peripherally). With ECG monitoring: up to 20–40 mmol/h via central line (max. 200 mmol/day)
Prednisolone	Orally active corticosteroid. Less mineralocorticoid action than hydrocortisone	Adrenal suppression, severe systemic infections	Dyspepsia and ulceration, osteoporosis, myopathy, psychosis, impaired healing, diabetes mellitus	PO: 1–2 mg/kg od. Croup: 2 mg/kg then 1 mg/kg tds	PO: 10–60 mg od, reduced to 2.5–15 mg od
Procyclidine	Antimuscarinic used in acute treatment of drug-induced dystonic reactions (except tardive dyskinesia)	Glaucoma, gastrointestinal obstruction	Urinary retention, dry mouth, blurred vision	IV: <2 years: 0.5–2 mg. 2–10 years: 2–5 mg	IV: 5 mg. IM: 5–10 mg repeat after 20 min if needed
Promethazine	Phenothiazine, antihistamine, anticholinergic, anti-emetic sedative. Paediatric sedation		Extrapyramidal reactions	>2 years Sedation/premed PO: 0.5–1 mg/kg.	PO/IM: 25–50 mg

IV = intravenous. IM = intramuscular. SC = subcutaneous. PO = per os (oral). SL = sublingual. ET = endotracheal. od = once daily. bd = twice daily. qds = four times daily. NR = not recommended. Doses are intravenous and dilutions in 0.9% saline unless otherwise stated. tds = three times daily.

Drug	Description and perioperative indications	Cautions and contraindications	Side-effects	Dose (paediatric)	Dose (adult)
Propranolol	Non-selective β-adrenergic antagonist. Controlled hypotension	Asthma, heart failure, AV block, verapamil treatment	Bradycardia, hypotension, AV block, bronchospasm	20–50 µg/kg over 5 min	1 mg increments up to 5–10 mg
Protamine	Basic protein produced from salmon sperm. Heparin antagonist	Weakly anticoagulant and marked histamine release. Risk of allergy	Severe hypotension, pulmonary hypertension, bronchospasm, flushing	Slow IV: 1 mg per 1 mg heparin (100 U) to be reversed	Slow IV: 1 mg per 1 mg heparin (100 U) to be reversed
Remifentanil	Ultra short-acting opioid used to supplement GA. Metabolized by non-specific esterases not plasma		Muscle rigidity, respiratory depression, hypotension, bradycardia	Slow bolus: up to 1 µg/kg. Infusion (IPPV): 0.1–0.5 µg/kg/min. Infusion (SV): 0.025–0.1 µg/kg/min	Slow bolus: up to 1 µg/kg. Infusion (IPPV): 0.1–0.5 µg/kg/min. Infusion (SV): 0.025–0.1 µg/kg/min
Salbutamol	β₂-receptor agonist. Treatment of bronchospasm.	Hypokalaemia possible	Tremor; vasodilatation, tachycardia	2–18yrs 15 µg/kg over 10min then 1–5 µg/kg/min	250 µg slow IV then 5 µg/min (up to 20 µg/min). Nebulizer: 2.5–5 mg prn
Suxamethonium	Depolarizing muscle relaxant. Rapid short-acting muscle paralysis. Phase II block develops with repeated doses (>8 mg/kg). Store at 2–8°C	Prolonged block in plasma cholinesterase deficiency; hypokalaemia, hypocalcaemia. Malignant hyperthermia, myopathies	Increased intraocular pressure. Increased serum potassium (normally 0.5 mmol/L— greater in burns, trauma, upper motor neuron injury). Bradycardia with second dose	1–2 mg/kg	1–1.5 mg/kg. Infusion: 0.5–10 mg/min

Teicoplanin	Glycopeptide antibiotic with activity against aerobic and anaerobic Gram-positive bacteria	Renal impairment	Ototoxicity, nephrotoxicity Blood disorders	10 mg/kg for 3 doses 12-hourly then 6 mg/kg od	IV/IM: 400 mg for 3 doses 12-hourly then 200 mg od
Thiopental	Short-acting thiobarbiturate. Induction of anaesthesia, anticonvulsant, cerebral protection. Recovery due to redistribution	Accumulation with repeated doses. Caution in hypovolaemia and elderly. Porphyria	Hypotension Necrosis if intra-arterial	Induction: neonate: 2–4 mg/kg child: 3–6 mg/kg	Induction/cerebral protection: 3–5 mg/kg. Anticonvulsant: 0.5–2 mg/kg prn
Tranexamic acid	Inhibits plasminogen activation reducing fibrin dissolution by plasmin. Reduced haemorrhage in prostatectomy or dental extraction	Avoid in thromboembolic disease, renal impairment and pregnancy	Dizziness, nausea	PO: 15–20 mg/kg tds	Slow IV: 0.5–1 g tds. PO: 15–25 mg/kg tds
Vancomycin	Glycopeptide antibiotic with activity against aerobic and anaerobic Gram-positive bacteria. Peak level <30 mg/L Trough level 5–10 mg/L	Avoid rapid infusion (hypotension, wheezing, urticaria, 'red man' syndrome). Reduce dose in renal impairment	Ototoxicity, nephrotoxicity, phlebitis, neutropenia	15 mg/kg IV tds	1 g over 100 min bd (check blood levels after third dose)
Vasopressin	ADH used in treatment of diabetes insipidus	Extreme caution in coronary vascular disease	Pallor, coronary vasoconstriction, water intoxication	Diabetes insipidus SC/IM: 2–10 U 4-hourly	Diabetes insipidus SC/IM: 5–20 U 4-hourly

IV = intravenous. IM = intramuscular. SC = subcutaneous. PO = per os (oral). SL = sublingual. ET = endotracheal. od = once daily. bd = twice daily. tds = three times daily. qds = four times daily. NR = not recommended. Doses are intravenous and dilutions in 0.9% saline unless otherwise stated.

Infusion regimes

Drug	Indication	Diluent	Dose	Suggested regime (60 kg adult)	Infusion range	Initial rate (adult)	Comments
Adrenaline	Treatment of hypotension	0.9% saline, 5% glucose	2–20 µg/min (0.04–0.4 µg/kg/min)	5 mg/50mL (100 µg/mL)	1.2–12+ mL/h	5 mL/h	Via central catheter. Suggest 1 mg/50 mL for initial intra-op. use (or 1 mg/500mL if no central access)
Aminophylline	Bronchodilatation	0.9% saline, 5% glucose	0.5 mg/kg/h	250 mg/50 mL (5 mg/mL)	6 mL/h	6 mL/h	After 5 mg/kg slow IV bolus over 30 min
Amiodarone	Treatment of arrhythmias	5% glucose only	Loading infusion 5 mg/kg over 1–2 h, then if required 900 mg over 24 h	300 mg/50 mL (6 mg/mL)	25–50 mL/h then 6 mL/h	25 mL/h	Via central line peripherally in extremis. Maximum 1.2 g in 24 h
Bicarbonate (sodium)	Acidosis	[weight (kg) × base deficit × 0.3] mmol	Undiluted (8.4% solution)				8.4% = 1000 mmol/L. Via central line if possible
Digoxin	Rapid control of ventricular rate	0.9% saline, 5% glucose	250–500 µg over 30–60 min	250–500 µg/50 mL	0–100 mL/h	50 mL/h	ECG monitoring suggested
Dobutamine	Cardiac failure/inotrope	0.9% saline, 5% glucose	2.5–10 µg/kg/min	250 mg/50 mL (5 mg/mL)	2–7 mL/h	2 mL/h	May be given via large peripheral vein
Dopamine	Inotrope	0.9% saline, 5% glucose	2–10 µg/kg/min	200 mg/50 mL (4 mg/mL)	2–9 mL/h	2 mL/h	Via central line

Drug	Indication	Diluent	Dose	Concentration	Rate range	Rate	Notes
Dopexamine	Inotrope	0.9% saline, 5% glucose	0.5–6 µg/kg/min	50 mg/50 mL (1 mg/mL)	2–22 mL/h	2 mL/h	May be given via large peripheral vein
Doxapram	Respiratory stimulant	0.9% saline, 5% glucose	2–4 mg/min	200 mg/50 mL (4 mg/mL)	30–60 mL/h	30 mL/h	Maximum dose 4 mg/kg
Enoximone	Inodilator	0.9% saline only	90 µg/kg/min for 10–30 min, then 5–20 µg/kg/min	100 mg/50 mL (2 mg/mL)	9–36 mL/h	162 mL/h for 10–30 min	Max. 24 mg/kg/day
Esmolol	Beta-blocker	0.9% saline, 5% glucose	50–200 µg/kg/min	2.5 g/50 mL (50 mg/mL)	3–15 mL/h	3 mL/h	ECG monitoring
Glyceryl trinitrate	Controlled hypotension	0.9% saline, 5% glucose	0.5–12 mg/h	50 mg/50 mL (1 mg/mL)	0.5–12 mL/h	5 mL/h	
Heparin	Anticoagulation	0.9% saline, 5% glucose	24000–48000 U per 24 h	50000 U/50 mL (1000 U/mL)	1–2 mL/h	2 mL/h	Check APTT after 12 h
Insulin (soluble)	Diabetes mellitus	0.9% saline	Sliding scale	50 U/50 mL (1 U/mL)	Sliding scale	Sliding scale	
Isoprenaline	Treatment of heart block or bradycardia	5% glucose, D =glucose saline	0.5–10 µg/min	1 mg/50 mL (20 µg/mL)	1.5–30 mL/h	7 mL/h	

Alternative regimes for any infusion: 3 mg/kg/50 mL then 1 mL/h = 1 µg/kg/min
3 mg/50 mL then 1 mL/h = 1 µg/min

Drug	Indication	Diluent	Dose	Suggested regime (60 kg adult)	Infusion range	Initial rate (adult)	Comments
Ketamine	General anaesthesia	0.9% saline, 5% glucose	1–3 mg/kg/h	500 mg/50 mL (10 mg/mL)	6–18 mL/h	10 mL/h	Induction 0.5–2 mg/kg
Ketamine	'Trauma' mixture	0.9% saline	0.5 mL/kg/h	50 mL mixture (4 mg/mL ketamine)	15–45 mL/h	30 mL/h	200 mg ketamine 10 mg midazolam + 10 mg vecuronium in 50 mL
Lidocaine	Ventricular arrhythmias	0.9% saline	4 mg/min for 30 min, 2 mg/min for 2 h, then 1 mg/min for 24 h	500 mg/50 mL (10 mg/mL = 1%)	6–24 mL/h	24 mL/h	After 50–100 mg slow IV bolus. ECG monitoring
Milrinone	Inodilator	0.9% saline, 5% glucose	50 µg/kg over 10 min, then 0.375–0.75 µg/kg/min	10 mg/50 mL (0.2 mg/mL)	7–14 mL/h	90 mL/h for 10 min	Maximum 1.13 mg/kg/day
Naloxone	Opioid antagonist	0.9% saline, 5% glucose	>1 µg/kg/h	2 mg/500 mL (4 µg/mL)		100 mL/h	Rate adjusted according to response
Nimodipine	Prevention of vasospasm after SAH	0.9% saline, 5% glucose	1 mg/h increasing to 2 mg/h after 2 h	Undiluted (0.2 mg/mL)	5–10 mL/h	5 mL/h	Via central line. Incompatible with polyvinyl chloride

Drug	Indication	Diluent	Dose	Concentration	Infusion rate	Starting rate	Notes
Nitroprusside (sodium)	Controlled hypotension	5% glucose	0.3–1.5 µg/kg/min	25 mg/50 mL (500 µg/mL)	2–10 mL	5 mL/h	Maximum dose 1.5 mg/kg. Protect from light
Noradrenaline	Treatment of hypotension	5% glucose	2–20 µg/min (0.04–0.4 µg/kg/min)	4 mg/40 mL (100 µg/mL)	1.2–12+ mL/h	5 mL/h	Via central line
Octreotide	Somatostatin analogue	0.9% saline	25–50 µg/h	500 µg/50 mL (10 µg/mL)	2–5 mL/h	5 mL/h	Use in variceal bleeding, unlicensed
Oxytocin	Prevention of uterine atony	5% glucose	0.02–0.04 U/min	20 U in 500 mL (0.04 U/mL)	30–60 mL/h	60 mL/h	Individual unit protocols vary
Phenytoin	Anticonvulsant prophylaxis	0.9% saline	18 mg/kg	1000 mg/100 mL (administer through 0.22–0.5 µm filter)	Up to 50 mg/min	180 mL/h	ECG and BP monitoring. Complete within 1 h of preparation
Salbutamol	Bronchospasm	5% glucose	5–20 µg/min	1 mg/50 mL (20 µg/mL)	15–60 mL/h	30 mL/h	After 250 µg slow IV bolus

Alternative regimes for any infusion: 3 mg/kg/50 mL then 1 mL/h = 1 µg/kg/min
3 mg/50 mL then 1 mL/h = 1 µg/min

Appendix 2: Checklist

Checklist for anaesthetic equipment 2004[1]

Use this guidance in association with the manufacturer's instructions for checking your specific anaesthesia machine—certain models should not have the common gas outlet occluded (see Check 5).

The following checks should be made prior to each operating session. In addition, checks 2, 6, and 9 should be made prior to each new patient during a session.

1. Check that the anaesthetic machine is connected to the electricity supply (if appropriate) and switched on

NB: Some anaesthetic workstations may enter an integral self-test program when switched on; those functions tested by such a program need not be retested.

- Take note of any information or labelling on the anaesthetic machine referring to the current status of the machine. Particular attention should be paid to recent servicing. Servicing labels should be fixed in the service logbook.

2. Check that all monitoring devices, in particular the oxygen analyser, pulse oximeter, and capnograph, are functioning and have appropriate alarm limits

- Check that gas sampling lines are properly attached and free of obstructions.
- Check that an appropriate frequency of recording non-invasive blood pressure is selected.

(Some monitors need to be in stand-by mode to avoid unnecessary alarms before being connected to the patient.)

3. Check with a 'tug test' that each pipeline is correctly inserted into the appropriate gas supply terminal

NB: Carbon dioxide cylinders should not be present on the anaesthetic machine unless requested by the anaesthetist. A blanking plug should be fitted to any empty cylinder yoke.

- Check that the anaesthetic machine is connected to a supply of oxygen and that an adequate supply of oxygen is available from a reserve oxygen cylinder.
- Check that adequate supplies of other gases (nitrous oxide, air) are available and connected as appropriate.
- Check that all pipeline pressure gauges in use on the anaesthetic machine indicate 400–500 kPa.

4. Check the operation of flowmeters (where fitted)

- Check that each flow valve operates smoothly and that the bobbin moves freely throughout its range.
- Check the anti-hypoxia device is working correctly.
- Check the operation of the emergency oxygen bypass control.

[1] This checklist is an abbreviated version of the Association of Anaesthetists publication 'Checking Anaesthetic Equipment 3 2004' (Endorsed by the Chief Medical Officer and the Royal College of Anaesthetists).

5. Check the vaporizer(s)

- Check that each vaporizer is adequately, but not over, filled.
- Check that each vaporizer is correctly seated on the back bar and not tilted.
- Check the vaporizer for leaks (with vaporizer on and off) by temporarily occluding the common gas outlet.
- Turn the vaporizer(s) off when checks are completed.
- Repeat the leak test immediately after changing any vaporizer.

6. Check the breathing system to be employed

NB: A new single-use bacterial/viral filter and angle-piece/catheter mount must be used for each patient. Packaging should not be removed until point of use.

- Inspect the system for correct configuration. All connections should be secured by 'push and twist'.
- Perform a pressure leak test on the breathing system by occluding the patient-end and compressing the reservoir bag. Bain-type co-axial systems should have the inner tube occluded for the leak test.
- Check the correct operation of all valves, including unidirectional valves within a circle, and all exhaust valves.
- Check for patency and flow of gas through the whole breathing system, including the filter and anglepiece/catheter mount.

7. Check that the ventilator is configured appropriately for its intended use

- Check that the ventilator tubing is correctly configured and securely attached.
- Set the controls for use and ensure that an adequate pressure is generated during the inspiratory phase.
- Check the pressure relief valve functions.
- Check that the disconnect alarms function correctly.
- Ensure that an alternative means to ventilate the patient's lungs is available.

8. Check that the anaesthetic gas scavenging system is switched on and is functioning correctly

- Check that the tubing is attached to the appropriate exhaust port of the breathing system, ventilator, or workstation.

9. Check that all ancillary equipment which may be needed is present and working

- This includes laryngoscopes, intubation aids, intubation forceps, bougies, etc., and appropriately sized facemasks, airways, tracheal tubes, and connectors, which must be checked for patency.
- Check that the suction apparatus is functioning and that all connectors are secure.
- Check that the patient trolley, bed, or operating table can be rapidly tilted head down.

10. Check that an alternative means to ventilate the patient is immediately available (e.g. self-inflating bag and oxygen cylinder)

- Check that the self-inflating bag and cylinder of oxygen are functioning correctly and the cylinder contains an adequate supply of oxygen.

11. Recording

- Sign and date the logbook kept with the anaesthetic machine to confirm that the machine has been checked.
- Record on each patient's anaesthetic chart that the anaesthetic machine, breathing system, and monitoring has been checked.

Index

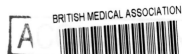